REMOVABLE PARTIAL DENTURE DESIGN

OUTLINE SYLLABUS

ARTHUR J. KROL
D.D.S., F.A.C.D., F.I.C.D., F.A.C.P.

Adjunct Professor, University of California, School of Dentistry
San Francisco, California
Formerly Professor and Chairman, Department of Removable Prosthodontics
University of the Pacific, School of Dentistry
San Francisco, California and
Loyola University, School of Dentistry, Chicago, Illinois

THEODORE E. JACOBSON
D.D.S., F.A.C.D., F.A.D.I.

Associate Clinical Professor, University of California, School of Dentistry
San Francisco, California

FREDERICK C. FINZEN
D.D.S., F.A.C.D., F.A.C.P.

Chief of Predoctoral Prosthodontics
Associate Clinical Professor, University of California, School of Dentistry
San Francisco, California

Pg 33
Pg 39
Pg 51
Pg 54-55
Biomechanics

Copies of this syllabus may be obtained from the:

Bookstore
University of the Pacific
School of Dentistry
2155 Webster Street
San Francisco, CA 94115
(415) 929-6467

Published by
Indent
57 Ridgewood Drive
San Rafael, CA 94901

Printed in the United States of America.

ACKNOWLEDGEMENT

We would like to acknowledge our appreciation for the assistance of the individuals who helped us in the preparation of this syllabus: Marcel Kapulica, C.D.T., for his time and dedication in fabricating many of the new partial denture frameworks used in this fourth edition; Peter P. Keri, C.D.T., for his laboratory assistance; Vickie Leow, Senior Artist at the UCSF School of Dentistry for the new drawings and diagrams in this edition; Carol Albright for her dedication and sacrifices in preparing the manuscript; and Paul Lancour for his help in manuscript preparation.

A. J. K.

T. E. J.

F. C. F.

PREFACE

The design of removable partial dentures remains one of the more challenging aspects of dental practice. Surveys indicate that most practitioners request the dental laboratory to design as well as fabricate removable partial dentures with few, if any, instructions. This prevalent practice cannot be attributed simply to a lack of interest or concern on the part of the dentist, but, results from an inadequate base of knowledge which further diminishes with time. Reluctance to correct this mental posture, however, is not without a reasonable basis. A scientific approach to the development of sound concepts in all the various aspects of removable partial denture prosthodontics is lacking. Adherence to a particular technique or philosophy continues to be based more on the opinions of its advocates than on objective scientific information. Some aspects of the subject remain obscure, lacking the rationale upon which a practitioner may comfortably rely. Nevertheless, in spite of these listed deficiencies, there are a number of fundamental concepts of removable partial denture design that provide a rational basis upon which decisions may be made. An understanding of these concepts enhances the potential to select materials, techniques and designs which meet functional and esthetic demands.

Currently, there is a de-emphasis on removable prosthodontics in the curriculum of many dental schools. The accent on other areas of dentistry has resulted in a reduction of didactic, clinical and laboratory requirements necessary to adequately train clinicians in the understanding and performance of restorative and prosthodontic procedures. Preventive dentistry has made great strides toward improving the dental health of the world population in reducing the incidence of decayed, missing and restored teeth within various age groups. However, several recently published surveys have demonstrated an increasing need for removable prosthodontic services, now, and in the future. As the longevity of our population increases, greater numbers of partially edentulous elderly patients will require more complex fixed and removable prosthodontic treatment.

The confusion which pervades the field of removable partial prosthodontics is perpetuated by a negative attitude toward removable partial dentures by both practicing dentists and their patients. This attitude was generated, perhaps during the earlier years of the more formal educational process when removable partial dentures were taught as an alternative treatment reserved for those patients whose remaining abutment teeth could not biomechanically support a fixed prosthesis or when financial constraints prohibited the more "ideal" treatment. This frame of mind is reinforced through many continuing education programs and is naturally passed on to the patient population. Unfortunately, for many practitioners, this negativism may be compounded by an inequitable monetary reward for the meticulous procedures required to fabricate a superior removable prosthesis. There, certainly, are many clinical conditions, that, when alternative treatment plans exist biomechanically and financially, the removable partial denture should be the treatment of choice.

FORWARD

The objectives of removable partial denture design have been well established. They include the restoration of function, enhancement of esthetics and most importantly the preservation of the remaining teeth and peridental structures. The preservation of these structures in the partially edentulous patient requires an emphasis on periodontal considerations. Positive correlation between the presence of bacterial plaque and periodontal disease has been well documented in the periodontal and prosthodontic literature. The effect of functional and parafunctional forces on the teeth and peridental structures, in the presence of periodontal disease, is now generally accepted. Mechanical forces act as an aggravating or accelerating factor in the progression of periodontal disease, but, not as the primary causative agent. The control of mechanical forces also plays an important part in the preservation of residual ridges under extension base partial dentures, especially in those patients who demonstrate a high susceptibility to pressure induced resorptive changes.

Two main concepts underlie the philosophy presented in this syllabus. The first is the concept of minimal tooth coverage and minimal gingival coverage to reduce the potential for plaque accumulation. Plaque has been identified as the primary cause of caries, gingivitis and periodontitis. Its control is essential for long term success of removable partial dentures. The second is the concept of equitable distribution of functional forces in extension base partial dentures. The term "equitable" is used to imply fair or optimum distribution of forces to the abutment teeth and to the edentulous ridge in accord with their potential to resist these forces. An attempt should be made to incorporate these concepts in attaining the clearly defined objectives of removable partial denture design.

This syllabus deals primarily with the partial denture framework and base design does not cover other equally important considerations such as maxillomandibular records and occlusion. References are included to provide the reader with various sources of information. As in the first three editions, the outline format is retained to make the book less onerous and more appealing to the reader and permits quick reference to the various topics.

TABLE OF CONTENTS

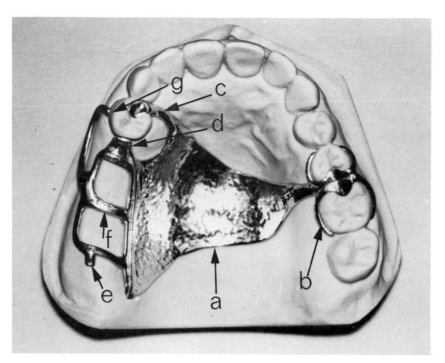

Fig. 1-1 Maxillary removable partial denture. Letters indicate various components. (a) Modified palatal plate major connector. (b) Lingual arm of a cast circumferential clasp. (c) Minor connector. (d) Proximal plate. (e) Metal stop. (f) Retentive strut for plastic resin. (g) "I" bar clasp arm.

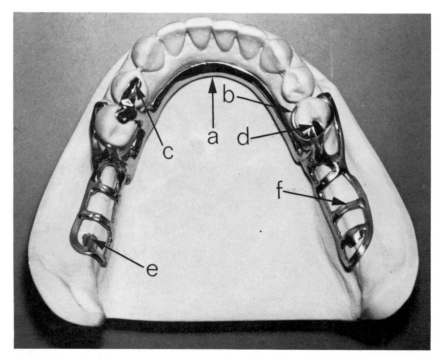

Fig. 1-2 Mandibular removable partial denture. Letters indicate various components. (a) Lingual bar major connector. (b) Lingual circumferential clasp arm. (c) Extended occlusal rest acting as an indirect retainer. (d) Conventional occlusal rest. (e) Metal stop. (f) Retentive strut for plastic resin.

Chapter I

COMPONENTS OF A REMOVABLE PARTIAL DENTURE

This chapter defines the various components of a removable partial denture (RPD) as used throughout this syllabus. Wherever possible the nomenclature and definitions adhere to the "Glossary of Prosthodontic Terms". An abbreviated glossary is located in the back of this book for reference.

DIRECT RETAINER

A clasp or attachment applied to an abutment tooth for the purpose of retaining a removable partial denture. It is directly responsible for the retention of the prosthesis.

A. CLASPS.

   1. Cast circumferential (Suprabulge). (Fig. 1–1 & 3)

   2. Cast bar (Infrabulge). (Figs. 1–1 & 3)

   3. Combination.

     a. Cast circumferential and cast bar. (Fig. 1–4)

     b. Cast circumferential and wrought wire. (Fig. 1–5)

B. ATTACHMENTS. (SEE CHAPTER XXII)

   1. Intracoronal.

   2. Extracoronal.

   3. Precision.

   4. Rigid.

   5. Non-rigid.

MAJOR CONNECTOR

A plate, strap or bar that connects the components of the partial denture on one side of the arch with those on the opposite side.

A. MAXILLARY.

   1. Anterior palatal strap.

   2. Posterior palatal (midpalatal) strap.

   3. Anteroposterior palatal strap.

   4. Modified palatal plate. (Fig. 1–1)

   5. Complete palatal plate. (Fig. 1–5)

B. MANDIBULAR.

   1. Lingual bar. (Fig. 1–2)

   2. Sublingual bar.

   3. Lingual plate. (Fig. 1–6)

   4. Labial bar. (Fig. 1–8)

MINOR CONNECTOR

A rigid component which links the major connector or base and other components of the partial denture, such as rests, indirect retainers, and clasps. (Fig. 1–1)

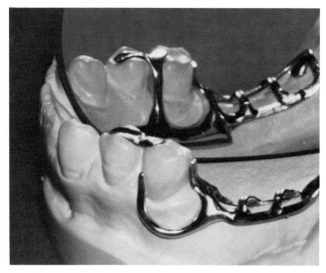

Fig. 1-3 Buccal and lingual (mirror) view of the clasp on the left second premolar of Fig. 1-2. An "I" bar infrabulge clasp arm is located on the buccal surface. Note absence of clasp arm on the lingual surface.

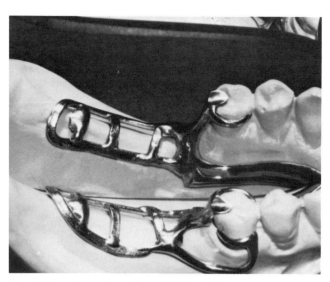

Fig. 1-4 Buccal and lingual (mirror) view of the clasp on the right second premolar of Fig. 1-2. A modified "T" bar clasp arm is located on the buccal surface. A circumferential clasp arm is located on the lingual surface.

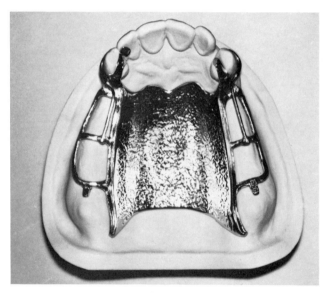

Fig. 1-5 A maxillary removable partial denture with complete palatal plate major connector and wrought wire facial clasp arms. Cingulum rests serve as lingual clasp arms. Note extension of rest onto lateral incisor. The extension acts as an indirect retainer and third point of reference.

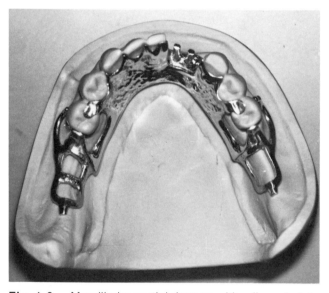

Fig. 1-6 Mandibular partial denture with a lingual plate major connector. Posts are used to increase retention of the artificial teeth that will replace the incisors.

REST

A rigid extension of a partial denture that prevents movement towards the mucosa and transmits functional forces to the teeth.

A. OCCLUSAL.

    1. Conventional. (Figs. 1–1 & 2)

    2. Extended. (Figs. 1–2 & 8)

    3. Overlay.

B. INCISAL. (Fig. 1–8)

C. LINGUAL.

    1. Cingulum. (Fig. 1–5)

    2. Ball.

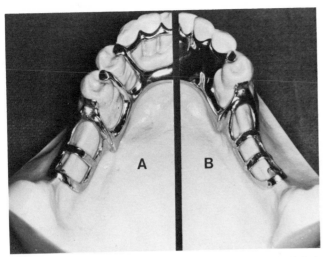

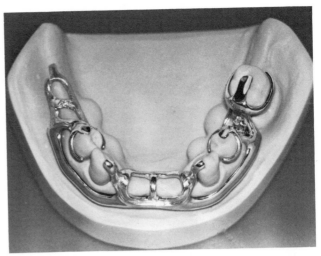

Fig. 1-7 Mandibular partial denture framework fabricated for demonstration purposes only. Side (A) shows a lingual bar major connector with a continuous bar connector (Kennedy bar) above. Side (B) shows a lingual plate as the major connector.

Fig. 1-8 Mandibular removable partial denture with labial bar major connector and incisal rests on canines. An extended occlusal rest is present on the molar.

PROXIMAL PLATE

A plate of metal in contact with the proximal surface of an abutment tooth. (Fig. 1–1)

INDIRECT RETAINER

A component of a removable partial denture, located on the opposite side of the fulcrum line, that assists the direct retainer in preventing displacement of an extension base through mechanical leverage.

A. RESTS. (Figs. 1–2 & 9)

B. MINOR CONNECTORS AND PROXIMAL PLATES.

C. OTHER.

    1. Lingual plate. (Fig. 1–6)

    2. Continuous bar (Kennedy bar) connector. (Fig. 1–7)

PLASTIC RETENTION AREA

That part of the framework to which the resin base is attached.

A. OPEN LATTICE. (Figs. 1–1 & 2)

B. MESH. (Fig. 1–9)

C. POSTS, LOOPS OR BEADS. (Fig. 1–6)

D. METAL STOP. A small projection of metal at the distal end of an extension base framework that contacts the cast and prevents downward movement of the plastic retention area during the packing with resin. (Figs. 1–1 & 2)

DENTURE BASE

The component of a removable partial that contacts the oral mucosa, to which the artificial teeth are attached.

A. PLASTIC RESIN. Resin base is attached to the framework by means of open lattice or mesh. (Figs. 1–1,2,5,6)

B. METAL. Teeth are attached by means of posts, loops or beads. (Fig. 1–6)

TEETH

A. DENTURE TEETH.

    1. Porcelain. (Figs. 1–10 & 11)

    2. Plastic.

B. METAL.

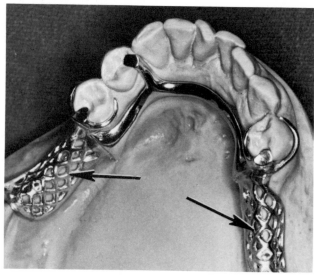

Fig. 1-9 Mandibular partial denture framework with retention mesh for attachment of denture bases. Note occlusal rest as an indirect retainer on left first premolar.

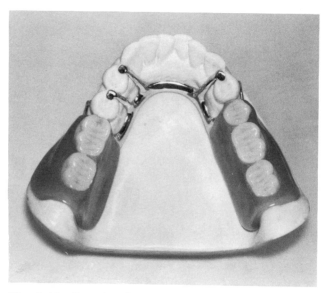

Fig. 1-10 Completed mandibular partial denture framework with plastic resin bases and artificial teeth.

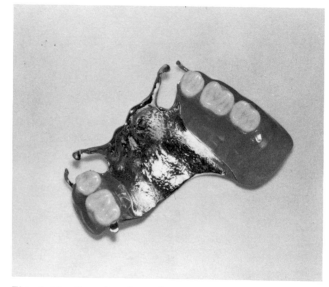

Fig. 1-11 Completed maxillary partial denture with resin bases and artificial teeth.

Chapter II

EXAMINATION, DIAGNOSIS AND TREATMENT PLANNING

Since this syllabus is primarily concerned with removable partial denture design, this chapter is presented in brief form. It highlights the role of the bone index, which is often misunderstood or overlooked during examination, diagnosis, and treatment planning.

INDICATIONS FOR A REMOVABLE PARTIAL DENTURE IN PREFERENCE TO A FIXED PARTIAL DENTURE

A. EDENTULOUS AREAS TOO LONG FOR A FIXED PROSTHESIS.

B. NEED TO RESTORE SOFT AND HARD TISSUE CONTOURS.

C. ABSENCE OF ADEQUATE PERIODONTAL SUPPORT.

D. STRUCTURALLY OR ANATOMICALLY COMPROMISED ABUTMENT TEETH.

1. Lack of clinical crown height.

2. Lack of sound tooth structure.

3. Unfavorable position, contour or inclination.

E. NEED FOR CROSS-ARCH STABILIZATION.

F. NEED FOR AN EXTENSION BASE.

G. ANTERIOR ESTHETICS.

H. AGE.

I. PHYSICAL AND EMOTIONAL PROBLEMS PRECLUDING FIXED PARTIAL DENTURES.

J. ATTITUDE AND DESIRES OF PATIENT.

K. EASE OF PLAQUE REMOVAL FROM NATURAL TEETH AND PARTIAL DENTURE.

EXAMINATION

A. VISUAL, DIGITAL AND EXPLORATORY.

1. Number and position of remaining teeth.

2. Caries present.

3. Restorations present.

4. Presence of facets.

5. Hypersensitivity of teeth.

6. Mobility of teeth.

7. Condition of soft tissues.

8. Level of oral hygiene.

9. Periodontal pocket depth.

10. Quantity of attached gingiva.

11. Action of muscle and frenal attachments.

12. Vestibular depth and undercuts.

13. Residual ridge conformation.

14. Presence of bony exostoses or tori.

15. Quantity and quality of saliva.

16. Occlusion, occlusal plane and articulation.

17. Occlusal vertical dimension.

18. Interarch distance.

19. Horizontal relationships of mandible to maxillae in centric occlusion and eccentric relations, including normal functional mandibular movements.

20. Elevator muscle development.

21. Lip length and mobility.

22. Phonetics.

23. Temporomandibular joint evaluation.

24. Design possibilities related to esthetics and function.

B. ROENTGENOGRAPHIC.

1. Pathology.

2. Caries.

3. Amount of bone support. Quantity of bone.

   a. Alveolar.

   b. Residual ridge.

   c. Basal.

4. Quality of bone. (Figs. 2–1 to 6).

   a. Bone index. The bone index is an assessment of the relative response of bone to stimulation or irritation. This assessment is made by analyzing bone index areas. Bone index areas are those areas of bony support which disclose the reaction of bone to increased force, e.g. areas of bone around abutment teeth or any other teeth subjected to increased loading. These areas are compared to areas of bone around teeth in normal function without increased loading. A similar consideration may be given to the residual ridge or an edentulous area of bone supporting a complete or an extension base removable partial denture. Evaluation of past response is important in predicting the future potential for dento-alveolar (abutment teeth) and muco-osseous (ridge) resistance to forces transmitted by an RPD. The bone index is difficult to determine from radiographs alone. The history of the patient is important in evaluating the rate of resorption that may be expected based on previous occurrences. The length of time from previous extractions together with morphological changes in the residual ridge gives some indication of the host response to various forces.

   b. Denser bone (more highly calcified) offers greater resistance to resorption. The reduced rate of resorption of cortical bone compared to cancellous bone is likely due to the remaining tensional stimuli, the degree of cellularity and mineralization, as well as to the extrinsic and intrinsic bone factors. These factors appear to account for the pattern of resorption of the residual ridges in the edentulous or partially edentulous patient. In the mandibular arch the external oblique ridge, the mylohyoid ridge and the genial tubercles, which are areas of muscle attachments, continue to resist resorption even when the residual ridge is greatly resorbed.

   The presence of dense cortical bone is usually the result of applied forces arising from ligamentous or muscle attachments which provide tension to the underlying bone.

   c. Extrinsic bone factors. Localized forces applied to bone.

      i. Pressure—Bone tends to resorb under localized compressive forces. The rate of resorption most likely depends on the intrinsic bone factors or on the interaction of pressure and tension.

      ii. Tension—Bone under tensional stimuli tends to increase in density and in some instances may increase in size. The lamina dura is a response to tensional forces produced by the periodontal ligament. Orthodontic movement of teeth is a good example of the pressure-tension theory.

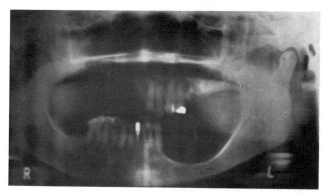

Fig. 2-1 Panoramic radiograph showing various levels of bone resorption with the wearing of removable partial dentures. Note the difference in the resorption between the right and left sides of the mandible. The difference is due to the presence of maxillary posterior teeth on the left side which increased the forces exerted on the mandibular residual ridge causing more resorption as compared to the mandibular ridge on the right side. On the right side the opposite condition exists. Mandibular posterior teeth are present on the right side with no opposing natural teeth in the maxillary arch. Note the greater resorption of the maxillary ridge on the patient's right side as compared to the left side.

The lamina dura resorbs on the pressure side and bone apposition occurs on the opposite side.

    d. Intrinsic bone factors. May influence the rate of resorption.

        i. Genetic.

       ii. Hormonal.

     iii. Nutritional.

     iv. Pathologic.

      v. Biochemical.

     vi. Other.

C. HISTORICAL.

    1. Physical health.

    2. Psychological health.

    3. Frequency of dental examinations.

    4. Previous dental treatment (especially previous removable partial denture experience).

    5. Presence of parafunctional habits.

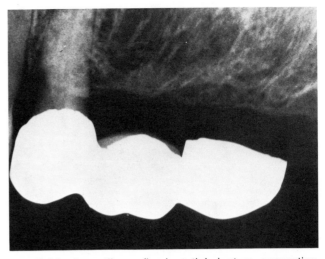

Fig. 2-2A A cantilever fixed partial denture supporting two molar pontics and retained by the second premolar for 28 years. Bone support around the secondary premolar root indicates an excellent bone index.

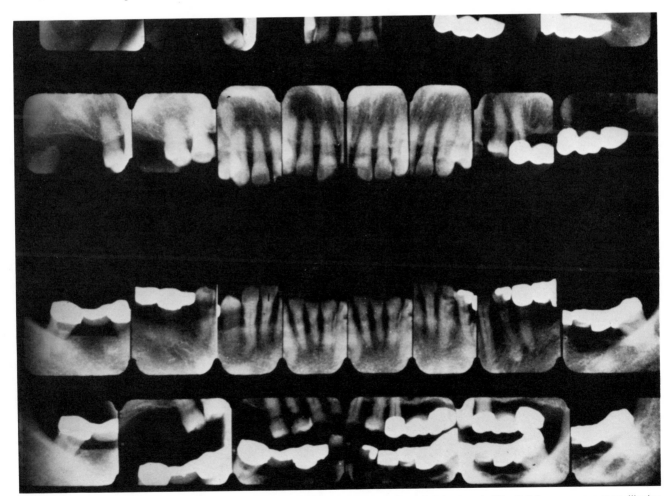

Fig. 2-2B Complete mouth radiographs indicate that the cantilever fixed partial denture in Fig. 2-2A opposes a mandibular fixed partial denture in function.

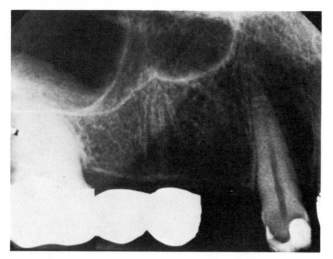

Fig. 2-3A Radiograph of molar supporting a cantilever fixed partial denture for 12 years. Bone surrounding molar root indicates an excellent bone index.

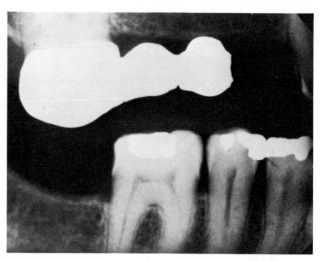

Fig. 2-3B Radiograph of cantilever fixed partial denture in Fig. 2-3A opposing natural teeth.

D. MOUNTED DIAGNOSTIC CASTS (Fig. 2–7). These will supplement the previously listed data and aid in demonstrating or determining the following:

1. Assist in preliminary design of the partial denture.

2. Aid in determining sequence of treatment.

3. Analysis of path of placement and removal (dislodgement).

4. Unfavorable tooth position, contours or inclinations requiring modification.

5. Unfavorable bony or soft tissues requiring modification.

6. Retentive and nonretentive areas of abutment teeth.

7. Development of undercuts accomplished by preparing dimples or grooves.

8. Development of rest seat preparations.

9. Embrasure clearance.

10. Occlusion, occlusal plane and articulation.

11. Need for occlusal adjustment.

12. Interarch distance.

E. ASSESSMENT OF POTENTIAL OF APPLIED FORCES (See Chapter III).

1. Opposing occlusion.

2. Muscular force potential. Elevator muscle development.

3. Presence of parafunctional habits.

a. Clenching.

b. Bruxing.

4. Length of edentulous span.

5. History of prosthesis failure.

a. Solder joint failure.

b. Porcelain failure.

c. Fractured RPD components.

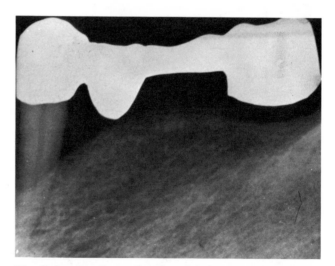

Fig. 2-4 Cantilever fixed partial denture supported by the mandibular first premolar for 18 years. This fixed prosthesis functioned in occlusion. Bone surrounding the premolar root shows marked degree of resorption, but, due to the 18 year period in which it supported the fixed partial denture the bone index would have to be considered favorable.

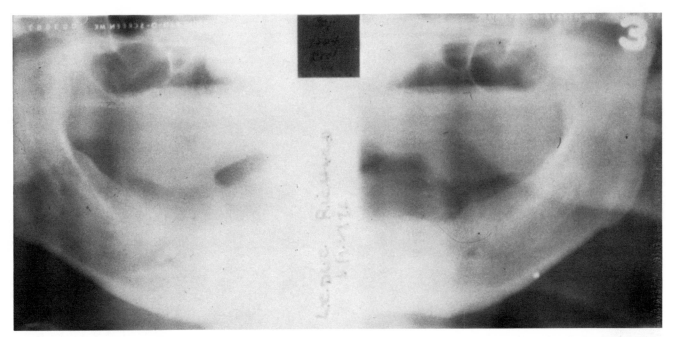

Fig. 2-5   Panoramic radiographic of a patient having worn complete dentures for 31 years. Note that limited resorption of the residual ridges has occurred indicating an excellent bone index.

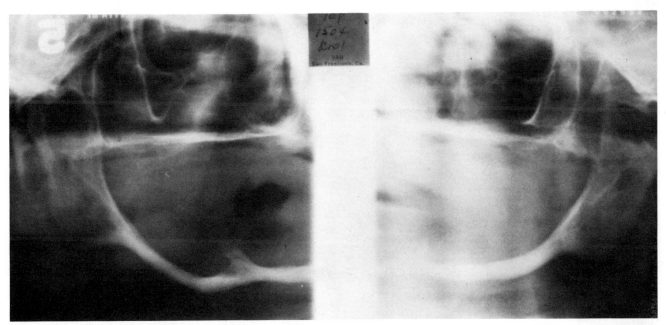

Fig. 2-6   Panoramic radiograph of a patient having worn complete dentures for 33 years. Note extensive resroption of residual ridges indicating a poor bone index.

6. History of poor tissue tolerance.

    a. Chronic sore spots.

    b. Excessive bone resorption.

    c. Abutment tooth mobility.

    d. Fracture or attrition of natural teeth.

F. ASSESSMENT OF PATIENT MOTIVATION, ATTITUDE AND HOME CARE.

BASIC CRITERIA FOR PATIENT SELECTION

A. ACCEPTABLE EMOTIONAL AND PHYSICAL HEALTH.

   1. Basic health observations.

   2. Complete health history.

B. GENERAL PHYSICAL AND MENTAL CAPACITY TO TOLERATE A PROSTHESIS.

   1. Previous number of prostheses.

   2. Physical handicaps.

C. DEGREE OF PATIENT MOTIVATION.

   1. General personal appearance.

   2. Past oral hygiene habits and response to suggested change.

   3. Patient's desire to preserve remaining teeth and surrounding structures.

   4. Physical and mental capabilities to augment motivation.

   5. Patient's response to scientific evidence.

D. PATIENT'S COMPREHENSION OF POTENTIAL SUCCESS OR FAILURE OF TREATMENT.

E. TYPES AND AMOUNTS OF DRUGS THE PATIENT CONSUMES INCLUDING ALCOHOL AND TOBACCO.

F. PATIENT'S DIETARY HABITS.

G. PERIODONTAL HEALTH.

H. ORAL INDICES OF TISSUE TOLERANCE. Indicate the capacity of supporting structures to resist mechanical forces.

   1. Muco-osseous (ridge) resistance. Bone index of the residual ridge (reaction of bone after extraction and ridge loading). (Figs. 2–1 to 2–6)

   2. Dento-alveolar (abutment) resistance. Bone index around the abutment teeth (reaction of bone to increased force).

   3. Soft tissue pressure and abrasion tolerance.

I. ORAL MANIFESTATIONS OF PATHOLOGY.

   1. Acute.

   2. Chronic.

   3. Systemic.

   4. Local.

   5. Chemical.

   6. Traumatic.

   7. Fistulas.

   8. Temporomandibular joint dysfunction.

   9. Head and neck.

      a. Lymphatics.

      b. Swellings.

      c. Asymmetries.

   10. Tumors.

   11. Abnormalities of any other type.

J. CONSULTATIONS WITH OTHER MEDICAL AND DENTAL SPECIALISTS.

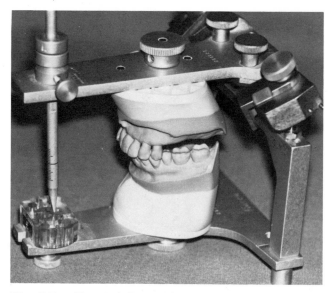

Fig. 2-7   Mounted diagnostic casts.

INSTRUCTIONS IN ORAL HYGIENE

A. INSTRUCTIONS ON PLAQUE REMOVAL TO AID IN DETERMINING PROGNOSIS.

(See Chapter XIX).

B. RE-EVALUATE PATIENT AT SUBSEQUENT APPOINTMENTS TO DETERMINE IMPLEMENTATION OF INSTRUCTION. PLAQUE CONTROL INSTRUCTIONS MAY HAVE TO BE REINFORCED.

IMPLEMENTATION OF DIAGNOSTIC AIDS

A. RADIOGRAPHS.

   1. Complete mouth periapical and bite-wing survey.

   2. Panoramic.

   3. Obtain previous radiographs if possible for purpose of comparison.

   4. Indicate oral pathology.

   5. Used in determining bone indices.

6. Used in discussing the treatment plan with patient.

7. Pretreatment records.

B. DIAGNOSTIC CASTS.

   1. Mounted casts. (Fig. 2–7)

      a. Centric occlusion (at centric maxillo-mandibular relation).

      b. Maximum intercuspation.

   2. Used in discussing the treatment plan with patient.

   3. Pretreatment records.

   4. Fabrication of custom impression trays.

C. PHOTOGRAPHS.

   1. Extraoral.

   2. Intraoral.

   3. May be of value in discussing the treatment plan with the patient.

   4. Pretreatment records.

PRELIMINARY DESIGN OF THE PARTIAL DENTURE

A. SHOULD BE MADE AFTER MOUNTING DIAGNOSTIC CASTS ON AN ARTICULATOR AND BEFORE INITIATING TREATMENT.

B. MAY DETERMINE NEED FOR PRE-PROSTHETIC SURGERY OR OTHER MOUTH PREPARATION.

C. MAY DETERMINE NEED FOR RESTORATION OF THE ABUTMENT TEETH.

D. MAY INFLUENCE THE SEQUENCE OF TREATMENT.

E. IMPORTANT FOR CONSULTATION WITH THE PATIENT.

CONSULTATION WITH THE PATIENT

A. THE PATIENT SHOULD BE MADE AWARE OF THE FOLLOWING.

   1. The nature and severity of the existing dental problems.

   2. Any limitation in function, phonetics, esthetics, and longevity provided by the prosthesis.

   3. The physical aspects of the prosthesis with regard to bulk and tissue coverage.

   4. Any treatment options that may be considered.

B. PATIENT MUST UNDERSTAND AND ACCEPT RESPONSIBILITY FOR PREVENTIVE HOME CARE AND RECALL VISITS.

Chapter III

BIOMECHANICS OF REMOVABLE PARTIAL DENTURES

Biomechanics may be defined as the application of the principles of mechanical engineering in the living organism. An understanding of the biological response to mechanical stimuli is of paramount importance for promoting long term success of removable partial dentures. Mechanical forces exerted on removable partial dentures during functional and parafunctional mandibular movements should be properly directed to the supporting tissues to elicit the most favorable response. The manner in which alveolar bone surrounding the natural teeth responds to forces differs markedly from that of the residual bone remaining after the extraction of teeth. The natural teeth are attached to bone by means of a periodontal ligament which converts much of the masticatory compressive force to tensional force, favorably stimulating the alveolar bone. This is especially true of forces which are directed along the long axes of the teeth. The mucosa of the residual ridge transmits compressive force through the submucosa to the underlying bone without changing the nature of the force frequently resulting in pressure induced resorption. Regardless of biomechanical classification, all removable partial dentures direct mechanical forces to bone which is the ultimate supporting tissue.

FORCES ACTING ON REMOVABLE PARTIAL DENTURES

A. VERTICAL (Dislodging).

B. HORIZONTAL (Lateral).

C. TORSIONAL (Rotational, or twisting).

D. VERTICAL (Seating).

REQUIREMENTS OF A REMOVABLE PARTIAL DENTURE

A. RETENTION. Resistance to vertical dislodging forces.

1. Direct retainers.

2. Indirect retainers.

B. STABILITY (Bracing). Resistance to horizontal, lateral, or torsional forces.

1. Minor connectors.

2. Proximal plates.

3. Bracing clasp arms and shoulders of circumferential retentive clasp arms.

4. Lingual plates.

5. Rests—When the walls of the rest seat are relatively parallel to the path of placement (e.g. channel rests).

6. Denture bases—In long span tooth-mucosa borne prostheses.

C. SUPPORT. Resistance to vertical seating forces.

   1. Rests. All RPDs.

   2. Major connectors—Maxillary tooth-mucosa borne RPDs.

   3. Denture bases—Maxillary and mandibular tooth-mucosa borne RPDs.

BIOMECHANICAL CLASSIFICATION OF REMOVABLE PARTIAL DENTURES

Based on the nature of the supporting structures.

A. TOOTH BORNE (Dento-alveolar supported). (Fig. 3–1)

   1. Abutment teeth border all edentulous areas where tooth replacement is planned.

   2. Functional forces are transmitted through abutment teeth to bone.

B. TOOTH-MUCOSA BORNE (Dento-alveolar and muco-osseous supported). (Fig. 3–2)

   1. Exhibits one or more edentulous areas which are not bordered by abutment teeth (extension base RPDs).

   2. Functional forces are transmitted through abutment teeth and mucosa to bone.

   3. The majority of these are distal extension RPDs.

   4. This category may also apply to tooth bordered situations when excessive abutment tooth mobility is present or when long span tooth bordered edentulous areas are present precluding total tooth support. (Fig. 3–3)

C. MUCOSA BORNE (Muco-osseous supported).

   1. Regardless of the natural teeth present, support is derived entirely from the muco-osseous segment.

   2. This category includes prostheses fabricated from hard, or combinations of resilient and hard denture base materials such as stayplates which function as interim, provisional, or transitional prostheses.

   3. These prostheses usually do not contain a metal framework and usually should not be considered definitive treatment.

   4. This syllabus discusses principles which apply to definitive tooth borne and tooth-mucosa borne prostheses.

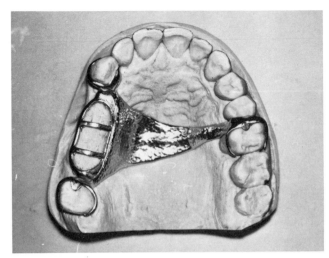

Fig. 3-1   Framework of a tooth borne RPD.

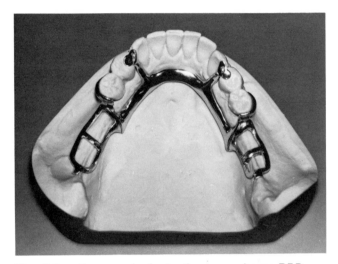

Fig. 3-2   Framework of a tooth-mucosa borne RPD.

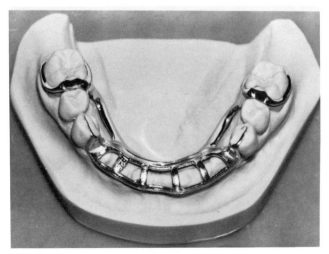

Fig. 3-3   Although tooth bounded, the edentulous space requires tooth and mucosal support.

14

KENNEDY CLASSIFICATION.

Based on the location and number of edentulous areas.

A. FOUR MAIN CLASSES.

Class I. Bilateral edentulous areas located posterior to the remaining natural teeth.

Class II. A unilateral edentulous area located posterior to the natural teeth.

Class III. A unilateral edentulous area with natural teeth both anterior and posterior to the area.

Class IV. A single but bilateral (crossing the midline) edentulous area located anterior to the remaining natural teeth.

B. MODIFICATION SPACES.

1. Edentulous areas other than those determining the main classes are modification spaces and are designated by the number of spaces present.

2. Class IV has no modifications because if more than one space is present in the dental arch it would fall into one of the other classifications.

KENNEDY CLASSIFICATION

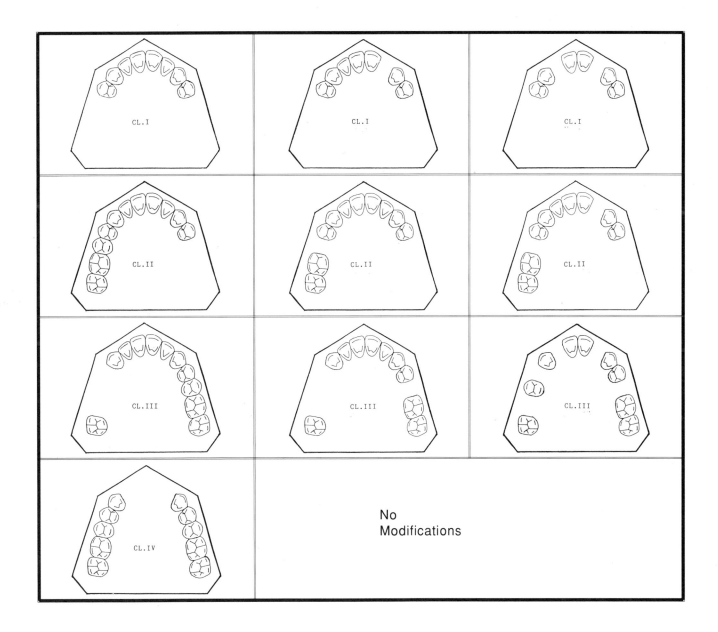

RESPONSE OF FORCE BEARING TISSUES TO MECHANICAL LOADING

The forces directed to the supporting tissues will be partially absorbed and partially transmitted to adjacent tissues. The percentage of force absorbed or transmitted will vary depending upon which tissue is involved. Bone is the tissue which ultimately absorbs the greatest amount of the force applied to both the muco-osseous and dento-alveolar segments.

A. DENTO-ALVEOLAR SEGMENT. (Fig. 3–4)

   1. Tooth.

      a. Structurally sound vital teeth are capable of withstanding normal functional forces.

      b. Excessive forces may result in adverse effects.

         i. Structural failure (tooth fracture).

         ii. Tooth movement.

         iii. Pulpal irritation. Reversible pulpitis (hyperemia) or irreversible pulpitis.

      c. Structurally compromised teeth may fail in response to normal functional forces.

         i. Teeth with large intracoronal restorations.

         ii. Endodontically treated teeth.

   2. Periodontium (including sulcular epithelium, junctional epithelium, connective tissue attachment, cementum, and the periodontal ligament).

      a. A normal periodontium permits some force absorption without damaging effects.

      b. Excessive forces may increase the width of the periodontal ligament and result in increased tooth mobility.

      c. Plaque induced inflammation compromises the periodontium. It may lead to apical migration of the pocket epithelium and destruction of the fibroblasts and connective tissue attachment of the PDL. Normal functional forces may accelerate a pre-existing periodontal disease process.

   3. Alveolar bone.

      a. Pressure-tension theory. Bone tends to resorb in response to compressive force and to be stimulated by tensional force. In order to preserve remaining alveolar bone, it is important that functional forces be transmitted to bone primarily as tension rather than pressure whenever possible. In tooth borne situations the majority of functional forces are transmitted as tension to bone through proper rest design and rest seat preparation. In tooth-mucosa borne situations the vertical components of the functional forces are transmitted as tension to bone through the rests. Lateral components

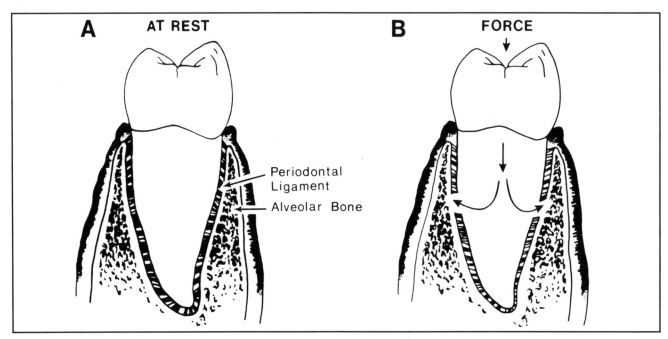

Fig. 3-4 (A) Dento-alveolar segment consists of the tooth, periodontium and alveolar bone. (B) During function, force is directed axially whenever possible and thereby transmitted through the tooth and periodontal ligament to the alveolar bone as tension.

of functional forces are transmitted as a combination of compressive and tensional forces to the alveolar bone (e.g. those forces directed through bracing clasp arms, proximal plates and minor connectors contacting proximal tooth surfaces and guiding planes). Vertical displacing forces are transmitted to bone as both compressive and tensional forces (e.g. sticky foods or retentive clasp arms engaging undercuts).

b. Bone index. The response of bone to pressure varies in terms of the rate of resorption depending on genetic, nutritional, hormonal and biochemical and other intrinsic factors. The bone index is determined by analyzing the previous response of bone to force (See Chapter II).

c. Cortical vs. cancellous bone. Lamina dura comprised of cortical bone responds to mechanical force more favorably than cancellous bone. Cortical bone is more highly mineralized, less cellular, and less metabolically dynamic.

d. Excessive forces which increase compressive components of forces transmitted to bone may increase the rate of bone resorption.

e. Periodontal disease. The presence of plaque induced periodontal disease is associated with a loss of bone height. Moderate forces may accelerate the disease process resulting in further bone loss, less bone support, and increased mobility.

B. MUCO-OSSEOUS SEGMENT. (Fig. 3–5)

1. Mucosa.

   a. Normal, firmly bound, keratinized tissues withstand mechanical forces within physiologic limits.

   b. Excessive mechanical forces may cause mucosal ulceration (e.g. denture sore spots).

2. Submucosa.

   a. Provides an "hydraulic cushion" effect.

   b. Increased thickness of fatty or glandular tissue increases tolerance of the residual ridge to applied force.

3. Bone.

   a. Pressure-tension theory. The functional loading of a tooth-mucosa borne denture base transmits force to the bone of the muco-osseous segment almost exclusively as pressure which tends to cause resorptive changes. Resorption occurs in proportion to the bone index and the intensity, duration, and direction of the applied force. With some longer span tooth borne partial dentures or when excessive mobility of abutment teeth is present some force may also be delivered through the mucosa to the underlying bone as pressure.

   b. Bone index. The bone index of the alveolar bone surrounding natural teeth may differ from that of the bone comprising the residual ridges. (Fig. 3–6)

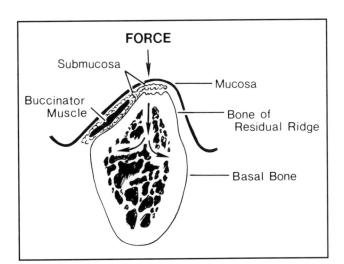

Fig. 3-5 Muco-osseous segment consists of the mucosa, submucosa, and bone of the residual ridge. During function, force is directed vertically toward the ridge area and transmitted through the mucosa and submucosa to the bone of the residual ridge as pressure.

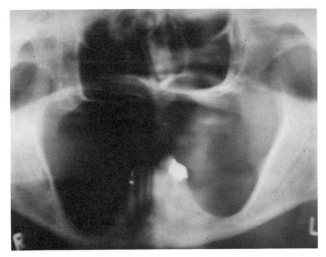

Fig. 3-6 Bone of the residual ridge demonstrates a poor bone index compared to the more favorable bone index of the alveolar bone supporting the teeth.

c. Cortical vs. cancellous bone. The residual ridge crest is comprised mainly of cancellous bone and is less resistant to resorption. The facial and lingual inclines of the residual ridges are comprised of cortical bone and are more resistant to remodelling. The rate of cancellous bone resorption has been described as being three times that of cortical bone.

d. Excessive forces may increase the rate of bone resorption.

e. Moderate forces may result in accelerated bone resorption when intrinsic factors, local abnormalities or systemic disorders compromise the bone index of the individual.

CHARACTERISTICS OF FAVORABLE DENTO-ALVEOLAR SUPPORT

A. TEETH.

1. Structurally sound.

2. Anatomically favorable.

   a. Root surface area.

   b. Root morphology.

   c. Presence of multiple roots.

   d. Presence of divergent roots.

   e. Crown to root ratio.

   f. Axial inclination.

B. PERIODONTIUM.

1. Normal (absence of periodontal disease).

   a. Pocket depths within normal limits.

   b. Absence of increasing mobility or hypermobility.

   c. Absence of inflammation.

2. Anatomically favorable.

   a. Normal epithelial and connective tissue attachment.

   b. Adequate zone of attached gingiva.

C. ALVEOLAR BONE.

1. Favorable bone index.

2. Anatomically normal.

   a. Bone height.

   b. Degree of mineralization.

   c. Presence of lamina dura (cortical bone).

CHARACTERISTICS OF FAVORABLE MUCO-OSSEOUS SUPPORT

A. MUCOSA.

1. Normal.

2. Keratinized.

3. Firmly bound.

B. SUBMUCOSA.

1. Normal submucosa serves as an "hydraulic cushion".

2. Firmly bound and dense.

C. BONE.

1. Cortical bone.

2. Favorable bone index.

3. Presence of muscle attachments which direct tension to bone (or the equivalent in terms of resistance to pressure induced resorption).

OPTIMAL FORCE BEARING MUCO-OSSEOUS ANATOMIC REGIONS

A. MAXILLARY. (Fig. 3–7)

1. Horizontal hard palate. (Fig. 3–8)

   a. Keratinized mucosa.

   b. Presence of fatty (anterior) and glandular (posterior) submucosa.

   c. Cortical bone.

   d. Longitudinal studies have demonstrated a high resistance to resorptive changes.

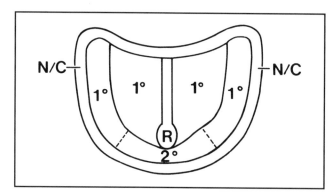

Fig. 3-7 Maxillary primary (1°) supporting areas are the horizontal hard palate and posterior ridge crest. The periphery of the denture bearing area is non-contributory (N/C). The midline suture often requires relief (R) and the anterior ridge crest serves as a secondary (2°) supporting area.

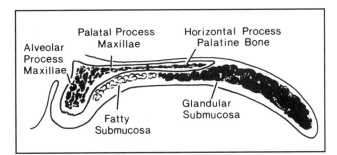

Fig. 3-8 The horizontal portion of the hard palate demonstrates keratinized mucosa overlying submucosa and cortical bone.

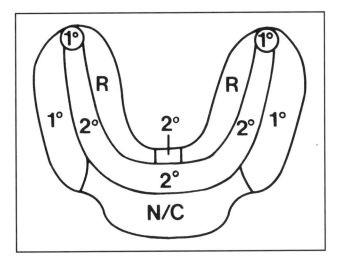

Fig. 3-9 Mandibular primary (1°) supporting areas are the buccal shelf and pear-shaped pad. The anterior facial incline of the ridge is non-contributory (N/C). The lingual ridge inclines may require relief (R) and the genial tubercle area and ridge crest serve as secondary (2°) supporting areas.

    2. Posterior ridge crest.

        a. Keratinized mucosa.

        b. Presence of dense firmly bound submucosal connective tissue which may contribute to clinically observed resistance to resorptive changes.

B. MANDIBULAR. (Fig. 3–9)

    1. Buccal shelf. The area between the external oblique ridge and the lateral border of the mandible. (Fig. 3–10)

        a. Presence of submucosa.

        b. Cortical bone.

        c. Buccinator muscle attachment. The longitudinally directed fibers provide tension but do not dislodge the denture base during contraction.

    2. Pear-shaped pad. The most distal extension of keratinized tissue covering the ridge crest. It is formed by the scarring pattern following the extraction of the most distal mandibular molar. It should be differentiated from the more posterior retromolar pad during clinical examination. (Fig. 3–11)

        a. Keratinized mucosa.

        b. Presence of dense firmly bound submucosa.

        c. Medial tendon of the temporalis muscle inserts lingually in the area of the apices of the mandibular third molars and provides tensional stimuli.

DESIGN OF TOOTH BORNE (DENTO-ALVEOLAR SUPPORTED) RPDs

A. OBJECTIVE: To transmit and axially direct functional forces to the abutment teeth. Virtually all functional forces are absorbed by the dento-alveolar segment.

B. DESIGN CONSIDERATIONS. (Fig. 3–12)

    1. Rigid connectors.

        a. Major connectors. Provide cross-arch force transmission (contributes to cross-arch stability and support).

        b. Minor connectors. Transfer forces to and from abutment teeth.

    2. Cast circumferential clasps. Bilateral bracing is provided by the bracing arm and rigid proximal or shoulder portion of retentive arm which promote effective force transmission from the artificial to the natural tooth.

    3. Proximate rests. Rests adjacent to edentulous areas transfer forces from artificial to natural teeth. (Fig. 3–13)

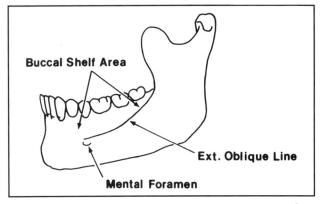

Fig. 3-10 The buccal shelf extends between the roots of the molar teeth and the external oblique ridge.

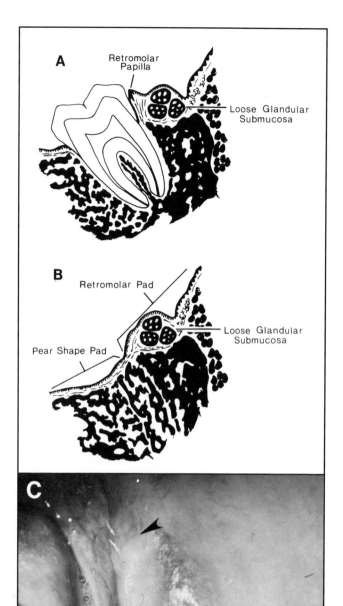

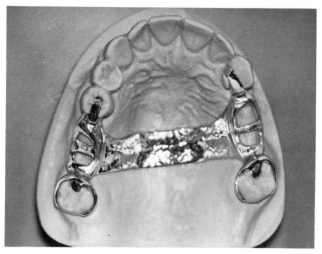

Fig. 3-12 Tooth supported framework with rigid connectors, cast circumferential clasps, and proximate rests.

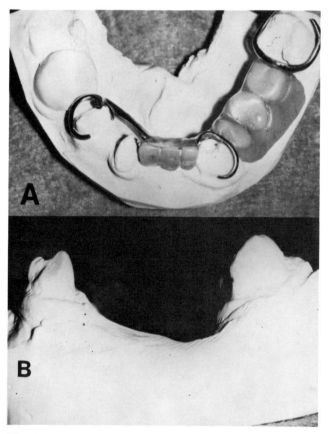

Fig. 3-11 (A) Pear-shaped pad is formed by the scarring pattern which follows the extraction of the mandibular third molar. (B) Retromolar papilla and extraction site form the pear-shaped pad. The retromolar pad contains loose glandular and vascular connective tissue. It is differentiated clinically by observing the color change associated with the more vascular tissues distal to the pear-shaped pad. (C) Arrow indicates demarcation between pear-shaped and retromolar pads.

Fig. 3-13 (A) Partial denture for a tooth supported situation improperly designed without rests. (B) In the absence of tooth support, functional forces directed to the mandibular ridge crest have resulted in accelerated resorption of the bone of the residual ridge.

DESIGN OF TOOTH-MUCOSA BORNE (DENTO-ALVEOLAR AND MUCO-OSSEOUS SUPPORTED) RPDs

A. OBJECTIVE: To transmit functional forces equitably to the dento-alveolar and muco-osseous segments. Equitable distribution of forces does not necessarily mean equal. It refers to an optimal distribution based upon the potential of tissue to withstand forces. Muco-osseous tissues have been described as being approximately 25 times more displaceable than the dento-alveolar tissues.

1. Evaluate muco-osseous and dento-alveolar tissue support potential. Review of history, diagnostic casts, radiographs, and clinical findings may indicate future trends based on present condition and past response. (See "Response of Force Bearing Tissues to Mechanical Loading").

2. Evaluate the potential magnitude of applied forces involved. The functional requirements of a prosthesis in each individual is unique. The anticipated magnitude of the functional forces of occlusion may vary (i.e. two casts from two different patients demonstrating the same missing teeth may require two different designs depending upon their functional requirements).

   a. Opposing occlusion.

      i. Mucosa borne (Complete dentures). Exert the least force during function.

      ii. Tooth-mucosa borne. (Extension base RPDs) The anticipated force during function usually will be more than provided by complete dentures but less than provided by tooth borne prostheses.

      iii. Tooth borne (Tooth borne RPDs, fixed partial dentures or natural dentition). Usually exert the greatest force during function.

   b. Muscular force potential. Elevator muscle development (strength).

      i. Masseter and temporalis. Evaluated by visualization and palpation.

      ii. Medial pterygoid. Difficult to evaluate.

      iii. Frankfort mandibular plane angle (FMA). It has been suggested that patients with more acute gonial angles (FMA less than $24°$) may demonstrate improved efficiency of the elevator musculature since fiber direction is more perpendicular to the occlusal plane. Such efficiency together with enhanced muscle development may increase muscular force potential. (Fig. 3-14)

   c. Parafunctional habits. Increased forces directed by musculature to the prosthesis.

      i. Bruxing

      ii. Clenching

   d. Length of edentulous span being replaced with articulating artificial teeth. Increased mechanical leverage of longer spans on abutment teeth may require emphasis on mucosal support.

   e. History of prosthesis failure.

      i. Solder joint failure.

      ii. Porcelain failure.

      iii. Fractured RPD components.

   f. History of poor tissue tolerance.

      i. Chronic sore spots.

      ii. Excessive bone resorption.

      iii. Abutment tooth mobility.

      iv. Fracture or attrition of natural teeth.

3. Determine the relative distribution of force to the various supporting tissues. Based upon the amount of force involved and tissue potential to absorb and transmit force within physiologic limits in each patient.

4. Reduce potential for denture base movement (**maximize support**). Apply those concepts and procedures which will reduce the movement of the tooth-mucosa borne prostheses during loading and resist long term resorptive changes.

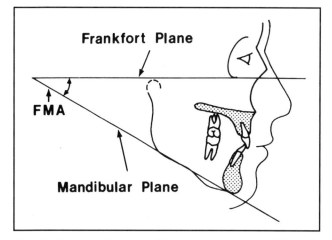

Fig. 3-14 Frankfort mandibular plane angle (FMA) is formed by the intersection of the mandibular plane with the Frankfort plane.

5. Recognize and compensate for denture base movement. Some movement will occur around the various axes of rotation during occlusal loading of the mucosa borne areas. Designs which permit base movement to occur with minimal adverse response of the supporting structures should be incorporated.

    a. Vertical axis. (Fig. 3–15)

        i. Passes at 90 degrees to the occlusal plane.

        ii. Horizontal (lateral) masticatory forces may cause a buccolingual movement of the partial denture around a vertical axis.

    b. Longitudinal axis. (Fig. 3–16)

        i. Passes along the edentulous ridge crest.

        ii. Unilateral loading causes tissueward movement on the loaded side and dislodging of the base on the opposite side.

    c. Fulcrum line axis. (Fig. 3–17)

        i. Passes through any two rests closest to the edentulous area depending upon the location of the force applied. While some rotational movement is inevitable during occlusal loading, excessive movement is undesirable.

        ii. A mandibular bilateral distal extension RPD fabricated without a corrected impression procedure (altered cast) may permit excessive rotational movement of the base in a tissueward direction during function due to the absence of adequate muco-osseous support.

6. Fulcrum line considerations.

    a. Fulcrum line generally passes through the two rests in closest proximity to the tooth-mucosa borne edentulous area. (Fig. 3–18)

    b. Distal extension base. Posterior to fulcrum line all components move gingivally and anterior to fulcrum line all components move occlusally. (Fig. 3–17)

    c. Mesial extension base. Anterior to fulcrum line all components move gingivally and posterior to fulcrum line all components move occlusally. (Fig. 3–3)

    d. Rigid elements of an RPD contacting abutment teeth occlusal to the survey line may result in torquing forces during occlusal

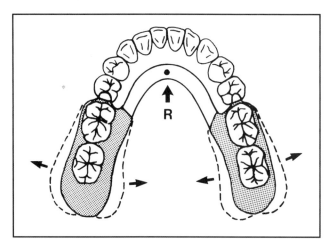

Fig. 3-15 Example of a vertical rotational axis. Arrows indicate potential direction of movement around rotational axis (R).

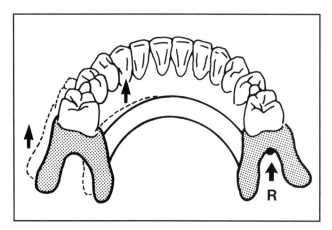

Fig. 3-16 Example of a longitudinal rotational axis. Arrows indicate potential direction of movement around rotational axis (R).

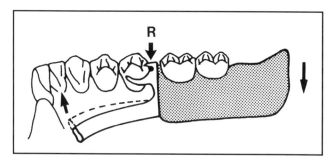

Fig. 3-17 Example of a horizontal rotational axis or fulcrum line. Arrows indicate potential direction of movement around rotational axis (R).

loading when present on the side of fulcrum line which moves gingivally.

e. Flexible elements engaging undercut areas of abutment teeth gingival to the survey line may result in torquing forces during occlusal loading when present on the side of the fulcrum line which moves occlusally.

f. Clasp design and evaluation of component movement is achieved following the identification of the fulcrum line.

B. DESIGN CONSIDERATIONS.

1. Rigid connectors.

   a. Major connector. Promotes cross-arch force transmission (contributes to cross-arch stability and support).

   b. Minor connectors. Transfer forces to and from abutment teeth.

2. Maxillary major connectors incorporate horizontal hard palate coverage to provide mucoosseous support as required. (Fig. 3–19)

3. Direct retainer designs for control of forces (minimize lateral and torsional forces to abut-

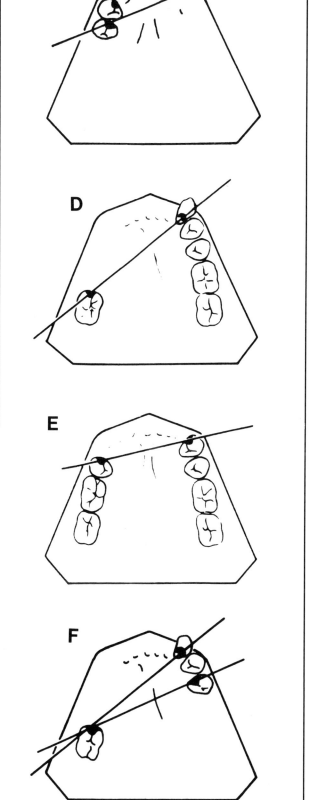

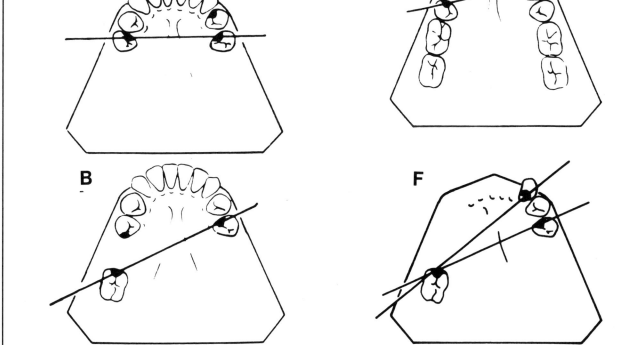

Fig. 3-18 (A,B,C) Fulcrum line axes indicated on distal extension RPD. (D,E) Fulcrum line axes indicated on mesial extension RPD. (F) Dual fulcrum lines indicated for a combined mesial and distal extension RPD.

ment teeth). Usually stress releasing designs are preferred.

    a. Stress director attachments. (See Chapter XXII)

    b. Wrought wire clasps. (See Chapter X)

    c. Remote rest and other conventional clasps. (See Chapter X)

    d. Split major connectors—permit more rigid clasp designs. (See Chapter V)

4. Rests provide dento-alveolar support.

    a. Although proximate rests may provide efficient force transmission to abutment teeth, remote rest clasp designs are usually more desirable since they may decrease unfavorable torquing forces on abutment teeth.

    b. Adequate tooth modification for rest seats promotes apically directed forces on abutment teeth.

5. Denture base extension provides muco-osseous support.

    a. Maximum soft tissue coverage as limited by movable tissues (i.e. snowshoe effect).

    b. Coverage of primary force bearing areas.

        i. Posterior maxillary ridge.

        ii. Buccal shelf.

        iii. Pear-shaped pad.

    c. Consequences of improper base extension. (Fig. 3–20)

6. Impression procedures. Application of selective pressure recording of the soft tissue to promote support. (See Chapter XVII).

    a. Dual stage selective pressure impression (altered cast impression).

    b. Reline at delivery.

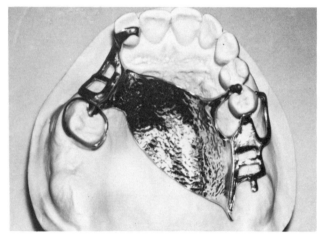

Fig. 3-19 Extent of major connector coverage of the horizontal palate depends upon the required support. Muco-osseous support is required on the tooth-mucosa borne segment indicating an expansion of the width of the major connector approaching that side of the arch.

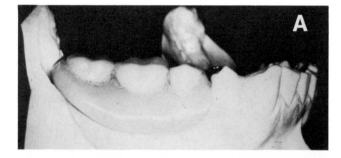

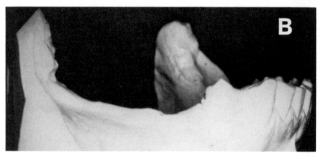

Fig. 3-20 (A) Denture base is under-extended without proper coverage of the pear-shaped pad and buccal shelf. (B) The accelerated resorption pattern is typical of denture bases which direct functional forces as pressure on the crest of the residual ridge crest.

Chapter IV

SURVEYING

Whenever possible, casts should be surveyed with the occlusal plane parallel to the base of the surveyor so that the path of placement is perpendicular to the occlusal plane. This position usually demonstrates favorable tooth contours which permit the development of an acceptable design. This neutral or zero degree tilt facilitates the development of a path of placement which may be easily managed by the patient. Unfortunately, most patients will tend to seat the partial denture under the force of occlusion. If the path of placement is other than perpendicular to the occlusal plane, such seating may deform the clasps.

DEFINITIONS

A. DENTAL SURVEYOR. A paralleling instrument used in the fabrication of a removable partial denture. (Fig. 4–1)

B. SURVEYING. The procedure of analyzing and delineating the contours of the abutment teeth and associated structures before designing a removable partial denture. (Fig. 4–2)

C. PATH OF PLACEMENT. The specific direction in which a prosthesis is placed upon the abutment teeth.

COMPONENTS OF A DENTAL SURVEYOR (Fig.4–3)

A. BASE.

B. VERTICAL ARM.

C. HORIZONTAL ARM.

D. MANDREL.

E. ADJUSTABLE TABLE.

F. ACCESSORIES.

   1. Analyzing rod.

   2. Carbon marker.

   3. Undercut gauges.

      a. 0.010 inch.

      b. 0.020 inch.

      c. 0.030 inch.

   4. Wax cutting instrument.

PURPOSE OF SURVEYING

A. DETERMINE MOST ACCEPTABLE PATH OF PLACEMENT AND REMOVAL. Whenever possible, the cast should be surveyed with its occlusal plane parallel to the base of the surveyor.

   1. Abutment tooth contours are usually favorable at this position.

   2. This facilitates the ease of placement and removal.

   3. Most patients will seat the partial denture under the force of occlusion. This directs the partial denture into place along a path perpendicular to the occlusal plane. If the partial denture was not surveyed with this same path of placement, the clasps may undergo permanent deformation.

B. IDENTIFY PROXIMAL TOOTH SURFACES THAT MAY SERVE AS GUIDING PLANES.

Guiding planes are proximal tooth surfaces that are parallel to one another and act to define a path of placement, contribute to stability, and ensure positive clasp action. (Fig. 4–4)

C. LOCATE AND MEASURE UNDERCUT AREAS OF TEETH THAT MAY BE USED FOR RETENTION. An undercut area is that portion of

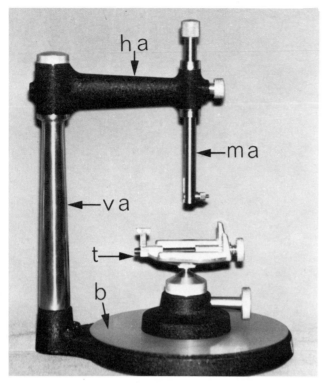

Fig. 4-1 Dental surveyor and surveying table. (b) Base; (va) vertical arm; (ha) horizontal arm; (ma) mandrel; (t) surveying table.

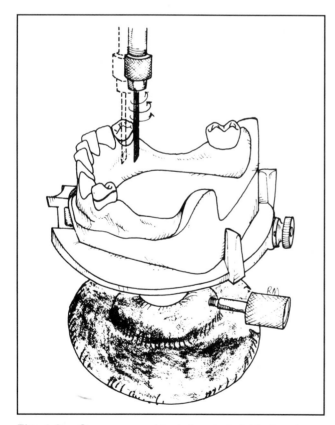

Fig. 4-2 Surveyor used to delineate height of contour.

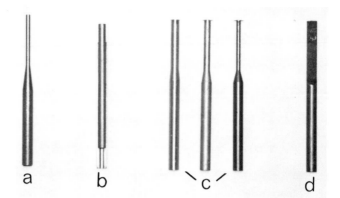

Fig. 4-3 Surveying accessories. (a) Analyzing rod; (b) carbon marker; (c) undercut gauges; (d) wax cutting instrument.

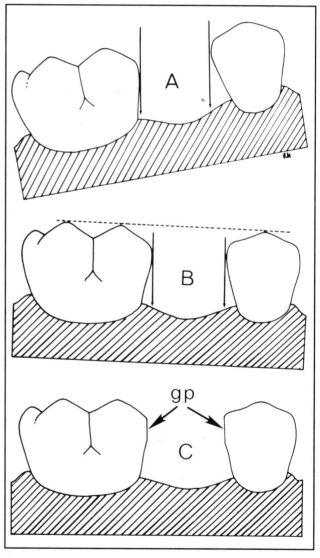

Fig. 4-4 Illustrations demonstrating the establishment of guiding planes. (A) Cast with occlusal plane not horizontal. (B) Cast surveyed with occlusal plane horizontal. (C) Guiding planes prepared on proximal surfaces of premolar and molar to define a path of placement.

a tooth which lies between the survey line (height of contour) and the free gingival margin. (Fig. 4–5)

D. EVALUATE TISSUE UNDERCUTS THAT WOULD ACT AS INTERFERENCES. (Fig. 4–6)

E. DETERMINE MOST SUITABLE PATH OF PLACEMENT FOR ESTHETICS. (Fig. 4–7)

F. ASSISTS IN DETERMINING RESTORATIVE PROCEDURES AND MOUTH PREPARATION.

G. DELINEATE HEIGHT OF CONTOUR (SURVEY LINE) ON THE ABUTMENT TEETH. The height of contour is a line encircling a tooth designating its greatest circumference at a selected position. (Fig. 4–5)

H. LOCATE UNDESIRABLE UNDERCUTS WHICH MAY NEED BLOCKING OUT PRIOR TO DUPLICATION.

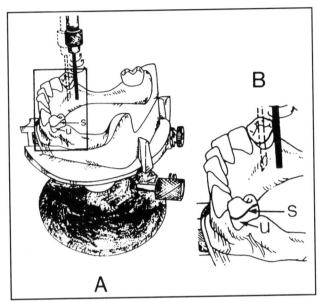

Fig. 4-5 Undercut area lies between the survey line (height of contour) and the free gingival margin. (A) Surveying table with cast in place. (B) Enlarged areas. (S) Survey line; (U) Undercut area.

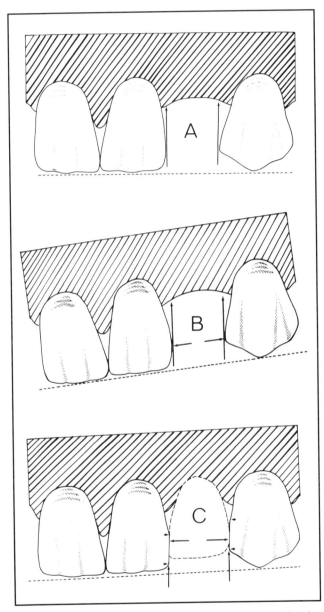

Fig. 4-7 Illustrations demonstrating a change in the path of placement for optimum esthetics. (A) Horizontal tilt would provide minimal interproximal space at the distal surface of the central incisor and excessive interproximal space at the mesial surface of the canine. (B) Cast tilted to distribute gingival embrasure space more favorably. (C) Guiding planes may be used to enhance esthetics where a wider tooth than permitted by the existing space would be indicated to provide symmetrical gingival embrasure space.

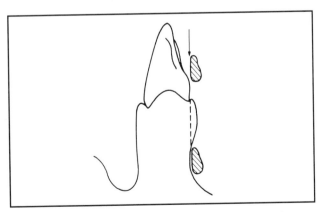

Fig. 4-6 Illustration indicating a soft tissue prominence that would interfere with the placement of a partial denture.

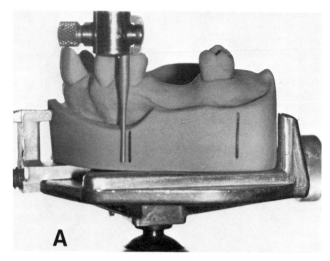

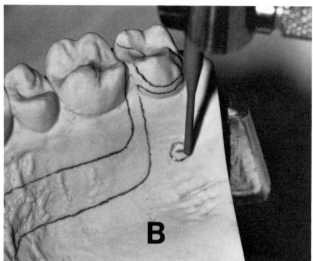

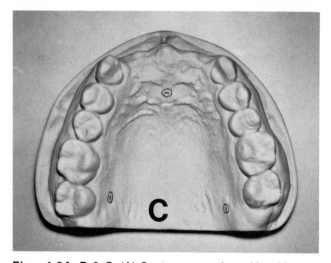

Figs. 4-8A, B & C (A) Cast on surveying table with analyzing rod indicating the path of placement. Three lines are placed on the sides of the cast to facilitate future repositioning. (B) Three marks placed on the tissue surface of the cast may be used in place of the lines. The marks are circled to make them more apparent. (C) An occlusal view of a maxillary tripodized cast.

I. RECORD THE CAST POSITION IN RELATION TO A SELECTED PATH OF PLACEMENT FOR FUTURE REFERENCE. Cast position can be recorded by tripodizing the cast by placement of three vertical lines widely separated on the sides of the cast, to permit its reorientation. (Fig. 4–8A) Three marks on the tissue surface may be used in place of the vertical lines. (Figs. 4–8B & C)

EFFECT OF TILTING A CAST ON A SURVEYOR

A. ALIGNS POTENTIAL GUIDING PLANE AREAS TO ALLOW A MORE FAVORABLE PATH OF PLACEMENT.

B. REDISTRIBUTES UNDERCUTS. (Figs. 4–9A & B)

C. FACILITATES THE USE OF A SPECIFIC TYPE OF CLASP FOR BETTER FUNCTION AND ESTHETICS.

D. DEVELOPMENT OF SYMMETRICAL GINGIVAL EMBRASURE SPACES FOR BETTER ESTHETICS.

E. MAY ELIMINATE SOFT TISSUE INTERFERENCES.

TYPES OF UNDERCUTS ESTABLISHED BY SURVEYING

A. TRUE. An undercut which is present in relation to the analyzing rod and to the path of placement or removal.

   1. CONTOUR—Due to natural contour of tooth.

   2. POSITIONAL—Due to tilt of cast.

B. FALSE. An apparent undercut which is present only in relation to the analyzing rod but not present in relation to a comparable undercut on the opposite side of the arch. (Fig. 4–10)

PROCEDURE FOR SURVEYING THE DIAGNOSITIC CAST

A. DETERMINING THE PATH OF PLACEMENT.

   1. Attach the cast to the adjustable surveying table and position the occlusal plane parallel to the platform of the surveyor.

   2. Place the analyzing rod in the surveyor mandrel and adjust the surveying table until the analyzing rod contacts the occlusal one third of the proximal surfaces of the proposed abutment teeth.

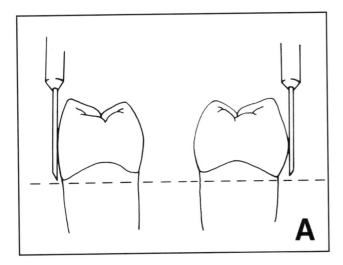

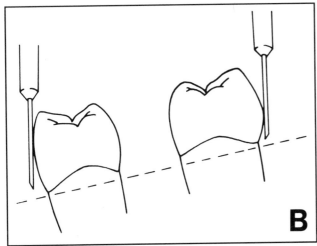

Fig. 4-9 Redistribution of undercuts by tilting the cast. (A) Cast surveyed with the teeth on the same horizontal level. (B) Cast tilted to redistribute undercuts.

3. Some tooth preparation usually is necessary to parallel these surfaces to one another, so they may serve as guiding planes. (Fig. 4–3)

4. These guiding plane surfaces will determine the path of placement.

B. ANALYZING THE UNDERCUT AREAS.

1. The analyzing rod is used to locate undercut areas. (Figs. 4–11 A & B)

2. The amount of undercut may be measured with undercut gauges provided with the surveyor. (Fig. 4–12)

3. The cast may be tilted to redistribute undercuts on the various abutment teeth. (Figs. 4–9A & B)

4. The locations of the undercuts must be suitable for the function and esthetics of the clasp.

5. Abutment teeth may have to be modified, or restored, to obtain proper contour. This may be indicated on the diagnostic cast.

6. Tissue undercuts that would act as interferences for any of the components of the partial denture should be evaluated on the diagnostic cast. A determination should be made to modify the design or to resort to surgical correction.

7. Lock the adjustable table in the most favorable position.

C. MARKING THE SURVEY LINES AND TRIPODIZING THE CAST.

1. Replace the analyzing rod with a carbon marker.

2. Mark the height of contour on the abutment teeth and other tissue prominences. (Fig. 4–5)

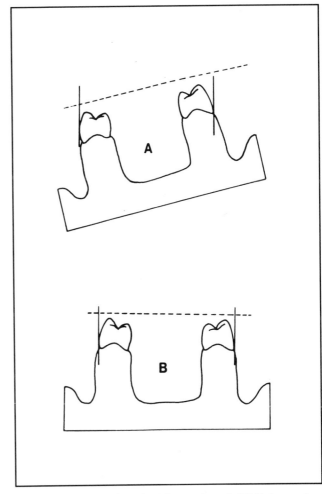

Fig. 4-10 Illustration of a false undercut. (A) False undercut produced by tilting. (B) Horizontal tilt indicates absence of contour undercuts. Utilizing false positional undercuts will not provide a retentive partial denture, since they are not present in relation to the path of placement or removal.

29

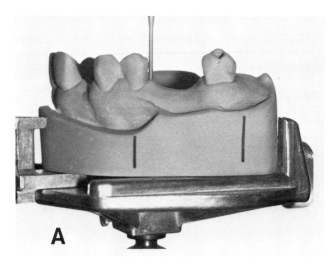

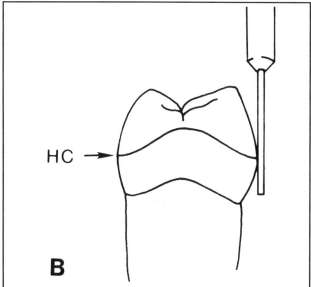

Fig. 4-11 (A) Analyzing rod used to locate undercut areas. (B) All the tooth surfaces gingival to the height of contour (HC) are undercut areas.

3. Record the cast position on the surveying table for future reference to this selected path of placement by marking it with three widely separated dots or lines. (Fig. 4–8)

D. SEQUENTIAL OUTLINING OF THE DESIGN ON THE DIAGNOSTIC CAST. (See Chapter XIII)

1. Rests.

2. Minor connectors and proximal plates.

3. Major connectors.

4. Clasp arms.

5. Bases.

6. Tooth modifications or restorations.

E. AN ADDITIONAL DIAGNOSTIC CAST MAY BE OBTAINED AFTER ALL MOUTH PREPARATION IS COMPLETED. This cast is surveyed to confirm the completed mouth preparation. It may be used to indicate the partial denture design to the laboratory.

PROCEDURE FOR SURVEYING THE MASTER CAST

A. ALIGN THE GUIDING PLANES. Which have been previously established.

B. DELINEATE THE HEIGHT OF CONTOUR (SURVEY LINE).

C. MARK THE UNDERCUTS. Indicate the precise location of the desired depth of undercut using a sharp line.

D. TRIPODIZE THE CAST.

Note: The final design may be drawn on the master cast or on a diagnostic cast which would accompany the master cast. A thin, clear, air dried cyanoacrylate coating may be applied to designed areas on abutment teeth of the master cast. This helps to protect the surface of the cast from abrasion and may improve casting adaptation.

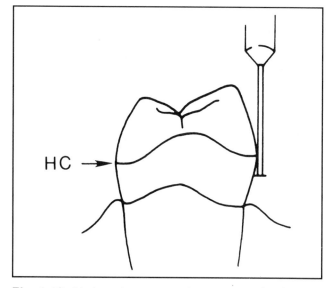

Fig. 4-12 Undercut gauge used to measure the depth of the undercut.

Chapter V

MAJOR AND MINOR CONNECTORS

Major and minor connectors serve to unite the various components of a removable partial denture. A major connector provides cross-arch stabilization by distributing forces from one side of the arch to the other. Maxillary major connectors may provide additional support for the tooth-mucosa borne partial denture by appropriate coverage of the hard palate. Whenever possible, major connectors should be designed to avoid gingival impingement and coverage.

MAJOR CONNECTORS

DEFINITION

A major connector is a plate, strap, or bar which connects the components on one side of the arch with those on the opposite side.

REQUIREMENTS OF MAJOR CONNECTORS

A. MUST BE SUFFICIENTLY RIGID TO TRANSMIT FORCES FROM ONE SIDE OF THE ARCH TO THE OTHER. This allows proper distribution of forces to supporting dento-alveolar and muco-osseous segments.

B. MUST BE PROPERLY LOCATED IN RELATION TO GINGIVAL AND MOVABLE SOFT TISSUES.

C. MUST NOT IMPINGE ON OR DEPEND ON THE MARGINAL GINGIVA FOR SUPPORT.

   1. Whenever feasible, major connectors which do not cover gingival tissues should be selected.

   2. Where gingival margins are covered, slight relief should be provided.

MAXILLARY MAJOR CONNECTORS— CRITERIA FOR SELECTION

A. THE LOCATION OF THE EDENTULOUS AREA(S). The major connector must connect the components of the partial denture.

B. THE AMOUNT OF SUPPORT REQUIRED. Maxillary tooth-mucosa borne partial dentures may derive support from the horizontal hard palate and maxillary residual ridge. The width of the major connector may be varied according to the amount of support required.

C. THE REQUIRED DEGREE OF RIGIDITY. The rigidity of the major connector may be increased by varying the thickness or by placing the metal in two different planes. Modifications may be limited by patient acceptance.

D. PATIENT PREFERENCE. Strap and plate type major connectors, because they can be made thinner, usually have a greater patient acceptance than the bar types. Some patients may find the increased palatal coverage uncomfortable due to alterations in gustatory, thermal or tactile perception. Generally, posterior (midpalatal) straps are less objectionable than anterior straps or bars.

E. ANTICIPATED LOSS OF NATURAL TEETH. The major connector may be designed to permit the future addition of artificial teeth to the partial denture.

F. LOCATION OF THE FULCRUM LINE. The extent of palatal coverage required for support may be influenced by the relation of the major connector to the fulcrum line. (Fig. 5–1)

MAXILLARY MAJOR CONNECTORS—DESIGN SPECIFICATIONS

A. THE BORDERS ARE PLACED AT LEAST 5 MM FROM THE GINGIVAL MARGINS. (Fig. 5–2)

B. WHEN A 6 MM DISTANCE FROM THE GINGIVAL MARGINS CANNOT BE OBTAINED, THE METAL MAY BE EXTENDED ONTO THE CINGULA OF ANTERIOR TEETH OR ONTO THE LINGUAL SURFACES OF THE POSTERIOR TEETH.

C. USUALLY NO RELIEF IS REQUIRED ON THE TISSUE SURFACE OF THE MAJOR CONNECTOR, EXCEPT WHEN IT CROSSES THE GINGIVAL MARGINS.

D. THE METAL SHOULD NOT BE HIGHLY POLISHED ON THE TISSUE SURFACE TO PRESERVE INTIMATE TISSUE CONTACT, EXCEPT WHERE IT CROSSES THE GINGIVAL MARGIN. When crossing the gingival margin, the tissue surface should be lightly relieved and highly polished.

E. ALL BORDERS SHOULD BE TAPERED SLIGHTLY TO BE LESS PERCEPTIBLE TO THE PATIENT.

F. THE FINISHED BORDERS SHOULD BE SMOOTHLY CURVED.

G. IN THE RUGAE REGION THE BORDER SHOULD PASS THROUGH THE VALLEYS OF THE RUGAE WHEN POSSIBLE.

H. THE POSTERIOR BORDER SHOULD NOT EXTEND ONTO THE MOVABLE SOFT PALATE.

I. THE BORDERS SHOULD BE BEADED.

1. A palatal major connector should have a specially prepared seal along the border of the connector where it contacts the soft tissue.

2. The seal is formed by a beading at the borders of the major connector that displaces the soft tissues slightly. This helps to prevent food from collecting under the connector and reduces patient awareness of the prosthesis. It is questionable whether or not the bead may contribute to the development of a peripheral seal that can significantly augment the physical retention.

3. The bead is produced by scribing a rounded groove on the master cast approximately 3/4 to 1 mm wide and deep at the edge of the design of the maxillary major connector. The groove must fade as it approaches within 6 mm of the gingival margins to prevent impingement. It should also fade over a hard midline suture or palatal torus. (Fig. 5–3)

J. THE PALATAL EXTENSION OF THE INTERNAL FINISH LINE IS DETERMINED PRIMARILY BY THE NEED TO RELINE THE PARTIAL DENTURE TO COMPENSATE FOR ANTICIPATED BONE RESORPTION.

1. For tooth borne partial dentures, the internal finish lines should be placed slightly palatal to the external finish lines. This staggered relationship contributes to increased framework strength and an adequate thickness of resin between the finish lines. Placement of the internal finish line more palatally is usually not indi-

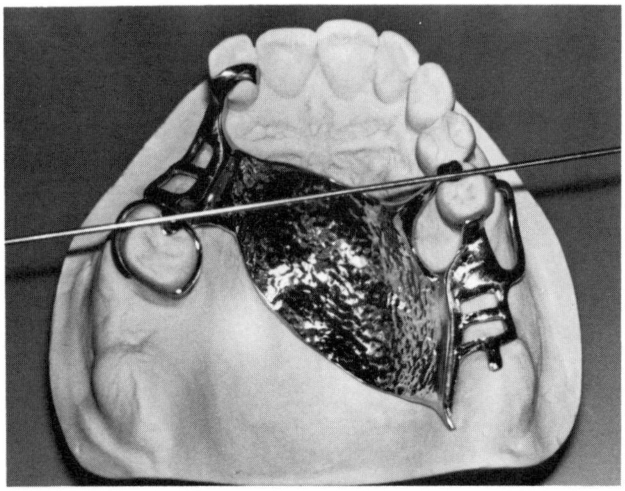

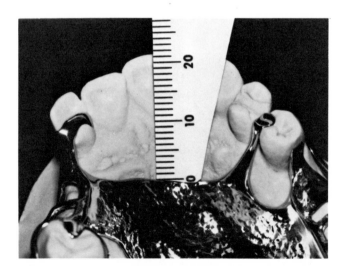

Fig. 5-1 Maxillary tooth-mucosa borne partial denture. The portion of the major connector located posterior to the indicated fulcrum line may provide muco-osseous support for the RPD.

Fig. 5-2 Maxillary major connector more than 6 mm from the gingival margin.

cated, since only minimal resorptive changes occur. (Fig. 5–4)

2. For tooth-mucosa borne partial dentures, the internal finish lines in the edentulous regions should be placed close to where the vertical and horizontal planes of the palate meet. This position is approximately 10 mm lingual to the previous position of the lingual gingival margins of the missing teeth. This permits proper relining, since bone resorption may occur up to this level. The horizontal portion of the hard palate is relatively resistant to pressure-induced resorptive changes. (Fig. 5–5)

L. WHEN FUTURE LOSS OF NATURAL TEETH IS ANTICIPATED A PLATE TYPE DESIGN MAY BE USED. The plate should extend onto the cingula of anterior teeth or onto the lingual surfaces of posterior teeth. (Fig. 5–6)

TYPES OF MAXILLARY MAJOR CONNECTORS

The term **strap** is used whenever the anteroposterior width of the major connector is in the 8 to 12 mm range. If the anteroposterior width exceeds 12 mm, the term **plate** is used. When the anteroposterior dimension covers the entire palate, the term **complete palatal plate** is used. Where the entire palate is not covered, the term **modified palatal plate** is applied. Since the thinner strap and plate designs usually have greater patient acceptance and biomechanical advantages, bar type maxillary major connectors are not described in this syllabus.

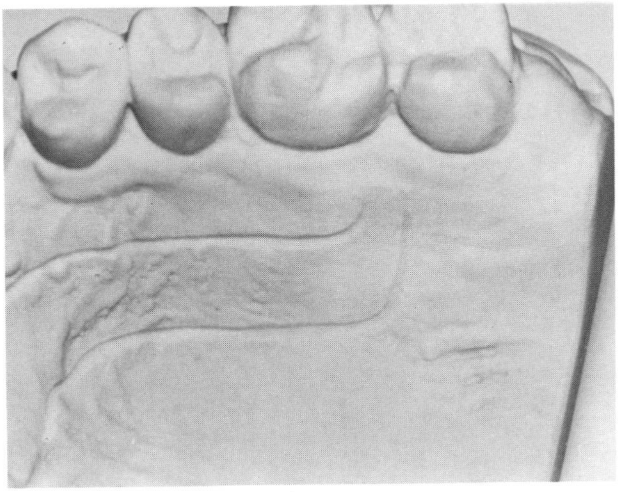

A. ANTERIOR PALATAL STRAP.

1. Indications.

a. May be used for tooth borne partial dentures when anterior teeth are missing. (Fig. 5–7)

b. May be used for tooth borne partial dentures when anterior and posterior teeth are missing. (Fig. 5–8)

c. May be used for partial dentures when a hard midline suture or palatal torus cannot be covered. (Fig. 5–8)

2. Additional factors.

a. Tends to be less rigid than other connectors as a buccolingual movement may occur in the posterior areas.

b. When increased rigidity is required, metal thickness in the central portion may be in-

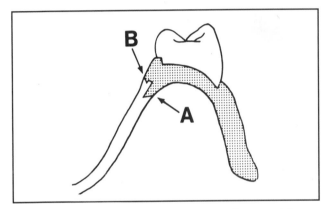

Fig. 5-4 Cross-sectional view of a maxillary tooth borne partial denture. The internal finish line indicated by arrow (A) is slightly palatal to the external finish line (B).

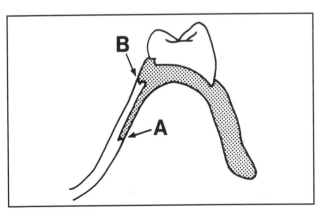

Fig. 5-5 Cross-sectional view of a maxillary tooth-mucosa borne partial denture. The internal finish line indicated by arrow (A) is placed approximately at the junction of the vertical and horizontal planes of the palate to permit relining. Arrow (B) indicates the external finish line.

Fig. 5-3 Maxillary cast grooved (scribed) to form a bead at the border of the major connector. The groove must fade as it approaches within 6 mm of the gingival margins.

creased to 1.5 mm, or the width of the strap can be increased to lie in two planes.

B. POSTERIOR PALATAL (MIDPALATAL) STRAP.

1. Indications.

   a. May be used for most maxillary tooth borne partial dentures when posterior teeth are missing. (Fig. 5–9)

   b. May be used for tooth-mucosa borne partial dentures when the extension base is short and minimal palatal support is required.

2. Additional factors.

   a. Anteroposterior width is within the 8–12 mm range. (Fig. 5–10)

   b. Rigidity may be increased by thickening the central portion to approximately 1.5 mm. (Fig. 5–10)

C. ANTEROPOSTERIOR PALATAL STRAP.

1. Indications.

   a. May be used for tooth borne, and tooth-mucosa borne partial dentures when replacement of anterior and posterior teeth

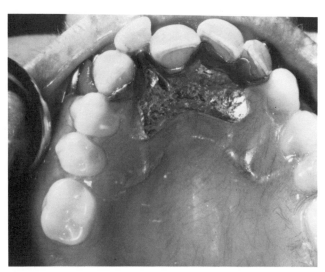

Fig. 5-6 Maxillary removable partial denture. Anterior teeth are plated to permit future addition of an artificial tooth to the RPD if a natural tooth is extracted.

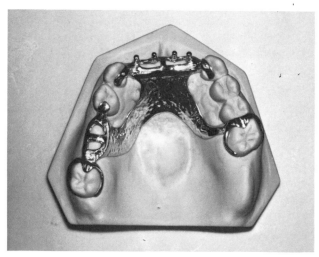

Fig. 5-8 Anterior palatal strap. This major connector may be used when anterior and posterior teeth are missing, or when a hard midline suture or palatal torus cannot be covered.

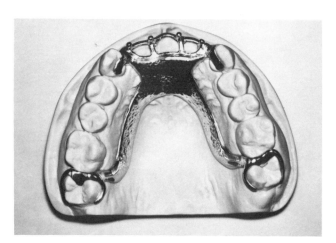

Fig. 5-7 Anterior palatal strap. This major connector may be used when anterior teeth are missing.

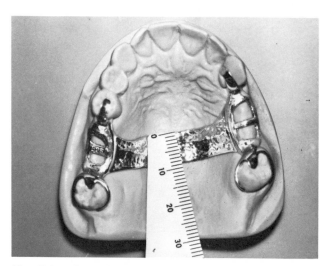

Fig. 5-9 Posterior palatal (midpalatal) strap. This major connector may be used for tooth borne partial dentures when posterior teeth are missing. The minimum width is 8 mm.

is required and greater rigidity than an anterior palatal strap is desired.

b. May be used when a palatal torus exists and rigidity is important. (Fig. 5–11)

2. Additional factors.

a. Straps lying in two different planes increase rigidity.

b. May lack muco-osseous support relative to the plate designs, since it covers less of the horizontal hard palate.

c. May compromise patient acceptance due to multiple borders.

D. MODIFIED PALATAL PLATE.

1. Indications.

a. May be used for tooth-mucosa borne partial dentures. (Fig. 5–12)

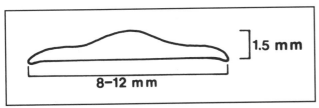

Fig. 5-10 Cross-sectional view of a posterior palatal (midpalatal) strap. The central portion may be thickened to increase rigidity.

b. May be used when complete palatal coverage is either not required or unacceptable to the patient.

2. Additional factors.

a. The width of the plate varies proportionally with the requirement for muco-osseous support. (Figs. 5–13 & 14)

i. The length of the edentulous span(s). A longer span generally requires a greater width for the required support, while a shorter span requires less width.

ii. Amount of anticipated occlusal forces. When the occlusion or muscular force potential indicates that a greater magnitude of force may be applied to the partial denture, the plate width should be increased.

iii. Periodontal status of abutment teeth. When the periodontal status of the abutment teeth is compromised, a wider plate is indicated to increase the support provided by the muco-osseous segment.

iv. Bone index of abutment teeth or the residual ridge(s). Poor bone indices indicate the need for a wider plate to increase the support provided by the horizontal hard palate.

b. Usually more acceptable to the patient than a complete palatal plate.

c. Usually provides greater support than any of the strap designs due to greater horizontal hard palate coverage.

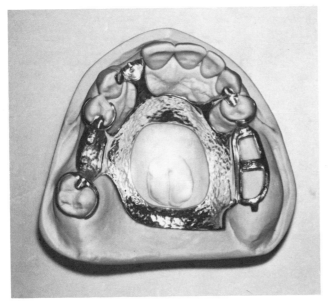

Fig. 5-11 Anteroposterior palatal strap. This major connector maybe used when a palatal torus exists and rigidity is important.

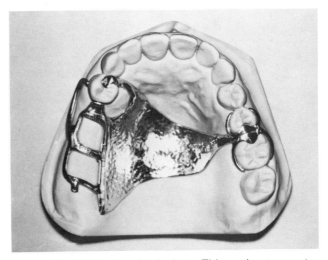

Fig. 5-12 Modified palatal plate. This major connector may be used for tooth-mucosa borne partial dentures.

E. COMPLETE PALATAL PLATE.

  1. Indications.

    a. May be used for long span bilateral tooth-mucosa borne partial dentures with or without anterior teeth replacement. (Fig. 5–15)

    b. Should be used whenever maximum muco-osseous support is desired.

    c. May be used in patients with palatal defects.

  2. Additional factors.

    a. Maximum palatal coverage should be considered whenever poor residual ridge conformation, periodontal disease, increased muscular forces or poor bone indices compromise abutment or ridge resistance.

    b. Often cannot be used in the presence of a palatal torus.

    c. Complete palatal coverage may alter gustatory, thermal, or tactile perception.

    d. Posterior border may be extended to the junction of movable and immovable soft palate to obtain maximum muco-osseous support.

  3. Types of complete palatal plates.

    a. Complete cast metal plate covering the entire palate. It may not be relined easily. (Fig. 5–16)

    b. Complete resin plate covering the entire palate. The resin areas may be relined or rebased.

    c. Combination of anterior metal with posterior resin areas. Permits the relining or rebasing of the resin areas. (Fig. 5–17)

F. SPLIT MAXILLARY MAJOR CONNECTORS. Permits a variable degree of independent movement of the muco-osseous supported segment of the RPD.

  1. Indications.

    a. May be used where some stress release from the abutment teeth is desired through the major connector. (Figs. 5–18 A, B, C, D)

    b. May be used in place of stress directors.

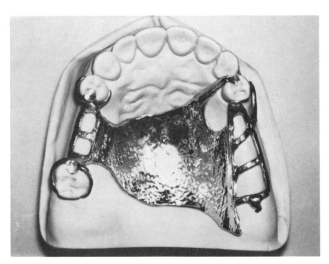

Fig. 5-13 Modified palatal plate. Broad palatal coverage provides optimum muco-osseous support.

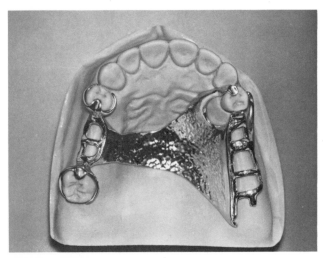

Fig. 5-14 Midpalatal strap. Narrow palatal coverage limits muco-osseous support provided by the major connector.

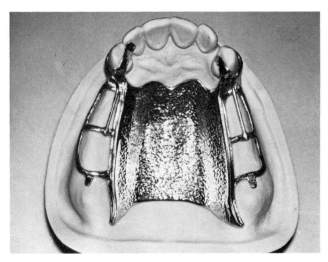

Fig. 5-15 Complete palatal plate. This major connector provides maximum muco-osseous support.

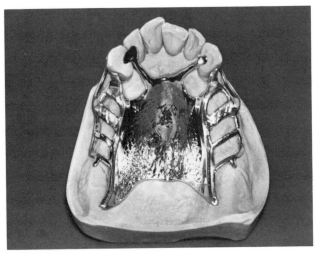

Fig. 5-16 Complete palatal plate. Palatal coverage with metal.

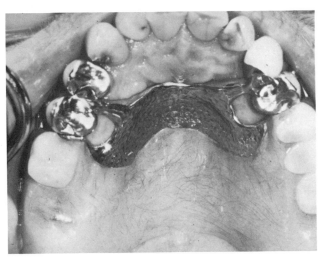

Fig. 5-17 Complete palatal plate. Posterior resin area facilitates relining.

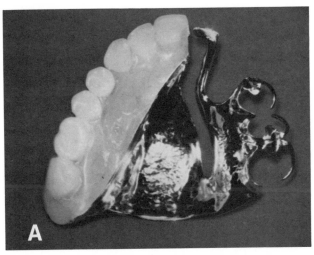

Fig. 5-18A Maxillary partial denture with split major connector.

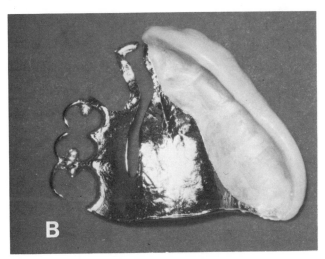

Fig. 5-18B Tissue surface of partial denture in Fig. 5-18A.

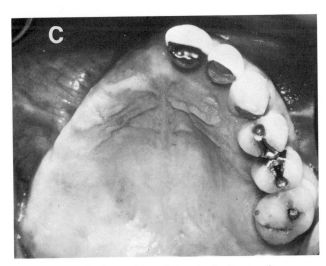

Fig. 5-18C Patient with unilateral missing teeth.

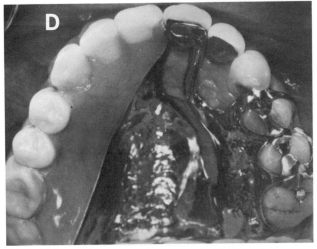

Fig. 5-18D Patient with partial denture in place.

2. Additional factors.

   a. Degree of stress release is determined by the width and thickness of the connection remaining and by the type of metal used.

   b. Separation of the segments should be wide enough or very narrow to avoid pinching the tongue or palatal mucosa. (Fig. 5–18A)

   c. The cast framework can flex in a single plane without work hardening and eventual fracture.

MANDIBULAR MAJOR CONNECTORS— CRITERIA FOR SELECTION

A. THE LOCATION OF THE EDENTULOUS AREA(S). The major connector must connect the components of the partial denture.

B. FUNCTIONAL DEPTH OF THE LINGUAL VESTIBULE (often referred to as the floor of the mouth). The major connector should not contact the mucosa at rest nor interfere with its movement during function.

C. ANTICIPATED LOSS OF NATURAL TEETH. The major connector may be designed to permit the future addition of artificial teeth to the partial denture.

D. INCLINATION OF REMAINING TEETH. Severe lingual inclinations may necessitate the use of a labial major connector.

MANDIBULAR MAJOR CONNECTORS— DESIGN SPECIFICATIONS

A. THE SUPERIOR BORDERS ARE PLACED AT LEAST 3 MM FROM THE GINGIVAL MARGINS. (Fig. 5-19)

B. WHERE A 3 MM DISTANCE FROM THE GINGIVAL MARGINS CANNOT BE OBTAINED, THE METAL SHOULD EXTEND ON TO THE CINGULA OF ANTERIOR TEETH OR ONTO THE LINGUAL SURFACES OF THE POSTERIOR TEETH.

C. RELIEF OF THE TISSUE SURFACE OF THE MAJOR CONNECTOR IS REQURIED TO PREVENT TISSUE IMPINGEMENT AT REST OR DURING FUNCTION.

   1. Relief is required for tooth borne partial dentures (30 gauge, 0.010 inch).

   2. More relief is required for tooth-mucosa borne partial dentures to accommodate for movement during function.

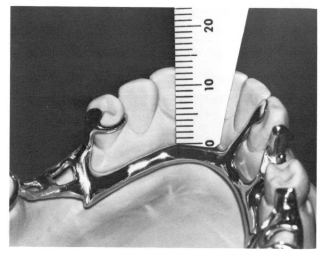

Fig. 5-19 Lingual bar major connector. The superior border is located more than 3 mm from the gingival margins.

   a. Relationship of the fulcrum line to the major connector.

      i. When the fulcrum line is posterior to the major connector less relief is usually required (28 gauge, 0.013 inch to 26 gauge, 0.016 inch). (Figs. 5–20A & B)

      ii. When the fulcrum line is anterior to the major connector more relief is usually required (26 gauge, 0.016 inch to 24 gauge, 0.020 inch). (Figs. 5–21A &B)

   b. Shape of the adjacent alveolar ridge. When the major connector moves tissueward, the lingual slope of the alveolar ridge may influence the amount of relief required (when the fulcrum line is posterior to the major connector). (Fig. 5–22)

      i. When the ridge has a vertical orientation, more relief may be required.

      ii. When the ridge has an anterior inclination, less relief may be required.

      iii. When the ridge has a posterior inclination (undercut), blockout of this undercut may provide sufficient relief.

      iv. Lingual tori require more relief.

   c. Quality of supporting tissues.

      i. Periodontal status of the abutment teeth. Increased mobility of the abutment teeth requires more relief of the major connector.

      ii. Quality of the muco-osseous supporting tissues. Residual ridges with displaceable tissues require more relief of the major connector.

iii. Bone index. Where the residual ridge exhibits a poor bone index, more relief may be required to compensate for resorptive changes occuring prior to anticipated relining.

iv. Movement of the dento-alveolar segment. When the anterior teeth have a pronounced labial inclination, more relief may be required. It may not be possible to direct the occlusal forces along the long axes of the teeth. With such an inclination, a continued labial migration of the teeth may occur. The labial migration may result in the major connector impinging on the soft tissues. (Fig. 5–23)

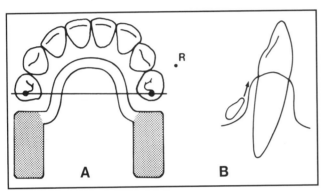

Fig. 5-20A & B (A) Fulcrum line located posterior to lingual bar. (B) Lingual bar rotates around fulcrum line axis (R). Rotation of bar parallels gingival tissue contour. Minimal relief is required.

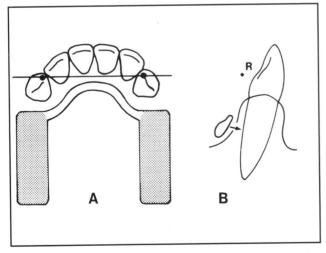

Fig. 5-21A & B (A) Fulcrum line located anterior to lingual bar. (B) Lingual bar rotates around fulcrum line axis (R). Bar rotates toward gingival tissues. Increased relief is required to prevent impingement.

D. THE METAL SHOULD BE HIGHLY POLISHED ON THE TISSUE SIDE TO MINIMIZE PLAQUE ACCUMULATION.

TYPES OF MANDIBULAR MAJOR CONNECTORS

A. LINGUAL BAR.

1. Indications.

   a. May be used when the functional depth of the lingual vestibule equals or exceeds 7 mm. (Fig. 5–24)

   b. May be used whenever gingival exposure is desired.

2. Additional factors.

   a. Should be half pear-shaped in cross-section. Superior-inferior dimension is 4 mm, and anteroposterior dimension is 2 mm. (Fig. 5–25)

   b. The superior border of the bar should be located at least 3 mm from the gingival margins of all adjacent teeth. (Fig. 5–25)

   c. The inferior border may be placed at the functional depth of the lingual vestibule. May require a functional impression to accurately register the lingual vestibule position and contour.

   d. Simplest mandibular major connector with highest patient acceptance.

B. SUBLINGUAL BAR.

1. Indications.

   a. May be used when the functional depth of the lingual vestibule is within the 5 to 7 mm range. (Fig. 5–26)

   b. May be used whenever gingival exposure is desired and a lingual bar cannot be used because of a lack of vestibular depth. (Figs. 5–27A & B)

2. Additional factors.

   a. The sublingual bar is essentially a lingual bar rotated 45 to 90 degrees. (Figs. 5–27A & B)

   b. The superior border of the bar should be located at least 3 mm from the gingival margins of all adjacent teeth. (Figs. 5–28 A, B & C)

   c. A functional impression of the lingual vestibule is required to accurately register the position and contour of the vestibule.

   d. Generally more rigid than a lingual bar in the horizontal plane.

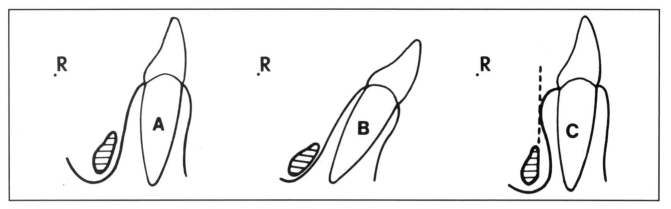

Fig. 5-22 Alveolar ridges of various shapes. (A) Vertical orientation, more relief may be required. (B) Anterior inclination, less relief may be required. (C) Posterior inclination (undercut), blockout of undercut may provide sufficient relief.

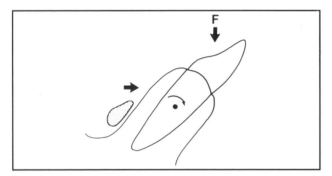

Fig. 5-23 Loading force (F) applied to tooth. Force is not directed along long axis, tooth may move labially. Lingual bar may impinge on soft tissues.

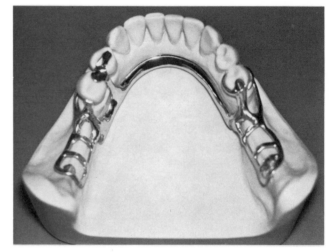

Fig. 5-24 Lingual bar. The lingual bar permits exposure of gingival tissues.

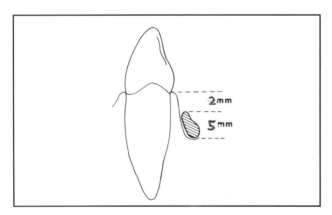

Fig. 5- 25 Lingual bar. Bar is 5 mm in height, 2 mm in width. Superior border is at least 2 mm from gingival margins.

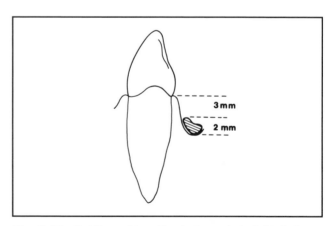

Fig. 5-26 Sublingual bar. Bar is 2 mm in height, 3-4 mm in width. Superior border is at least 3 mm from gingival margins.

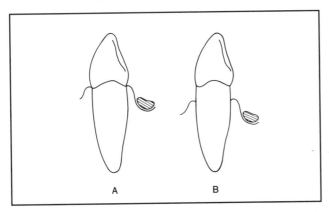

Fig. 5-27A & B Sublingual bar used when lingual vestibule is shallow. Sublingual bar used when gingival recession would contraindicate use of a lingual bar.

C. LINGUAL PLATE.

 1. Indications.

  a. May be used when the functional depth of the lingual vestibule is less than 5 mm. (Fig. 5–29)

  b. May be used when future loss of natural teeth is anticipated to facilitate addition of artificial teeth to the partial denture.

  c. May be used in combination with a labial bar, multiple clasps, or channel rests for splinting of teeth. (Figs. 5–30 A & B)

  d. May be used when lingual tori are present.

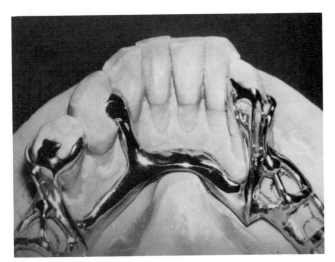

Fig. 5-28A Sublingual bar used posterior to incisors.

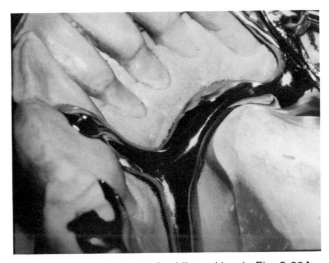

Fig. 5-28B Lateral view of sublingual bar in Fig. 5-28A.

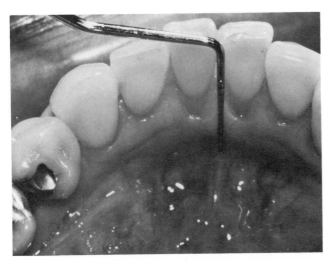

Fig. 5-28C Periodontal probe used to measure functional depth of the lingual vestibule (floor of mouth). A sublingual bar may be used when the depth is within the 5 to 7 mm range.

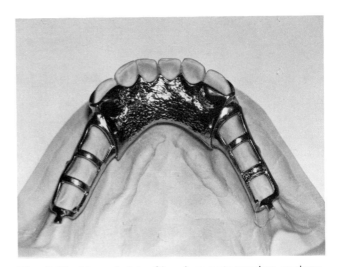

Fig. 5-29 Lingual plate. Cingulum rests used on canines.

2. Additional factors.

    a. Covers more tooth and gingival tissues than other mandibular major connectors.

    b. The superior border must positively contact the lingual surfaces of the teeth at or above the survey line to avoid food entrapment. The border should be as thin as possible without sharp edges to enhance patient comfort.

    c. The superior border should be positioned near the junction of the middle and gingival one thirds and extend interdentally to the contact points.

    d. In extension base partial dentures, the lingual plate should have a positive vertical stop (rest) on each side to prevent labial movement of the teeth.

    e. The inferior portion is shaped like a lingual bar, but may be thicker to increase rigidity. (Fig. 5–31)

    f. May deflect food from impacting on lingual tissues.

    g. May prevent or minimize extrusion of anterior teeth.

D. LABIAL BAR.

1. Indications.

    a. May be used when the mandibular teeth are so severely inclined lingually as to prevent the use of a lingual major connector. (Fig. 5–32)

    b. May be used when large lingual tori exist and their removal is contraindicated. (Figs. 5–33A & B)

2. Additional factors.

    a. Labial vestibular depth should be adequate to allow the superior border to be placed at least 3 mm below the free gingival margins.

    b. The labial bar tends to lack rigidity since it is considerably longer than a lingual bar.

E. SPLIT MANDIBULAR MAJOR CONNECTORS. Permits a variable degree of independent movement of the muco-osseous supported segment of the RPD.

1. Indications.

    a. May be used where some stress release from the abutment teeth is desired through the major connector.

    b. May be used in place of stress directors.

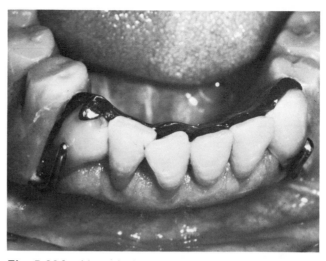

Fig. 5-30A Lingual plate major connector. Teeth have migrated labially. Lingual plate without rests or facial bracing components on all teeth may fail to prevent tooth movement.

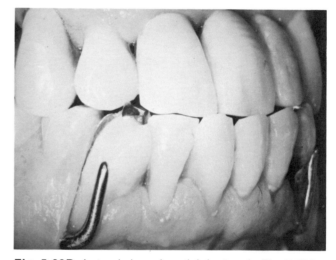

Fig. 5-30B Lateral view of partial denture in Fig. 5-30A.

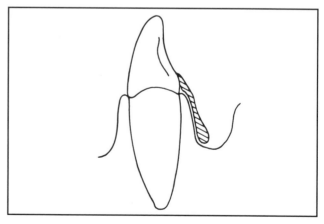

Fig. 5-31 Cross-sectional view of lingual plate. Inferior portion is shaped like a lingual bar. Note relief between tissue surface of plate and soft tissues.

2. Additional factors.

    a. May be fabricated in a single casting or in combination with a soldered wrought wire of large diameter.

    b. Due to the stress concentration, there is a tendency to fracture at the union of the bars, especially when a single casting is used.

MINOR CONNECTORS
DEFINITION

A minor connector is a rigid component that links the major connector or base and other components of the partial denture such as rests, indirect retainers and clasps.

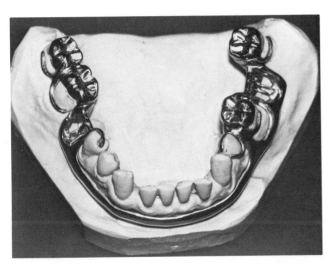

Fig. 5-32 Labial bar. Labial bar used where teeth are severely lingually inclined. Length of bar compromises rigidity.

REQUIREMENTS OF MINOR CONNECTORS

A. MUST BE SUFFICIENTLY RIGID TO TRANSMIT FORCES BETWEEN THE LINKED COMPONENTS.

B. MUST NOT IMPINGE ON MARGINAL GINGIVAL TISSUES.

DESIGN SPECIFICATIONS

A. THE MINOR CONNECTOR SHOULD HAVE SUFFICIENT THICKNESS FOR RIGIDITY.

B. WHERE THE MINOR CONNECTOR JOINS A REST, A MINIMUM METAL THICKNESS OF 1.5 MM AT THE JUNCTION IS REQUIRED FOR BASE METAL ALLOYS (2 MM FOR GOLD ALLOYS). (Fig. 5–34)

C. MINOR CONNECTORS SHOULD EXHIBIT MINIMAL GINGIVAL COVERAGE.

1. Lingual minor connectors should cross the gingival tissues directly, joining the major connector at a right angle. (Fig. 5–35)

2. The base of mesial and distal minor connectors and proximal plates adjacent to edentulous areas should swing back to join the major connector in a rounded acute angle in order to increase gingival exposure. (Fig. 5–35)

3. Maximum gingival exposure may be provided for mesial and distal minor connectors and proximal plates by increasing the relief which exists gingival to their contact with the guiding plane. (Fig. 5–36)

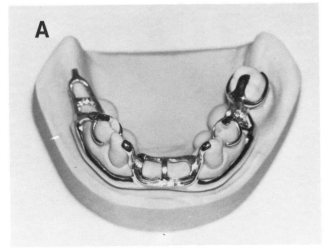
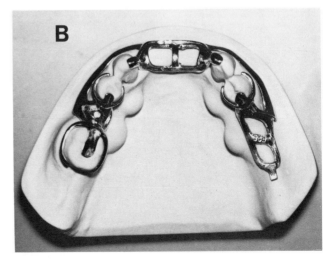

Fig. 5-33 (A) Labial bar. (B) Large tori prevent use of a lingual major connector.

D. RELIEF IS REQUIRED WHEN CROSSING GINGIVAL TISSUES.

1. Tooth-mucosa borne partial dentures. Slight relief (30 gauge) of minor connectors adjacent to extension base areas is required to prevent gingival impingement upon rotation of the partial denture during function. Other minor connectors require only minimal relief (32 gauge, 0.008 inch).

2. Tooth borne partial dentures. Only minimal relief (32 gauge) is required.

E. IN TOOTH-MUCOSA BORNE PARTIAL DENTURES, RELIEF SHOULD BE PROVIDED ON ADJACENT TEETH TO PERMIT MINOR CONNECTOR MOVEMENT DURING FUNCTION. (Fig. 5-37)

F. MINOR CONNECTORS WHICH CROSS GINGIVAL TISSUES SHOULD BE HIGHLY POLISHED TO MINIMIZE PLAQUE ACCUMULATION.

G. SHOULD BE LOCATED AT LEAST 5 MM FROM OTHER VERTICAL COMPONENTS. (Figs. 5-38 and 5-39)

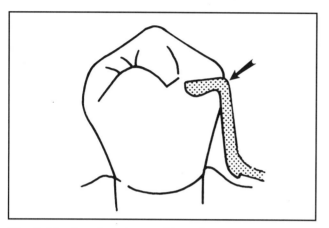

Fig. 5-34 Junction of rest with a minor connector should be a minimum of 1.5 mm thick.

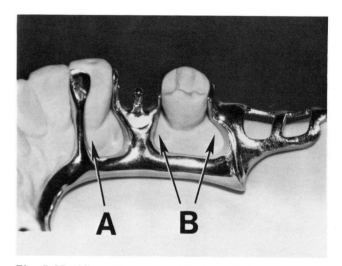

Fig. 5-35 Minor connectors. (A) Lingual minor connector from rest on canine crosses the gingival tissues directly, minimizing coverage. (B) Mesial and distal minor connectors swing back to increase gingival exposure.

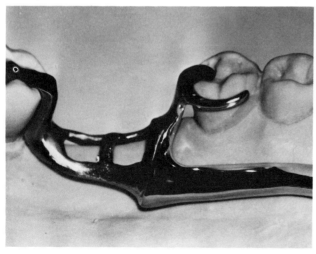

Fig. 5-36 Increased relief between minor connector and tooth maximizes gingival exposure.

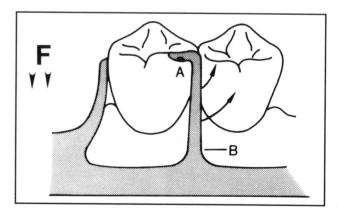

Fig. 5-37 Lingual view of RPI clasp during function. (A) Indicates center of rotation. Minor connector (B) rotates mesio-occlusally toward the adjacent tooth.

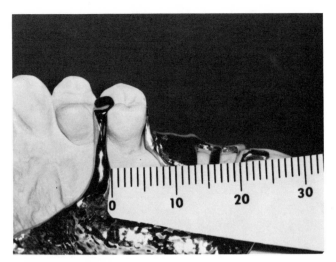

Fig. 5-38 Maxillary partial denture framework on cast. Minor connector should be located at least 5 mm from other vertical components.

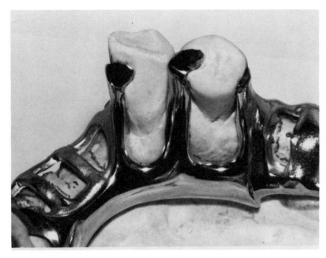

Fig. 5-39 Mandibular partial denture framework on cast. Note lack of exposure of gingival tissues. Minor connector from proximal plate should swing back distally, and minor connector from lingual rest should swing mesially. Compare with gingival exposure in Fig. 5-35.

Chapter VI

CLASPS AND INDIRECT RETAINERS

Clasps and indirect retainers are the components usually responsible for the retention of removable partial dentures. A great number of clasps have been described in the literature, creating confusion in the minds of many practitioners as to their indications. This chapter describes a limited variety of clasps that satisfy established biomechanical requirements for most partial denture designs.

CLASPS

DEFINITION

A clasp is an extracoronal direct retainer that engages an abutment tooth for retention, stability, and support of the partial denture.

CLASP COMPONENTS (Fig. 6–1)

A. REST. A rigid extension of a partial denture which contacts a remaining tooth in a prepared rest seat to transmit vertical and horizontal forces.

    1. Occlusal.

        a. Conventional.

        b. Extended.

        c. Overlay.

    2. Incisal.

    3. Lingual.

        a. Cingulum.

        b. Ball.

B. RETENTIVE COMPONENT. A clasp arm whose terminal portion engages an undercut area of an abutment tooth.

    1. Cast circumferential.

2. Cast bar.

3. Wrought wire circumferential.

C. BRACING (STABILIZING) COMPONENT. A rigid component that contacts a non-undercut area of an abutment tooth.

    1. Cast circumferential bracing clasp arm.

    2. Cast bar bracing clasp arm.

    3. Shoulder of circumferential retentive clasp arm.

    4. Minor connector.

    5. Proximal plate.

    6. Lingual plate.

    7. Rest.

REQUIREMENTS OF CLASPS

To fulfill the biomechanical requirements for a clasp, all components must contact a single abutment tooth (except splinted teeth).

A. RETENTION—Resistance to vertical dislodging forces.

    1. Provided by retentive clasp arms.

    2. Ordinarily, retentive areas on one side of the arch should be opposed by retentive areas similarly placed on the other side of the arch. For

example, a clasp with facial retention on the right side should be opposed by a clasp with facial retention on the left side. (Fig. 6–2)

3. Retention should be the minimum necessary to resist reasonable dislodging forces. This minimizes the possibility of deformation of the retentive clasp arms and facilitates placement and removal of the prosthesis.

B. BRACING (Stability)—Resistance to horizontal, lateral or torsional components of force.

   1. Provided by rigid portions of clasps or other rigid components.

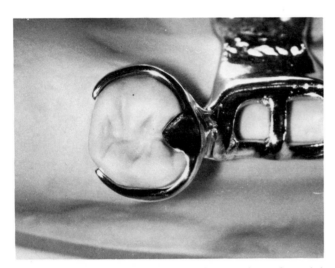

Fig. 6-1 Circlet (Akers) type of cast circumferential clasp. **Support** is provided by the occlusal rest; **bracing** is provided by the lingual cast circumferential bracing clasp arm, the shoulder of the buccal cast circumferential retentive clasp arm, the mesial minor connector and the occlusal rest; **retention** is provided by the retentive terminal of the buccal clasp arm; **reciprocation** is provided by the rigid lingual clasp arm; **adequate encirclement** is provided by the buccal and lingual arms engaging more than 180° of the circumference of the tooth.

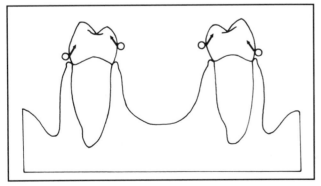

Fig. 6-2 Facial undercuts used bilaterally. Clasps resist vertical and lateral dislodging forces.

2. Bracing may be unilateral or bilateral.

   a. Unilateral bracing—when bracing component(s) contact(s) the facial **or** lingual surface of an abutment tooth.

   b. Bilateral bracing—when bracing components contact both facial **and** lingual surfaces of an abutment tooth.

C. SUPPORT—Resistance to vertical seating forces.

   1. Provided by the rest.

   2. Prevents trauma to peridental structures.

D. RECIPROCATION (Reciprocal action)—Resistance to horizontal forces exerted on a tooth by an active retentive element.

   1. Provided by rigid bracing components contacting the surface of the tooth opposite the retentive clasp arm.

   2. Opposes forces exerted by the retentive clasp arm terminal through its action distance during seating and unseating of the prosthesis. This type of reciprocation is relatively unimportant since the force exerted by the retentive terminal during seating and unseating is transient, limited in magnitude, and occurs infrequently. (Figs. 6–3A & B)

   3. Prevents tooth movement that may result from over adjustment of retentive clasp arms. This type of reciprocation is important. (Fig. 6–4)

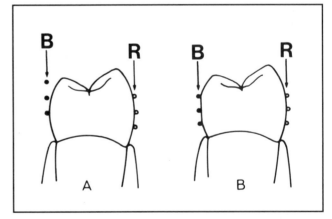

Fig. 6-3A (A) Circlet type clasp being placed on a tooth. (R) Retentive clasp arm, and (B) bracing clasp arm. Retentive clasp arm is not directly opposed by bracing clasp arm and exerts a mild, transient torquing force to the tooth until complete seating when the bracing clasp arm contacts the tooth.
Fig. 6-3B Surface of tooth modified to permit simultaneous contact of retentive and bracing clasp arms during placement. Retentive clasp arm is reciprocated minimizing torquing forces. This is accomplished with long guiding planes or ledged cast restorations, which are often not feasible.

4. Only one flexible retentive terminal should be used on each clasp, permitting the rigid component or components on the opposite side of the tooth to provide reciprocation and prevent tooth movement.

5. Rigid components do not engage undercuts unless a rotational path of placement is used.

E. ADEQUATE ENCIRCLEMENT—Prevents horizontal tooth movement from within the confines of the clasp.

1. May incorporate a minimum of three widely separated points of contact. (Fig. 6–5A)

2. May engage greater than 180 degrees (more than half the circumference). (Figs. 6–5B & C)

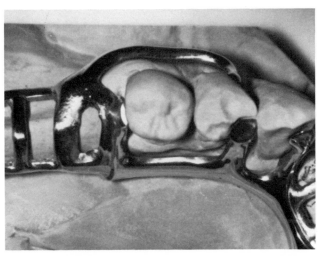

Fig. 6-4 Clasp on non-splinted mandibular premolars. Retentive "I" bar clasp arm is not opposed by a reciprocal component. Over-adjustment of the "I" bar may cause tooth movement.

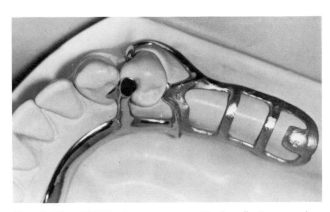

Fig. 6-5A "RPI" clasp on mandibular first premolar. Limited space between the three widely spaced components contacting the tooth prevents movement out of the clasp.

F. PASSIVITY—There should be no active force on the tooth when the clasp is in place. Its retentive function should be activated only when a dislodging force is applied. A force in an occlusal direction causes the retentive terminal to bind in the undercut from a gingival direction. The clasp should never "grip" the tooth.

CRITERIA FOR SELECTION OF CLASPS

A. TYPE OF SUPPORT (NATURE OF SUPPORTING TISSUES).

1. Tooth borne partial dentures. These partial dentures are supported by the dento-alveolar segment. Rests usually should be placed adjacent to edentulous areas minimizing or eliminating rotational movements of the partial denture during function. Clasps that are capable of directing forces to the muco-osseous segment are usually not indicated. All other criteria for the selection of clasps in this section apply.

2. Tooth-mucosa borne partial dentures. These partial dentures are supported by the dento-alveolar and muco-osseous segments. Due to the difference in displaceability between the segments the partial denture can be expected to rotate when forces are applied to the extension base. Clasps that direct forces equitably to the supporting segments are indicated.

B. MINIMAL TOOTH AND MINIMAL GINGIVAL COVERAGE. Clasps which minimize coverage of these tissues are preferred since they tend to reduce plaque accumulation.

C. LOCATION OF THE SURVEY LINE. The position of the height of contour (location of

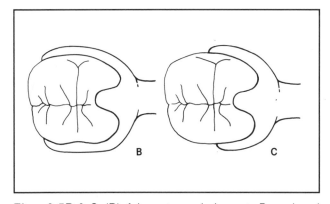

Figs. 6-5B & C (B) Adequate encirclement. Buccal and lingual clasp arms engage more than 180° of tooth circumference. Tooth cannot move horizontally away from clasp. (C) Inadequate encirclement. Buccal and lingual clasp arms do not engage more than 180° of tooth circumference. Tooth may move horizontally away from clasp.

undercuts) on the abutment tooth influences the selection of retentive and bracing components.

D. BILATERAL BRACING. When a broad distribution of forces is required, the use of clasps that provide bilateral bracing is indicated.

E. CONTOURS OF TISSUES ADJACENT TO THE ABUTMENT TOOTH. When the tissues surrounding the abutment tooth are undercut, or when the tooth is tilted relative to the path of placement, a bar type clasp arm may not be acceptable.

F. ANATOMIC LIMITATIONS. The occlusion, axial inclination, or overlapping of adjacent teeth may influence clasp selection.

G. ESTHETICS. The amount of the clasp arm visible during normal facial movements may be dependent upon the type of clasp selected. Most patients (95%) do not demonstrate the gingival one third of the mandibular canines and premolars during normal function. The figure is approximately 50% for the maxillary arch. Bar clasps, which usually contact less surface area and approach the undercut from the gingival direction, are often less conspicuous than circumferential clasps.

H. CLASPS ON PREVIOUS REMOVABLE PARTIAL DENTURE.

   1. May indicate esthetic awareness and demands of the patient.

   2. May indicate amount of retention necessary.

RETENTIVE CLASP ARM CONSIDERATIONS

A. CLASP ARM FLEXIBILITY IS INFLUENCED BY SEVERAL FACTORS.

   1. The cross-sectional size (diameter) of the arm. The smaller the diameter of the arm, the greater the flexibility.

   2. The length of the arm. The longer the arm, the greater the flexibility.

   3. The taper of the arm. Proper taper of the arm will increase flexibility.

     a. The clasp arm should taper uniformly in thickness and width.

     b. The thickness at the tip should be about one half the thickness at the attachment to the body. A clasp arm so tapered will have twice the flexibility of a non-tapered arm, and the greatest concentration of stress will be at the arm's thickest portion.

     c. Clasp arms which cross a groove on a tooth should follow the groove contour to main-

tain a uniform thickness. If a thin area were formed in the arm, stresses would concentrate in this area possibly leading to fracture. An increased thickness over the groove would impair flexibility.

     d. The tip of a clasp arm should be rounded and must not end in a sharp point.

   4. The metal alloy used. The flexibility of the arm varies with different alloys used for partial denture frameworks.

B. FACTORS DETERMINING THE DEPTH OF UNDERCUT ENGAGED.

   1. Amount of retention required. Little scientific evidence is available to determine the precise amount of retention required to promote optimal function, comfort and longevity.

   2. The number and location of retentive elements.

   3. Clasp flexibility. The more flexible the retentive arm of the clasp, the greater the amount of undercut which must be engaged to adequately retain the partial denture.

   4. Degree of gingival convergence. (Fig. 6–6)

   5. Presence of tripping action. Tripping action is attributed to clasp arms that engage the undercut directly from a gingival direction. These clasps tend to exert a pushing type of force during removal. Not all bar clasp arms exhibit tripping action, since the retentive terminal may actually engage the undercut from an occlusal direction, as is usually true with the "T"

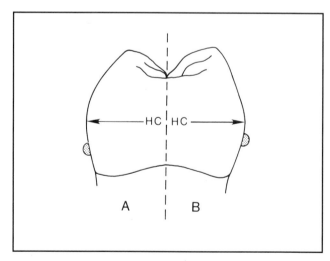

Fig. 6-6 Degrees of gingival convergence. Both clasps engage the same depth of undercut, but the distance to height of contour varies. (A) Less gingival covergence - less resistance to vertical dislodging forces. (B) More gingival convergence - more resistance to vertical dislodging forces.

bar or modified "T" bar. Clasps that do not demonstrate tripping action are termed pull type clasps.

CATEGORIES OF CLASPS

A. CAST CIRCUMFERENTIAL (SUPRABULGE). The retentive clasp arm originates from a minor connector or proximal plate, usually near the occlusal surface and approaches the undercut from an occlusal direction. Pull type clasps.

B. CAST BAR (INFRABULGE). The retentive arm originates from a major connector or denture base, passing adjacent to the soft tissues and approaching the tooth from a gingival direction. Some types (Push type, e.g. "I" bar) have a tripping action. Bar clasps are commonly named by the letter which most accurately describes the shape of the terminal portion.

C. COMBINATION.

1. Cast circumferential clasp arm and cast bar clasp arm.

2. Cast clasp arm and wrought wire clasp arm.

TYPES OF CIRCUMFERENTIAL (SUPRABULGE) CLASPS

A. CIRCLET CLASP (AKERS). The term circlet clasp is applied to what was previously known as an Akers clasp. (Figs. 6–7A & B)

1. Components.
   a. Rest.
   b. Minor connector.
   c. Cast circumferential retentive clasp arm.
   d. Cast circumferential bracing clasp arm.
2. Engages 0.010 - 0.020 inch undercut.
3. Provides bilateral bracing.
4. Commonly used in tooth borne segments.

B. EMBRASURE CLASP. Essentially two circlet clasps originating from a common minor connector. (Fig. 6–8)

1. Components.
   a. Two rests.
   b. One minor connector.
   c. Two cast circumferential retentive clasp arms.
   d. Two cast circumferential bracing clasp arms.
2. Engages 0.010 - 0.020 inch undercut.

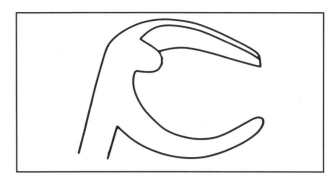

Fig. 6-7A Illustration of a circlet clasp.

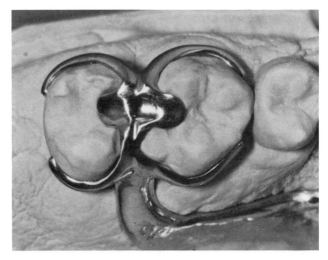

Fig. 6-7B Circlet clasp on a mandibular molar. The flexible lingual retentive arm is thinner than the rigid buccal bracing arm.

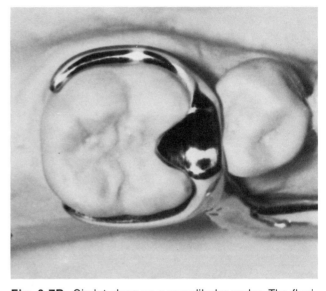

Fig. 6-8 Embrasure clasp on maxillary molars.

3. Provides bilateral bracing.

4. May be used when adjacent teeth are present on one side of the arch and additional retention and bracing are required.

5. Requires attention in rest seat preparation to ensure adequate metal thickness.

C. "RPC" ("RPA") CLASP. (Fig. 6–9)

1. Components.

    a. Rest.

    b. Minor connector.

    c. Proximal plate.

    d. Cast circumferential retentive clasp arm.

2. Engages 0.010 - 0.020 inch undercut.

3. Provides bilateral bracing.

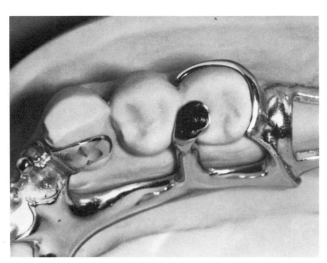

Fig. 6-9   "RPC" ("RPA") clasp on mandibular premolar.

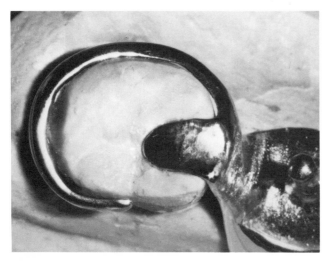

Fig. 6-10   Ring clasp on mandibular molar.

4. Commonly used in tooth-mucosa borne partial dentures where an "RPI" clasp cannot be used because of bar clasp arm contraindications.

D. RING CLASP. A single clasp arm which encircles nearly the entire circumference of the tooth. (Fig. 6–10)

1. Components.

    a. Rest(s).

    b. Minor connector.

    c. A single cast circumferential retentive clasp arm.

    d. Reinforcing component for retentive clasp arm (optional).

2. Engages 0.020 - 0.030 inch undercut.

3. Provides unilateral bracing.

4. May be used for tilted molars, although it is rarely indicated.

E. BACK ACTION CLASP. Similar to the ring clasp. (Fig. 6–11)

1. Components.

    a. Rest.

    b. Minor connector.

    c. A single cast circumferential retentive clasp arm which encircles nearly the entire circumference of the tooth.

    d. Does not have a reinforcing component for the clasp arm as the ring clasp usually does.

2. Engages 0.010 - 0.020 inch undercut.

3. Provides unilateral bracing.

4. May be used for premolars, though it is rarely indicated.

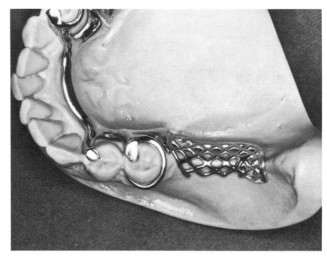

Fig. 6-11   Back action clasp on mandibular second premolar.

F. CIRCUMFERENTIAL "C" CLASP.
  (Figs. 6–12A & B)

  1. Components.

     a. Rest.

     b. Minor connector.

     c. Cast circumferential "C" retentive clasp arm.

     d. Cast circumferential bracing clasp arm.

  2. Engages 0.010 - 0.020 inch undercut.

  3. Provides bilateral bracing.

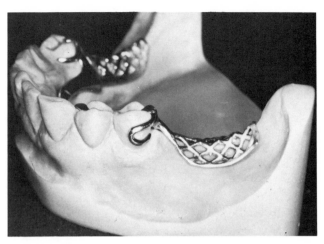

Fig. 6-12B Circumferential "C" clasp on mandibular second premolar.

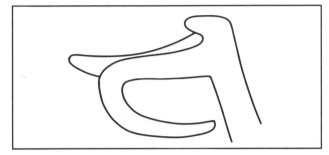

Fig. 6-12A Illustration of circumferential "C" clasp.

  4. May be used when a distofacial undercut exists, although it is rarely indicated, since the "C" clasp arm covers a large amount of tooth structure.

G. ADDITIONAL DESIGN CONSIDERATIONS FOR CAST CIRCUMFERENTIAL CLASPS.

  1. Only the terminal one third of the retentive clasp arm engages an undercut. (Fig. 6–13A)

  2. The retentive clasp arm terminus ideally should be located at the occlusal portion of the gingival one third of the tooth occlusogingivally. (Fig. 6–13A)

  3. The retentive clasp arm terminus should not contact the free gingival margin.

  4. For circumferential clasps, the proximal two thirds of the retentive clasp arm and the entire length of the bracing clasp arm should be located at the junction middle and gingival one third of the tooth occlusogingivally.

  5. Circumferential clasp arms located in the gingival one third of the tooth occlusogingivally may increase plaque accumulation apical to the clasp arms.

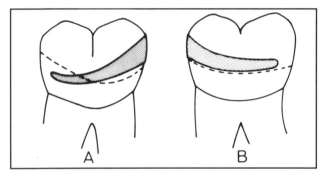

Figs. 6-13A & B (A) Retentive circumferential clasp arm. Terminal one third of clasp arm engages undercut. (B) Bracing circumferential clasp arm. Entire clasp arm is above height of contour.

  6. The bracing clasp arm should be slightly thicker than the retentive clasp arm to promote rigidity. (Fig. 6–13B)

TYPES OF BAR (INFRABULGE) CLASPS

A. "RII" CLASP. (Fig. 6–14)

  1. Components.

     a. Rest.

     b. Minor connector.

     c. Cast "I" bar retentive clasp arm.

     d. Cast "I" bar bracing clasp arm.

  2. Engages 0.010 inch undercut.

  3. Provides unilateral bracing.

  4. May be used for tooth borne segments. However, the additional gingival coverage may limit its use.

B. "RPI" CLASP. (Fig. 6–15)

1. Components.
   a. Rest.
   b. Minor connector.
   c. Proximal plate.
   d. Cast "I" bar retentive clasp arm.
2. Engages 0.010 inch undercut.
3. Provides unilateral bracing.
4. Commonly used for tooth-mucosa borne partial dentures.

C. ADDITIONAL DESIGN CONSIDERATIONS FOR BAR CLASPS.

1. The approach arm of a bar clasp must never impinge on soft tissue. The tissue surface of the metal should be smooth and polished with relief provided (30 gauge).
2. The superior border of the approach arm must be located at least 3 mm from the free gingival margin. (Fig. 6–16)

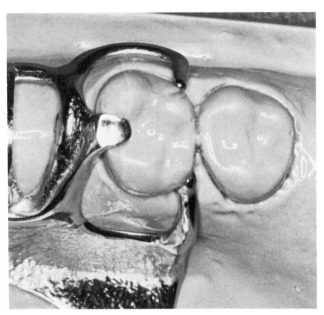

Fig. 6-14 "RII" clasp on maxillary molar.

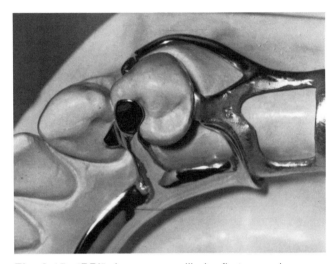

Fig. 6-15 "RPI" clasp on mandibular first premolar.

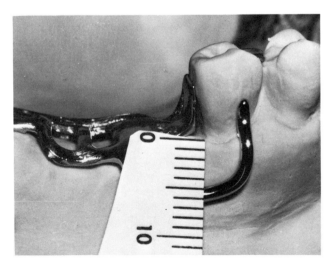

Fig. 6-16 Superior border of "I" bar approach arm located more than 3 mm from free gingival margin. Vertical portion of approach arm crosses gingival margin at 90° angle.

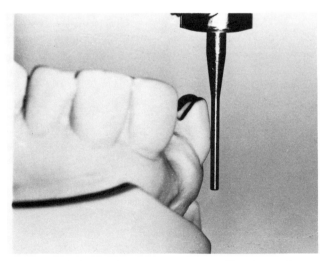

Fig. 6-17 Diagnostic cast on surveyor. Terminus of analyzing rod indicates position of approach arm for an infrabulge clasp. Note space between soft tissue area on cast and analyzing rod.

3. The approach arm should not be located over a deep tissue undercut since the great deal of relief required may form a food trap, interfere with patient comfort, or cause injury to the mucosa of the lip or cheek. Relief of 2 mm or more is considered excessive. Soft tissue undercuts are most accurately evaluated with a surveyor and a diagnostic cast. (Fig. 6–17)

4. The approach arm should not interfere with movable tissues. This requires a functional vestibular depth of at least 5 mm. This depth should be evaluated clinically by activating associated soft tissue attachments manually, since diagnostic casts do not accurately demonstrate soft tissue reflections.

5. The vertical portion of the approach arm should cross the gingival margin at a 90 degree angle. (Fig. 6–16)

6. The vertical portion approach arm should be located at least 5 mm from other vertical components. (Fig. 6–18)

TYPES OF COMBINATION CLASPS

A. CAST CIRCUMFERENTIAL AND CAST BAR CLASP. (Figs. 6 –19A & B)

1. Components.
   a. Rest.
   b. Minor connector.
   c. Cast bar retentive clasp arm.
   d. Cast circumferential bracing clasp arm.
2. Engages 0.010 - 0.020 inch undercut.
3. Provides unilateral bracing.

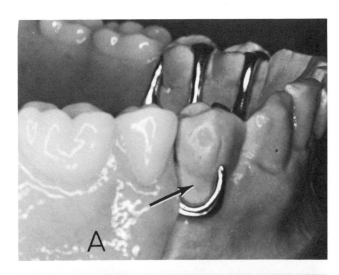

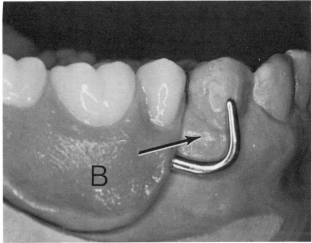

Fig. 6-18 Mandibular partial denture with acrylic resin base on cast. (A) Arrow indicates inadequate exposure of gingival tissue between denture base and approach arm of "I" bar. (B) Arrow indicates adequate exposure of gingival tissue.

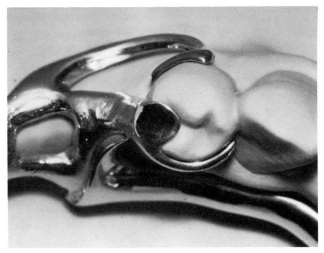

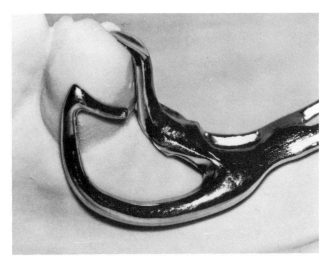

Figs. 6-19A & B (A) Occlusal view of combination clasp. Buccal modified "T" bar retentive clasp arm, lingual circumferential bracing clasp. (B) Buccal view of clasp from Fig. 6-19A.

4. Indications.

   a. Commonly used with "I" bar retentive clasp arm for tooth borne partial dentures when esthetics is important. (Fig. 6–20)

   b. May be used with modified "T" bar retentive clasp arm when a distofacial undercut exists. (Figs. 6–19A &B)

B. CAST CIRCUMFERENTIAL AND WROUGHT WIRE CIRCUMFERENTIAL CLASP.
(Figs. 6 –21A &B)

  1. Components.

   a. Rest.

   b. Minor connector.

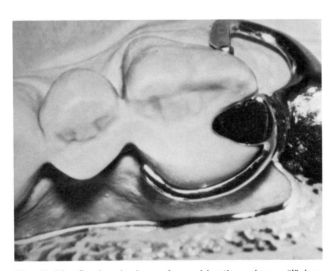

Fig. 6-20 Occlusal view of combination clasp. "I" bar retentive clasp arm engages a distobuccal undercut.

   c. Wrought wire circumferential retentive clasp arm.

   d. Cast circumferential bracing clasp arm.

  2. Engages 0.010 - 0.020 inch undercut.

  3. Provides bilateral bracing, but less than a cast circlet clasp.

  4. Commonly used for tooth-mucosa borne partial dentures.

C. ADDITIONAL DESIGN CONSIDERATIONS FOR WROUGHT WIRE CLASP ARMS.

  1. Selection of wrought wire clasps is determined primarily by the flexibility required. The flexibility is influenced by the gauge and composition of the wire. (See Chapter XV)

  2. The wrought wire should be attached to the framework at some distance from the minor connector to maintain flexibility and decrease fracture potential. (Figs. 6–21A & B)

INDIRECT RETAINERS

DEFINITION

An indirect retainer is a component of a tooth-mucosa borne partial denture which contacts an abutment tooth on the opposite side of the fulcrum line, assisting the direct retainers in preventing displacement of an extension base through mechanical leverage.
(Figs. 6–22A & B)

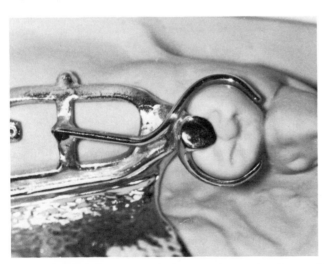

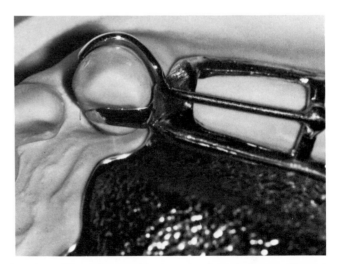

Figs. 6-21A & B (A) Occlusal view of wrought wire combination clasp. Buccal wrought wire retentive clasp arm, lingual cast bracing clasp arm. (B) Wrought wire clasp. Cingulum rest provides support, bracing and reciprocation. Note wrought wire is soldered to base area.

DESIGN CONSIDERATIONS FOR INDIRECT RETAINERS

A. THE EFFECTIVENESS OF INDIRECT RETAINERS IS THOUGHT TO BE DIRECTLY PROPORTIONAL TO THEIR DISTANCE FROM THE FULCRUM LINE. Several recent laboratory studies have questioned the effectiveness of conventional indirect retainers.

B. GUIDING PLANES PREPARED ON ABUTMENT TEETH ADJACENT TO THE EXTENSION BASE MAY PROVIDE THE MOST EFFECTIVE INDIRECT RETENTION. This may be due to the binding of the corresponding proximal plates or minor connectors. (Figs. 6–23A & B and 6–24A & B)

C. INDIRECT RETAINERS REQUIRE A POSITIVE VERTICAL STOP SUCH AS A PREPARED REST SEAT OR ROOT RETAINED FOR THIS PURPOSE.

TYPES OF INDIRECT RETAINERS

A. RESTS. The incorporation of a rest extending from a clasp may serve as an indirect retainer and permit the elimination of a minor connector. (Figs. 6–25 A, B & C)

B. MINOR CONNECTORS AND PROXIMAL PLATES.

C. OTHERS. Usually provide poor indirect retention unless positive rest seats are used.

1. Lingual plate.

2. Continuous bar (Kennedy bar) connector.

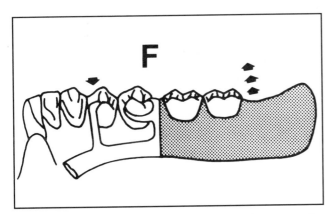

Fig. 6-22A Occlusal rest on mandibular first premolar located anterior to fulcrum (F) acts to resist lifting of denture base.

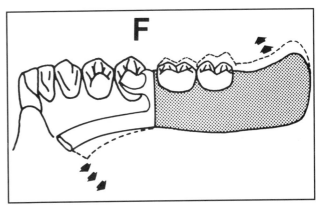

Fig. 6-22B Without an indirect retainer, the partial denture may rotate.

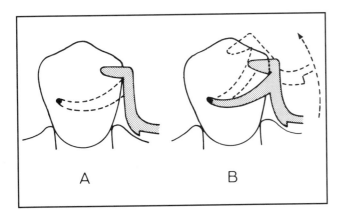

Figs. 6-23A & B (A) Cross-sectional view of a clasp on a tooth without a guiding plane.(B) Clasp may rotate during a vertical dislodging force as minor connector does not bind on guiding plane.

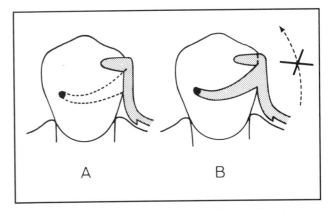

Figs. 6-24A & B (A) Cross-sectional view of a clasp on a tooth with a guiding plane. (B) Clasp rotation during a vertical dislodging force is restricted. Minor connector binds on guiding plane.

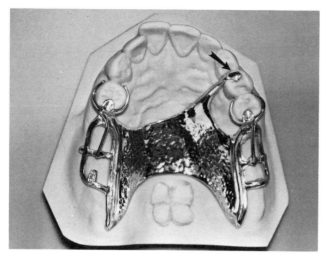

Fig. 6-25A Occlusal view of maxillary RPD. Arrow indicates indirect retainer.

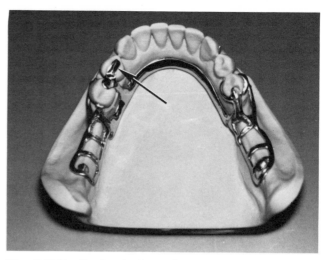

Fig. 6-25B Occlusal view of mandibular RPD. Arrow indicates indirect retainer.

ADDITIONAL FUNCTIONS OF INDIRECT RETAINERS

A. ENHANCE BRACING. Minor connectors associated with some indirect retainers may promote bracing, although this is questionable. Most indirect retainers move occlusally during function which may result in disengagement of the bracing component from the tooth.

B. IMPORTANT IN RELINE PROCEDURES FOR TOOTH-MUCOSA BORNE PARTIAL DENTURES AS A THIRD POINT OF REFERENCE. (Fig. 6–26)

1. When tooth-mucosa borne RPDs cause remodelling of the muco-osseous segment, the indirect retainer moves away from the tooth during function. An indirect retainer which moves away from its rest seat during seating forces may indicate a need for relining of the extension base.

2. During reline and impression procedures, the indirect retainers should be completely seated in their rest seats. This correctly orients the casting in relation to the teeth in three planes.

NOTE: Often maxillary complete dentures that oppose extension base partial dentures are erroneously relined or rebased when the problem lies in ridge resorption and subsequent settling of the partial denture. Indirect retainers may demonstrate this phenomenon and indicate the need for a reline procedure.

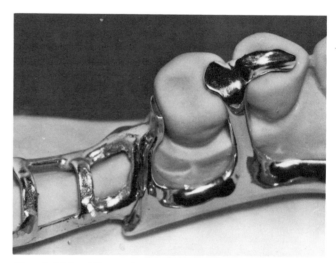

Fig. 6-25C View of indirect retainer in Fig. 6-25B. Extended rest from second to first premolar eliminates need for an additional minor connector, minimizing gingival coverage.

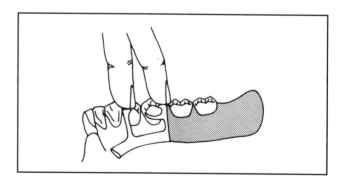

Fig. 6-26 The occlusal rest on the mandibular first premolar acts as a third point of reference. This allows the framework to be correctly oriented on the abutment teeth for a relining procedure.

Chapter VII

RESTS

Support derived from the dento-alveolar segment is provided by the rests. Surveys have indicated that a large percentage of removable partial dentures are fabricated without adequate rest seat preparation. Partial dentures that are well supported through proper rest design and rest seat preparation contribute to a favorable response of the dento-alveolar and muco-osseous supporting structures.

DEFINITION

A rest is a rigid extension of a partial denture which contacts a remaining tooth in a prepared rest seat to transmit vertical and horizontal forces.

REQUIREMENTS OF RESTS

A. SHOULD HAVE SUFFICIENT THICKNESS OF METAL TO PREVENT FRACTURE, ESPECIALLY AT THE JUNCTION OF THE REST AND MINOR CONNECTOR. (Fig. 7–1)

B. SHOULD BE PLACED ONLY ON SURFACES THAT WILL DIRECT FORCES ALONG THE LONG AXES OF TEETH. SHOULD NOT BE PLACED ON INCLINED SURFACES. Rest seat preparations are required to ensure axial force direction. (Fig. 7–2)

C. SHOULD BE EXTENDED AS CLOSE TO THE CENTER OF THE TOOTH (MESIODISTALLY) AS FEASIBLE TO PROMOTE AXIAL DIRECTION OF FORCES.

D. SHOULD BE PLACED IN REST SEATS WHICH DEMONSTRATE SMOOTH AND ROUNDED INTERNAL LINE ANGLES. For base metal alloys this improves the adaptation of the casting.

TYPES OF RESTS

A. OCCLUSAL. Used on the occlusal surface of a posterior tooth.

    1. Conventional. (Fig. 7–3)

    2. Extended. (Fig. 7–4)

    3. Overlay. (Fig. 7–5)

B. INCISAL. Used on the incisal surface of an anterior tooth. (Fig. 7–6)

C. LINGUAL. Used on the lingual surface of an anterior tooth.

    1. Cingulum. (Fig. 7–7)

    2. Ball. (Fig. 7–8)

DESIGN CONSIDERATIONS

A. OCCLUSAL RESTS.

    1. Conventional.

        a. The rest demonstrates a rounded triangular outline form when viewed from the occlusal.

        b. The tissue surface of the rest should be smooth and rounded. (Fig. 7–9)

        c. Should be one third the faciolingual width of the tooth or one half the width of the tooth measured at the cusp tips. (Fig. 7–10)

        d. Marginal ridge should be reduced 1.5 mm for base metal alloys, and 2 mm for gold alloys.

        e. Floor of the rest seat preparation should be spoon shaped and inclined apically as it approaches the center of the tooth. (Fig. 7–11)

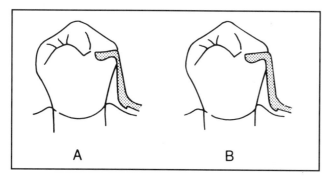

Fig. 7-1 Junction of rest and minor connector. (A) Inadequate thickness of metal at rest—minor connector junction. This may allow fracture of the rest. (B) Adequate thickness of metal at rest—minor connector junction.

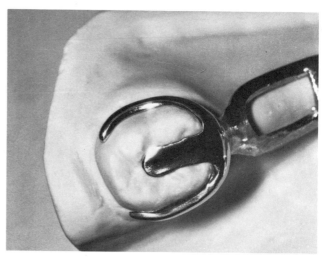

Fig. 7-4 Extended occlusal rest on mandibular molar.

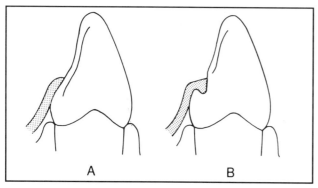

Fig. 7-2 Cingulum rests. (A) Cingulum rest placed on inclined surface of canine. Rest could move gingivally and cause a labial movement of the tooth. (B) Cingulum rest placed in a positive rest seat that prevents gingival movement of the rest.

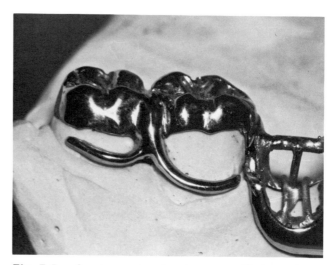

Fig. 7-5 Overlay occlusal rests on mandibular molars.

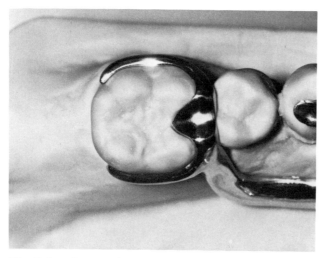

Fig. 7-3 Conventional occlusal rest on mandibular molar.

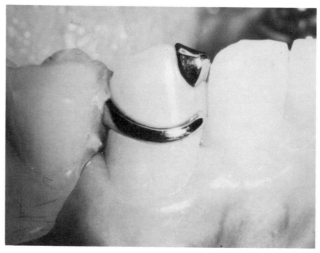

Fig. 7-6 Incisal rest on mandibular canine.

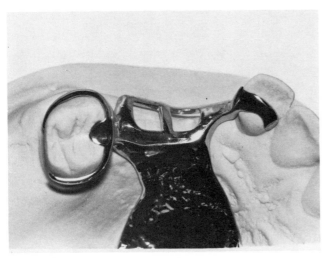

Fig. 7-7 Lingual cingulum rest on maxillary lateral incisor. Occlusal rest on molar.

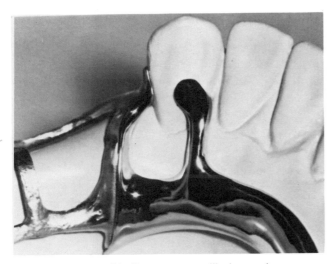

Fig. 7-8 Lingual ball rest on mandibular canine.

f. The angle between minor connector and rest should usually be less than 90 degrees. For distal rests on distal extension base partial dentures, the angle between the minor connector and rest should be 90 degrees. This permits release of the rests during function.

g. Rests for embrasure clasps are formed by two adjacent occlusal rests.

2. Extended.

a. For tooth borne segments of partial dentures, rests may be carried more than half way across the occlusal surface in order to promote axial force direction.

b. For tipped teeth, usually molars, extended occlusal rests should be designed to mini-

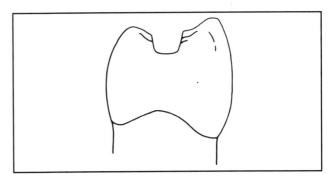

Fig. 7-9 Proximal view of occlusal rest seat preparation. Internal line angles are rounded.

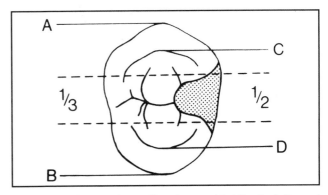

Fig. 7-10 Occlusal rest. Rest is one third the faciolingual width of the tooth (A-B) and one half the width of the tooth at the cusp tips (C-D).

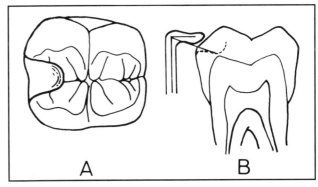

Fig. 7-11 Rest seat preparation on molar. (A) Occlusal view. (B) Lateral view.

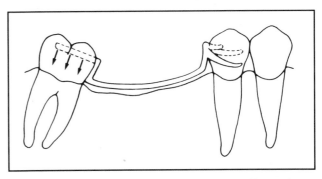

Fig. 7-12 Extended occlusal rest on molar. Floor of rest seat preparation is perpendicular to long axis of tooth.

mize further tipping, and should attempt to direct forces along the long axes of the teeth. (Fig. 7–12)

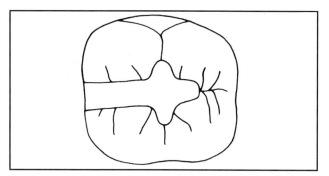

Fig. 7-13A Illustration of extended occlusal rest with irregular outline form.

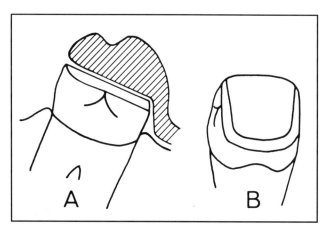

Fig. 7-13B Extended occlusal rest on mandibular molar.

c. An irregular occlusal outline form, or buccal and lingual dovetail extensions of the rest help to minimize rotation of the teeth. (Figs. 7–13A & B)

3. Overlay.

a. Cast restorations placed on tipped teeth may be fabricated with a flat occlusal surface perpendicular to the long axis. A bevel of 1 to 2 mm on the facial and lingual surfaces and a 2 to 3 mm guiding plane on the proximal surface will promote bilateral bracing and minimize further tipping of the tooth. (Figs. 7–14 A & B)

b. The occlusion is restored with a base metal or gold occlusal overlay as part of the partial denture framework. This type of rest takes advantage of the inclined plane effect, directing forces along the long axis of the tooth. It also serves to decrease the crown to root ratio of the abutment tooth. (Figs. 7–14A & B)

c. When overlay rests are placed over natural teeth, the facial and lingual bevels may be anatomically present in the form of cusp inclines. The proximal guiding plane should be prepared as in the cast restoration.

B. INCISAL RESTS.

1. Outline form of the rest seat is saddle shaped.

a. Concave when viewed from the facial. (Fig. 7–15)

b. Convex when viewed from the proximal. (Fig. 7–15)

2. The display of metal may be objectionable.

3. Greater mechanical leverage than lingual rests.

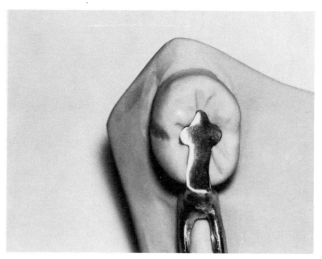

Fig. 7-14 Cast restoration on tipped molar. (A) Buccal view. (B) Mesial view.

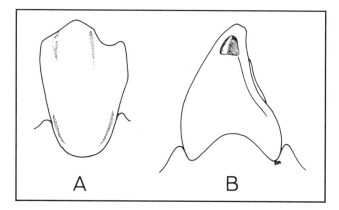

Fig. 7-15 Incisal rest seat preparation on canine. (A) Facial view. (B) Proximal view.

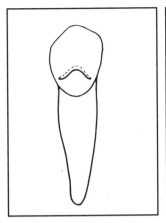

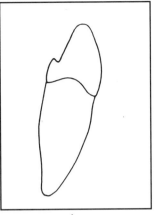

Fig. 7-16 Cingulum rest viewed from lingual.

Fig. 7-17 Cingulum rest viewed from proximal.

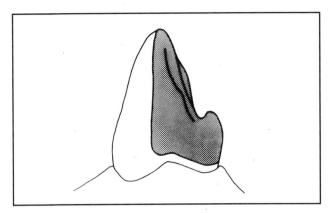

Fig. 7-18 Cingulum rest on partial veneer crown.

C. LINGUAL RESTS.

   1. Cingulum Rests.

      a. Inverted "V" or "U" shaped outline form when viewed from the lingual. (Fig. 7–16)

      b. Rest is "V" or "U" shaped when viewed from the proximal. (Fig. 7–17)

      c. Often difficult to obtain a positive apically inclined rest seat due to tooth angulation or anatomy. May require the use of a restoration to establish a definite rest seat. (Fig. 7–18)

      d. Precast etched metal cingulum rests have been described in the literature as an alter-

native when an adequate rest seat cannot be prepared in tooth structure.

   2. Ball Rests.

      a. Ball shaped rest with rounded outline form.

      b. Placed on the mesial or distal half of tooth, usually at the junction of middle and gingival one thirds. (Fig. 7–8)

      c. Preparation of a positive rest seat often results in dentin exposure. If the dentin is exposed the preparation may be modified to accept an amalgam or composite restoration. (Figs. 7– 19A & B)

      d. Ball shape permits rotational movements to occur during function of tooth-mucosa borne RPDs.

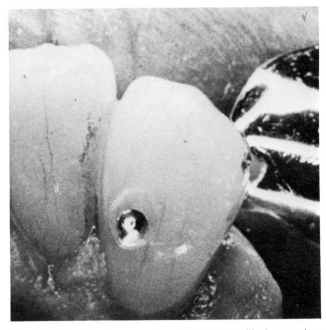

Fig. 7-19A Amalgam restoration in mandibular canine ball rest. Preparation of a positive rest seat resulted in dentin exposure.

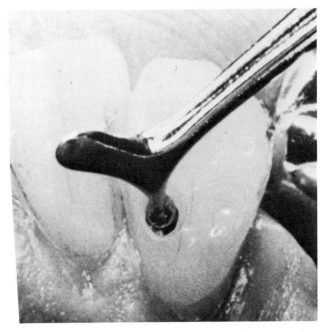

Fig. 7-19B Ball burnisher placed in rest seat preparation to verify contour. When an axially directed force is applied on the ball burnisher it should not slip out of the rest seat.

Chapter VIII

TOOTH BORNE REMOVABLE PARTIAL DENTURE DESIGN

The functional requirements of tooth borne fixed and removable partial dentures are similar. Support for the tooth borne partial denture is derived primarily from the dento-alveolar segment. Proximate rests are generally used on all abutment teeth adjacent to edentulous areas. Rotational movements of the partial denture in function are negligible. Selection of clasps is simplified and is based primarily on the periodontal status of the abutment teeth and esthetics.

ADVANTAGES OF A REMOVABLE PROSTHESIS

A. ABUTMENT TEETH MAY OFTEN BE UTILIZED WITHOUT REQUIRING CROWNS OR OTHER RESTORATIONS.

B. EASIER TO MAINTAIN ORAL HYGIENE.

C. CROSS-ARCH STABILIZATION IS READILY ACHIEVED.

D. USUALLY MORE ECONOMICAL ESPECIALLY WHEN MULTIPLE EDENTULOUS SPACES EXIST.

E. USUALLY MORE ESTHETICALLY ACCEPTABLE ESPECIALLY WHEN UTILIZING THE ROTATIONAL PATH OF PLACEMENT OR PRECISION ATTACHMENTS. (SEE CHAPTERS IX & XXII)

F. EASIER TO REPLACE LOST BONY AND SOFT TISSUE CONTOURS.

DISADVANTAGES OF A REMOVABLE PROSTHESIS

A. MAY BE PSYCHOLOGICALLY LESS ACCEPTABLE.

B. MAY BE DEFORMED IN CLEANING OR HANDLING.

C. MAY BE LESS ESTHETICALLY ACCEPTABLE WHEN UTILIZING CONVENTIONAL DESIGNS TO REPLACE ANTERIOR TEETH DUE TO DISPLAY OF CLASP ARMS.

D. MORE BULK IS PRESENT IN THE MOUTH.

FACTORS DETERMINING THE SELECTION OF MAJOR CONNECTORS

A. SUPPORT. The support for the tooth borne partial denture is derived almost exclusively from the dento-alveolar segment through the rests. Only in rare instances does the muco-osseous segment contribute support.

1. Maxillary major connectors. Strap designs are generally preferred. Plate designs which may derive support from the muco-osseous segment (horizontal hard palate) are seldom indicated.

2. Mandibular major connectors. Mandibular major connectors do not provide support since they do not contact the underlying mucosa. Minimal tissue relief is required since rotational movements are negligible.

B. LOCATION OF EDENTULOUS AREA(S). The major connector must connect the restored edentulous areas.

C. ANTICIPATED LOSS OF NATURAL TEETH.

   1. Plating the lingual surfaces of natural teeth facilitates the addition of artificial teeth to the partial denture. However, it requires unfavorable coverage of teeth and gingival tissues.

   2. A palatal plate major connector may be used if the anticipated loss of an abutment tooth will result in a tooth-mucosa borne partial denture. Plate designs provide more muco-osseous support than do strap designs.

D. FUNCTIONAL DEPTH OF THE LINGUAL VESTIBULE (FLOOR OF MOUTH). When inadequate depth exists for a lingual bar (less than 7 mm), a sublingual bar or a lingual plate may be used. (See Chapter V)

E. INCLINATION OF THE REMAINING TEETH. In rare situations when mandibular teeth are severely lingually inclined, a labial bar major connector may be required.

F. TISSUE RESTRICTIONS. Anatomic limitations such as palatal or mandibular tori, exostoses, or high lingual freni may affect the position or selection of the major connector.

G. PATIENT PREFERENCE. The major connector of the patient's previous partial denture should be noted, and the patient's acceptance should be evaluated. Those patients receiving an RPD for the first time usually prefer a lingual bar or a midpalatal strap.

FACTORS DETERMINING THE SELECTION OF CLASPS

A. SUPPORT. The support for the tooth borne partial denture is derived almost exclusively from the dento-alveolar segment. With supporting abutment teeth at both ends of the edentulous area(s), potentially destructive rotation of the partial denture under functional forces is virtually eliminated. Proximate rests adjacent to the edentulous areas are recommended to provide optimal support.

B. LOCATION OF UNDERCUTS. The location of true undercuts on abutment teeth will influence the choice of retentive clasp arms.

C. MINIMAL TOOTH AND MINIMAL GINGIVAL COVERAGE. Clasps which minimize coverage of these tissues are preferred since they tend to reduce plaque accumulation. (Figs. 8–1A & B and 8-2A &B)

D. ESTHETICS. The choice of a clasp arm may be influenced by its visibility during normal facial movements. Bar clasps, usually contact less surface area of the tooth, and are usually confined to the gingival one third of the tooth. Approaching the undercut from the gingival direction, they are often less conspicuous than circumferential clasps. (Fig. 8–3)

E. PERIODONTAL STATUS OF ABUTMENT TEETH. A broader distribution of vertical and

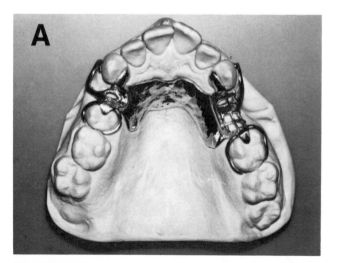 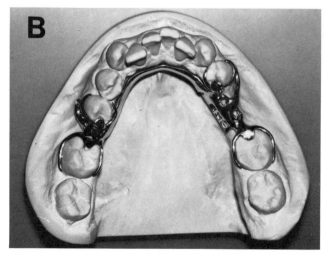

Fig. 8-1A & B Maxillary and mandibular arches with partial denture frameworks in place. Note the use of four clasps in each arch. With the edentulous spans being as short as they are clasping could be reduced. Either the rotational path or conventional path may be used reducing the clasp number from four to two to minimize tooth coverage and reduce plaque accumulation.

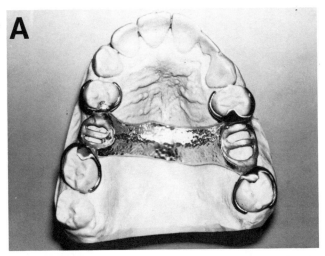

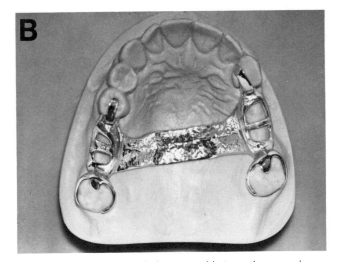

Fig. 8-2A & B (A) A maxillary partial denture using four clasps. (B) Maxillary partial denture with two clasps using a rotational path of placement. Note absence of clasp arms on the anterior abutments.

horizontal forces may be required when the periodontal status is compromised or when excessive tooth mobility is present.

1. A broad distribution of force may be accomplished by the use of multiple rests, lingual plates, and clasps that provide bilateral bracing.

2. Patient's oral hygiene and periodontal status must be carefully monitored since the additional number of components and increased tissue coverage may increase plaque accumulation.

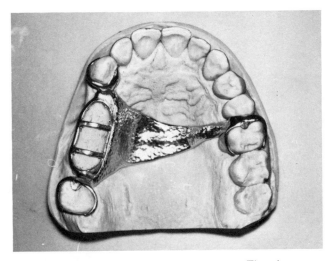

Fig. 8-3 A well designed partial denture. The clasp arm on the right canine could be eliminated if sufficient undercut exists on the distal surface of the canine permitting use of the rotational path.

F. ANTICIPATED LOSS OF ABUTMENT TEETH. Where the loss of an abutment tooth is anticipated and will result in a tooth-mucosa borne partial denture, clasps providing stress release should be considered for the retained abutment tooth. It should be noted that such a prognosis is difficult to make and may unnecessarily lead to a less than optimal design. Teeth that cannot be retained for the anticipated length of service of the RPD should usually be removed prior to prosthesis fabrication.

G. CLASPS ON PREVIOUS REMOVABLE PARTIAL DENTURE.

1. May indicate esthetic awareness and demands of the patient.

2. May indicate amount of retention necessary.

CLASPS COMMONLY USED FOR TOOTH BORNE REMOVABLE PARTIAL DENTURES

A. CAST CIRCLET CLASP (AKERS). Provides bilateral bracing.

B. CAST CIRCUMFERENTIAL AND CAST BAR CLASP. May provide better esthetics with a cast "I" bar retentive arm on the facial, and a cast circumferential bracing clasp arm on the lingual.

C. EMBRASURE CLASP. Provides increased bracing, support and retention.

FACTORS DETERMINING THE SELECTION OF DENTURE BASES

A. LENGTH OF SPAN.

  1. Long span bases. Denture base resin on metal framework.

     a. Facilitates restoration of lost tissue contours.

     b. Allows periodic relining to compensate for idiopathic or pressure induced resorptive changes.

  2. Short span bases. Metal base.

     a. Provides maximum strength with minimum bulk.

     b. Esthetics may limit use in anterior regions (See Chapter XI).

B. ANTICIPATED LOSS OF A DISTAL ABUTMENT TOOTH. A resin-metal base facilitates the addition of an artificial tooth to the denture base.

Chapter IX

ROTATIONAL PATH OF PLACEMENT FOR TOOTH BORNE PARTIAL DENTURES

The rotational path of placement differs substantially from the conventional or straight path. In the conventional path of placement, all the rests are seated more or less simultaneously. In the rotational path, one portion of the partial denture is placed first. This permits rigid portions of the framework to gain entry to undercut areas of abutment teeth which otherwise would not be accessible. The prosthesis is then rotated into its final position. The rotational path is limited primarily to tooth borne partial dentures. Its advantages are the elimination of anterior clasps to improve esthetics, and reduction of tooth coverage to minimize plaque accumulation. The most critical elements in utilizing the rotational path are the rest seat preparations and the development and maintenance of intimate contact between the rigid retainers and their corresponding tooth surfaces. If the proper form of the rest seat cannot be achieved, the rotational path design is contraindicated.*

GENERAL CONSIDERATIONS

A. WITH THE CONVENTIONAL PATH OF PLACEMENT, ALL OF THE RESTS ARE SEATED SIMULTANEOUSLY. (Figs. 9–1A & B) With the rotational path, one portion of the RPD must be seated first followed by rotation of the remainder of the partial denture into its final position. (Figs. 9–2A & B)

B. THE ROTATIONAL PATH CONCEPT CANNOT BE REDUCED SIMPLY TO A STRAIGHT PATH THAT DEVIATES MARKEDLY FROM THE PERPENDICULAR. (Fig. 9–3) A true rotational path partial denture cannot be seated along any straight path since the dimension between the cervical portions of the minor connectors in edentulous areas is greater than the distance between the corresponding marginal ridges. (Fig. 9–4)

C. PROPER USE OF THE ROTATIONAL PATH CONCEPT PERMITS THE ELIMINATION OF UNDESIRABLE OR UNESTHETIC CLASP ARMS WHILE STILL FULFILLING THE REQUIREMENTS OF SUPPORT, STABILITY, AND RETENTION.

---

* Many of the line drawings in this chapter have been reprinted from the International Journal of Prosthodontics, Volume 1, Nos. 1 & 2, 1988, with the permission of Quintessence Publishing Co., Inc., Lombard, Illinois.

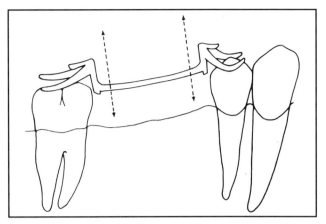

Fig. 9-1A Straight path of placement. Rests will seat simultaneously.

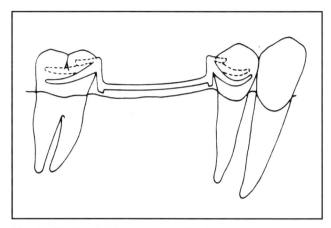

Fig. 9-1B Partial denture completely seated.

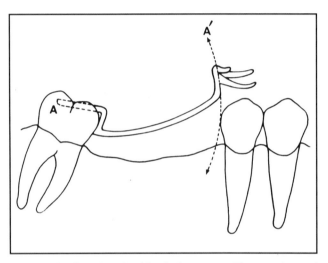

Fig. 9-2A Rotational path of placement. The terminus of the molar rest (A) is seated first followed by rotation of the premolar clasp along arc (A') into its final position.

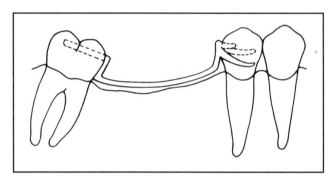

Fig. 9-2B Rotational path partial denture completely seated.

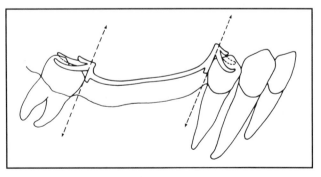

Fig. 9-3 Straight path of placement that deviates markedly from the perpendicular. Rests will still seat simultaneously.

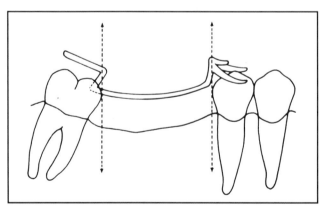

Fig. 9-4 A true rotational path partial denture cannot be seated along a straight path since the dimensions between the cervical portions of the minor connectors is greater than the distance between the corresponding marginal ridges.

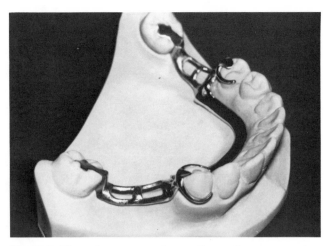

Fig. 9-5 The minor connector on the molar serves also as the rigid retentive component. Note contact of the minor connector along the mesial surface of the molar.

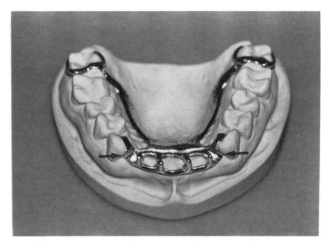

Fig. 9-6 Arrows indicate extensions of the minor connectors onto the mesial surfaces of the canines. These extensions act as the retentive elements (rigid retainers).

D. CONVENTIONAL CLASPS ARE REPLACED BY THE USE OF RIGID RETENTIVE UNITS IN COMBINATION WITH SPECIALLY DESIGNED RESTS (RIGID RETAINERS). Typically, each retainer consists of a rest and its retentive component. The retentive component may be a minor connector generally used on posterior teeth (Fig. 9–5) or an extension from a minor connector, generally used on anterior teeth (Fig. 9–6). The rigid retainers are designed to satisfy all of the biomechanical requirements for clasps.

E. THE RIGID RETENTIVE COMPONENTS ARE PLACED OR ROTATED INTO UNDERCUTS AND ARE MAINTAINED IN INTIMATE TOOTH CONTACT BY THEIR MODIFIED RESTS AND THE OTHER CONVENTIONAL CLASPS UTILIZED IN THE DESIGN.

F. FABRICATION OF ROTATIONAL PATH PARTIAL DENTURES PERMIT LITTLE TOLERANCE FOR ERROR. It requires appropriate knowledge on part of both the dentist and laboratory technician.

TYPES OF ROTATIONAL PATHS

A. Anteroposterior (AP)-Anterior segment seated first. (Fig. 9–7)

B. Posteroanterior (PA)-Posterior segment seated first. (Fig. 9–8)

C. Lateral. The edentulous side is seated first, followed by seating of the opposite side. (Fig. 9–9)

CATEGORIES OF ROTATIONAL PATH DESIGNS

A. CATEGORY I.

1. Rotational centers are located at the termini of the extended rests of the rigid retainers.

2. The rotational centers on each side of the arch determine the axis of rotation for placement of the partial denture. (Fig. 9–10)

3. The rotational centers are seated first then the prosthesis is rotated into place.

4. Includes AP and PA paths of rotation replacing missing posterior teeth, and lateral paths of rotation utilizing proximolingual undercuts.

B. CATEGORY II. (Sometimes referred to as dual path of placement.)

1. Rotational centers are located at the gingival extensions of the rigid retainers.

2. The rotational centers on each side of the arch determine the axis of rotation for final placement of the partial denture.

3. To gain access to the rotational centers, the segment with the rigid retainers is seated first along the straight path. The prosthesis is then rotated into place . (Figs. 9–11A)

4. Includes all AP paths of rotation replacing missing anterior teeth and all lateral paths of rotation utilizing proximofacial undercuts.

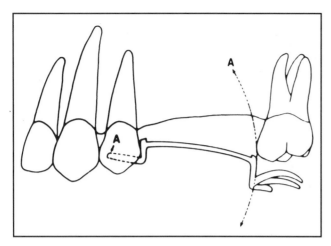

Fig. 9-7 Anteroposterior path of placement. Anterior segment is placed first. (A) is the center of rotation around which the partial denture rotates into position. (A') is the arc that the minor connector on the molar must follow for final placement.

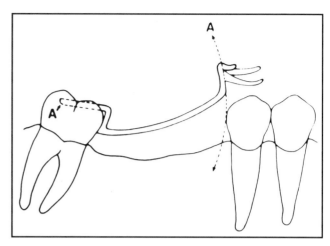

Fig. 9-8 Posteroanterior path of placement. Posterior segment is placed first. (A) is the center of rotation around which the partial denture rotates into position. (A') is the arc that the minor connector on the premolar must follow for final placement.

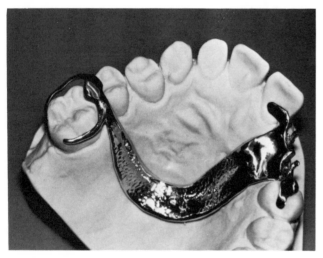

Fig. 9-9 Lateral path of placement. The side with the rigid retainers is placed first followed by seating the opposite side.

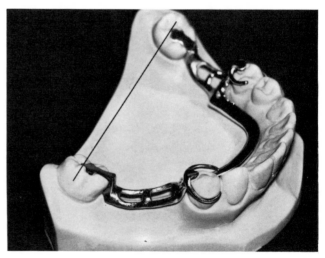

Fig. 9-10 The rotational centers on each side of the arch determine the axis of rotation for placement of the partial denture.

EXTENDED OCCLUSAL REST FOR THE RIGID RETAINER

A. THE REST SEAT PREPARATION MUST BE OF SUFFICIENT DEPTH TO ALLOW A REST THICKNESS OF 1.5 TO 2 MM.

B. THE FLOOR OF THE REST SEAT SHOULD BE PERPENDICULAR TO THE LONG AXIS OF THE TOOTH. (Fig. 9–12)

C. THE REST SEAT PREPARATION SHOULD EXTEND MORE THAN HALF THE MESIO-DISTAL DIMENSION OF THE ABUTMENT TOOTH WITH ITS FACIAL AND LINGUAL WALLS NEARLY PARALLEL. (Figs. 9–13A & B) The configuration and depth of the rest seat contributes to bracing, and axial distribution of forces.

D. RESTS SHOULD HAVE AN ASYMMETRICAL OUTLINE, DOVETAILS, ETC., WHICH WILL PROVIDE THE EQUIVALENT OF ADEQUATE ENCIRCLEMENT OF A CLASP. (Fig. 9–14) When a tooth is severely tipped a straight channel rest which minimizes further tipping may be indicated. (Fig. 9–13A)

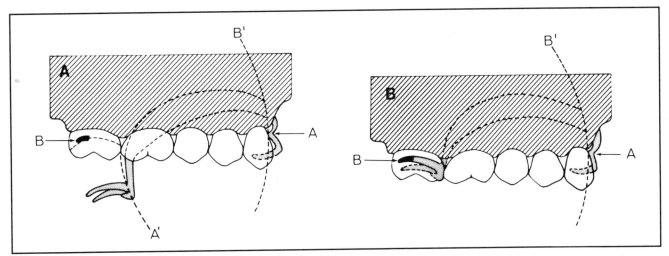

Figs. 9-11A & B (A) Category II rotational path. The segment with the rigid retainer is seated first along a straight path to gain access to the rotational center (A). The molar clasp is then rotated into place along the arc (A'). (B) indicates the retentive area for the molar clasp when the partial denture is seated. Displacement of the anterior segment would require the minor connector on the canine to pass through the mesial portion of the tooth.
(B) The partial denture completely seated.

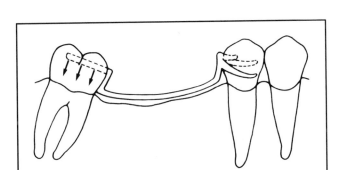

Fig. 9-12 The floor of the rest seat preparation in a mesiodistal direction is perpendicular to the long axis of the tooth.

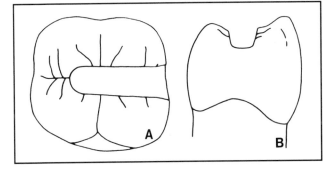

Figs. 9-13A & B (A) A straight channel rest preparation extends more than one half the mesiodistal dimension of the tooth.
(B) Facial and lingual walls are nearly parallel.

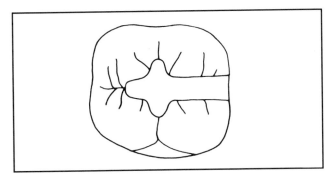

Fig. 9-14 Rests should have an asymmetrical outline form, dovetail etc. which will provide the equivalent of adequate encirclement of a clasp. If a tooth is severely tipped mesially a straight channel rest which minimizes further tipping is preferred (Fig. 9-13A).

E. THE FACIAL WALLS OF THE REST SEATS ALSO SHOULD BE BILATERALLY PARALLEL OR SLIGHTLY DIVERGENT. This is a critical factor in Category I PA path partial dentures when tipped molars are used for abutments. Because these abutments are frequently tipped mesially and lingually, care must be taken to ensure that the facial walls of the rest preparations are parallel or slightly divergent across the arch to permit seating of the rests. (Figs. 9–15A, B, & C)

F. INTIMATE CONTACT OF THE MINOR CONNECTOR AND REST WITH THEIR CORRESPONDING TOOTH SURFACES MUST BE PRESERVED. Caution must be taken while finishing or adjusting the rigid retainer. Loss of contact can render the retainer ineffective.

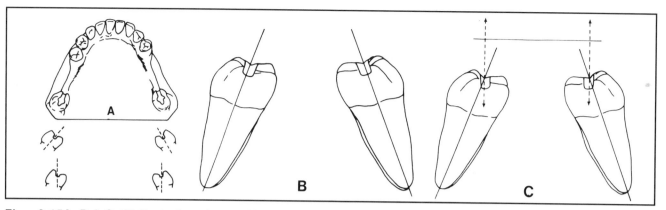

Figs. 9-15A, B & C (A) Illustration of a mandibular arch with molars tipped mesially and lingually.
(B) Occlusal rest seat preparations across the arch would not permit seating of the rests.
(C) The facial walls of the rest seat preparations across the arch must be parallel or slightly divergent to permit placement of the rests.

CINGULUM REST FOR THE RIGID RETAINER

A. THE REST SEAT PREPARATION MUST BE OF SUFFICIENT DEPTH TO ALLOW A REST THICKNESS OF 1.5 TO 2 MM.

B. REST SEAT PREPARATIONS ON THE INCISORS OR CANINES MAY REQUIRE A RESTORATION TO ACHIEVE AN ADEQUATE REST SEAT. A casting may be used to develop the rest seat. When a composite retained metal cingulum or a composite restoration is used, the floor of the rest seat preparation should be in enamel. This minimizes the transmission of vertical seating forces to the bonded restoration. The restoration serves primarily to prevent migration of the abutment. (Fig. 9–16)

C. THE MAXILLARY CINGULUM REST SEAT, WHEN VIEWED FROM THE LINGUAL, SHOULD HAVE A "V" OR "U" SHAPED CONFIGURATION. WHEN VIEWED FROM THE PROXIMAL, IT SHOULD HAVE THE SHAPE OF AN INVERTED "V" OR "U". THIS TYPE OF REST SEAT WILL ASSURE AXIAL DIRECTION OF FORCE. (Figs. 9–17A & B)

D. FOR CATEGORY II DESIGNS, THE PROXIMAL SURFACES THAT WILL BE USED FOR RETENTION AND THE WALLS OF THE REST SEAT SHOULD BE SO RELATED AS TO PERMIT AN INITIAL STRAIGHT PATH OF PLACEMENT.

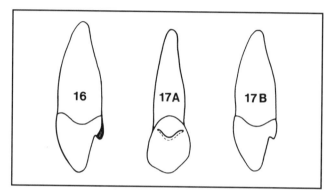

Fig. 9-16   The floor of the cingulum rest seat preparation should be in the enamel if possible. The restoration should serve primarily to prevent migration of the tooth.
Fig. 9-17A   Maxillary cingulum rest seat preparation, when viewed from the lingual should have a "V" or "U" shaped configuration.
Fig. 9-17B   When viewed from the proximal, it should have the shape of an inverted "V" or "U".

ADVANTAGES OF THE ROTATIONAL PATH

A. MINIMIZES NUMBER OF CLASPS, REDUCING TOOTH COVERAGE.

B. MAY REDUCE PLAQUE ACCUMULATION.

C. ANTERIOR CLASPS MAY OFTEN BE ELIMINATED, IMPROVING ESTHETICS.

D. MAY BE USED IN PREFERENCE TO AN ANTERIOR FIXED PROSTHESIS TO ATTAIN BETTER ESTHETICS.

E. MINIMAL TOOTH PREPARATION WHEN COMPARED TO A PRECISION ATTACHMENT OR A FIXED PROSTHESIS.

F. MAY OFTEN BE USED IN ABSENCE OF LINGUAL OR FACIAL UNDERCUTS.

G. DISTORTION OF RIGID RETENTIVE COMPONENTS IS UNLIKELY.

H. MAY PREVENT FURTHER TIPPING OF ABUTMENT TEETH CONTACTED BY RIGID RETAINER.

DISADVANTAGES OF THE ROTATIONAL PATH

A. ADJUSTMENT OF THE RIGID RETENTIVE COMPONENT IS DIFFICULT.

B. LESS TOLERANCE FOR ERROR.

C. REQUIRES WELL PREPARED REST SEATS. May require conservative restorative treatment to develop an acceptable rest seat.

PROCEDURES FOR VARIOUS ROTATIONAL PATHS

A. CATEGORY I—AP ROTATIONAL PATH REPLACING POSTERIOR TEETH. (Figs. 9–18 A-F)

1. In addition to the use of a surveyor to determine the undercut on the tooth to be clasped, a divider is helpful in determining the amount of blockout necessary to eliminate interference in seating the framework. (Fig. 9–19A)

2. One point of the divider is placed on the axis around which the framework will rotate into position. The other point is placed at the most cervical portion of the tooth on which the rigid retainer will be located. The cervical point of the divider is then rotated occlusally to determine that the minor connector is not in too deep an undercut. The point of the divider should be able to move occlusally without interference. (Figs. 9–19B & C)

3. One point of the divider is placed on the axis around which the framework will rotate into position. The other point is placed in contact with the height of contour of the tooth surface

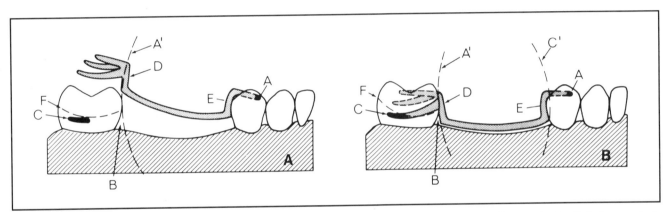

Figs. 9-18A & B (A) Illustration of a RPD utilizing an AP rotational path for replacement of posterior teeth being seated. (B) The partial denture completely seated. (A) point on the rotational axis of which (A') is the arc of rotation for the seating of the molar clasp and its minor connector (D);
(B) indicates amount of blockout necessary; (C) indicates the arc that the minor connector (E) would have to follow to be displaced when (C) becomes the rotational center; (F) indicates the survey line on the molar.

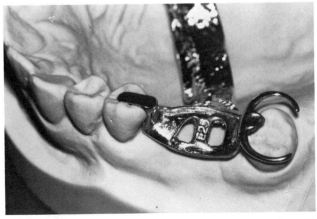

Fig. 9-18C Buccal view of an AP rotational path RPD being seated.

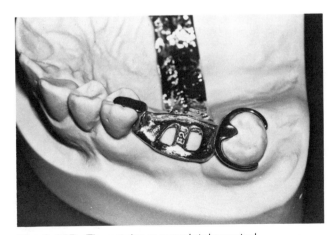

Fig. 9-18D The retainers completely seated.

75

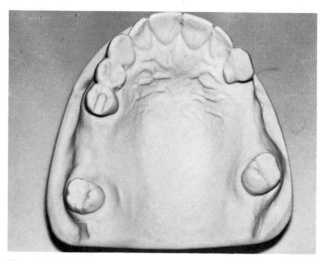

Fig. 9-18E Master cast.

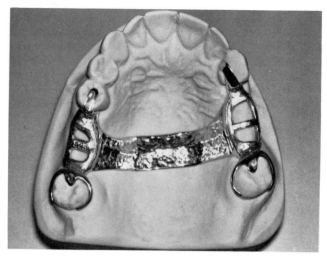

Fig. 9-18F Completed partial denture framework placed on master cast.

requiring relief. It is then rotated cervically to determine the amount of blockout. (Figs. 9–20A & B)

4. Surveying is done with a zero degree tilt to determine the proper undercut on the tooth to be clasped.

5. After the undercut to be utilized by the retentive clasp arm has been selected, the divider may be used to determine whether the undercut for the rigid retainer will be adequate. One point of the divider is placed at the proposed undercut area of the retentive clasp arm and the other point at the cervical portion of the area to be engaged by the rigid retainer. This latter point is rotated occlusally. If it does not contact the tooth, the undercut area is false in relation to the retentive clasp. (Figs. 9–21A, B, & C)

6. Another method for ascertaining if there is true and sufficient undercut for the rigid retainer, is to survey all abutments on the same horizontal plane. (Figs. 9–22 A & B)

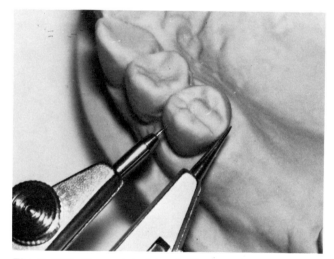

Fig. 9-19B One point of the divider is placed on the axis around which the framework will rotate into position. The other point is placed at the most cervical portion of the tooth where the rigid retainer will be located.

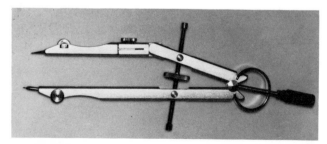

Fig. 9-19A Type of divider whose arm or arms may be adjusted to parallel one another is recommended.

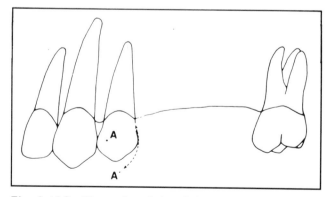

Fig. 9-19C The point of the divider should be able to move occlusally without interference.

B. CATEGORY I—PA ROTATIONAL PATH REPLACING POSTERIOR TEETH.
(Figs. 9–23A to F)

1. Used mainly for mesially tipped molars when clasping them would be difficult.

2. A procedure similar to that used in designing the AP path replacing posterior teeth is utilized except that the rigid retainer is placed on the molar and the clasp on the premolar.

C. CATEGORY II—AP ROTATIONAL PATH REPLACING ANTERIOR TEETH.
(Figs. 9–24A, B & C)

1. Diagnostic cast is surveyed with a zero degree tilt to determine adequacy of undercut on mesial surface of anterior abutments and distobuccal surfaces of posterior abutments. The

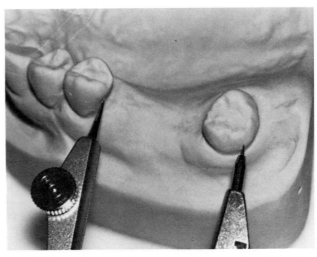

Fig. 9-21A Determining adequacy of undercut for the rigid retainer. One point of the divider is placed at the proposed undercut area of the retentive clasp arm and the other point at the cervical portion of the area to be engaged by the rigid retainer.

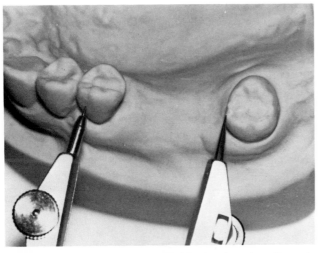

Fig. 9-20A One point of the divider is placed on the axis around which the framework will rotate into position. The other point is placed in contact with the height of contour of the tooth surface requiring relief.

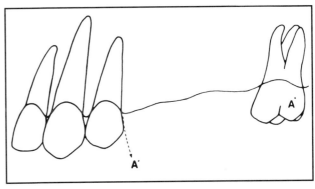

Fig. 9-21B This latter point is rotated occlusally. If it is able to escape the tooth, the undercut is false in relation to the retentive clasp.

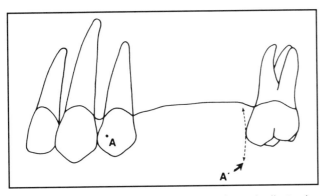

Fig. 9-20B This second point is rotated cervically to determine the amount of blockout.

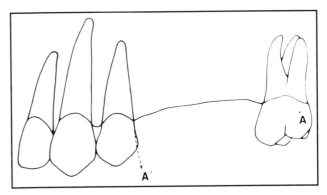

Fig. 9-21C Indicates the presence of a slight undercut which would cause the divider arm to bind since the molar is at a lower level in the arch. The undercut may be increased somewhat to insure positive retention.

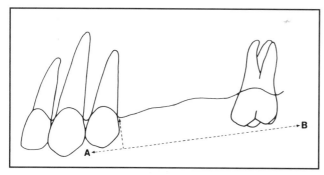

Fig. 9-22A All abutments are surveyed on a horizontal plane with the analyzing rod perpendicular to the plane. No undercut is present on the distal surface of the first premolar as in Fig. 9-21C.

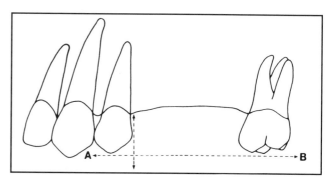

Fig. 9-22B A slight undercut is present as in Fig. 9-21C. The undercut may be increased to ensure adequate retention.

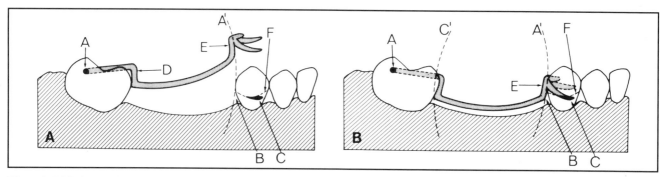

Figs. 9-23A & B (A) Illustration of a RPD utilizing a PA path of rotation for replacement of posterior teeth being seated. (B) The partial denture completely seated.
(B) The distal portion of the molar rest (A) is positioned first. The remainder of the partial denture is rotated into its final position. (A') arc of rotation upon placement; (b) space indicating the amount of blockout for the minor connector (E) to permit premolar clasp to seat; (D) minor connector moves into intimate contact with the mesial surface of the molar; (C) center of rotation of arc (C') that the minor connector (D) would have to follow to be displaced; (F) indicates survey line.

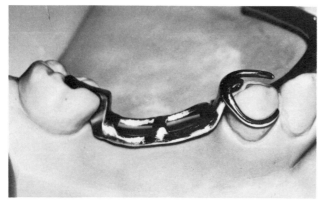

Fig. 9-23C Partial dentures using a PA path of placement being seated. The minor connector on the molar engages its mesial surface while the clasps on the premolar is being seated.

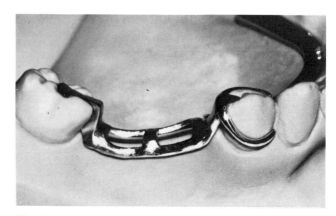

Fig. 9-23D The partial denture completely seated.

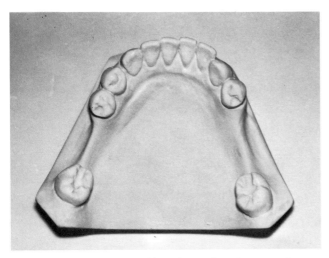

Fig. 9-23E Master cast. Note dovetail rest preparation on the molar abutments.

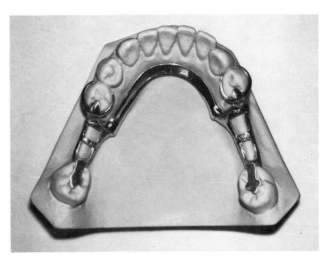

Fig. 9-23F Partial denture completely seated.

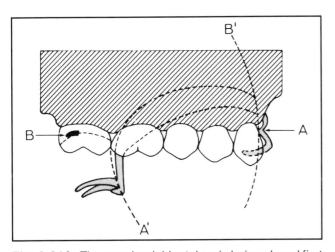

Fig. 9-24A The anterior rigid retainer is being placed first along a straight path to gain access to the rotational center (A) located on the mesial surface of the canine.

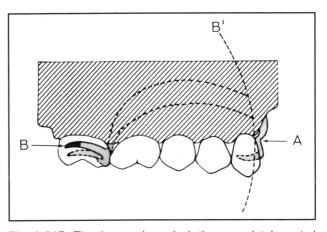

Fig. 9-24B The clasp on the molar is then completely seated along arc (A'). (B) represents the retentive area for the molar clasp and (B') the arc along which the rigid retainer on the canine would have to move to be displaced.

amount of undercut anteriorly should be at least 0.020 inch (Fig. 9–25). The undercut on the molar is determined by the type of clasp selected to attain optimum retention. (Fig. 9–26)

2. The cast is then tilted upward anteriorly until the undercuts on the mesial surfaces of the anterior abutments are eliminated.
(Figs. 9–27A, B, & C)

3. The analyzing rod is then used to determine if access still exists for the rest to be seated. (Figs. 9–28A & B) If it does not exist, addi-

tional tooth modification in addition to the rest preparation is necessary. There must be no interference for placement of the anterior segment of the casting along the determined initial straight path.

4. A preliminary outline is drawn on the diagnostic cast indicating rest seat areas and any additional tooth modifications. (Fig. 9–29)

5. Rest seats and other tooth modifications are completed on the patient and a master cast is obtained.

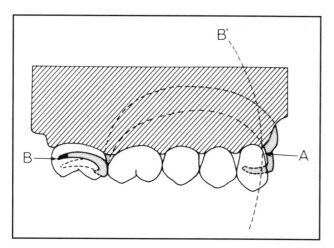

Fig. 9-24C Arrow indicates a slight space between the minor connector and the mesial surface of the canine which may result from excessive finishing or adjusting the framework. Such a space reduces the effectiveness of the rigid retainer.

6. The master cast is resurveyed as before. (Figs. 9–30A, B, C, & D)

7. The cast is tripodized for each position on the surveyor. (Figs. 9–31A & B)

8. The final casting is positioned anteriorly first, then the posterior segment is seated. (Figs. 9–32A, B &C)

9. Resistance to vertical displacement of the anterior segment may be increased by the use of proximal plates or other rigid components on the distal surfaces of the molars (Fig. 9–33).

This diminishes horizontal movement in an anterior direction, reducing the possibility of anterior vertical displacement.

D. CATEGORY I AND II — LATERAL ROTATIONAL PATH FOR REPLACING TEETH UNILATERALLY.

1. May be used for unilateral replacement of anterior or posterior teeth, or both.

2. A thorough understanding of the AP and PA paths of rotation permits application of the same concepts to the lateral path of rotation. (Figs. 9–34A to D)

IMPORTANT FACTORS IN THE USE OF THE ROTATIONAL PATH

A. MULTIPLE EDENTULOUS AREAS.

1. As the number of minor connectors increases, so does the potential difficulty of rotating the framework into place.

2. Adequate blockout of interferences generated by the rotational path of placement must be provided for all minor connectors. This may readily be determined by the use of a divider in analyzing all edentulous areas and the amount of blockout necessary for each minor connector to be seated.

3. The further the minor connector is from the axis of rotation, the straighter the arc that it must follow. The closer the minor connector is to the axis of rotation, the greater the curvature of the arc that it must follow, requiring more blockout. (Figs. 9–35 & 9–36)

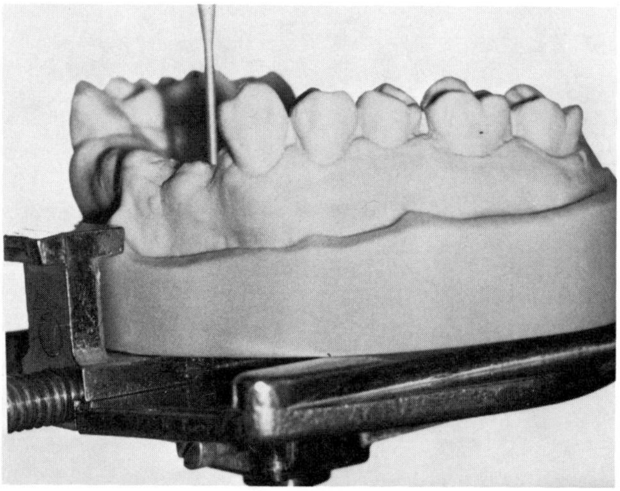

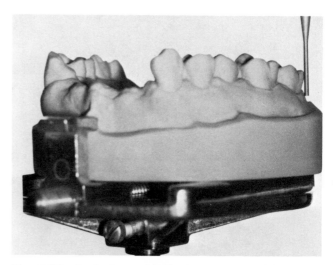

Fig. 9-25 Diagnostic cast being surveyed at a zero degree tilt. Analyzing rod indicates an adequate undercut on the mesial surface of the canine.

Fig. 9-26 Analyzing rod indicates an acceptable undercut on the distobuccal surface of the molar. The amount of undercut utilized will depend on the type of clasp selected.

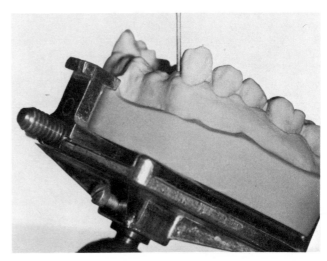

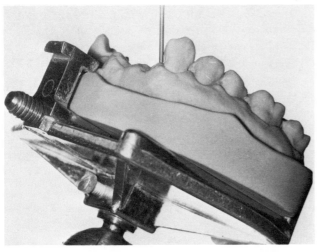

Figs. 9-27A & B   (A) The cast is tilted upward anteriorly until the undercuts on the mesial surfaces of the anterior abutments are eliminated. In this photo, a slight space exists between the analyzing rod and the mesial surface of the canine which can best be eliminated by judicious reduction of the tooth.
(B) Analyzing rod now indicates absence of undercut.

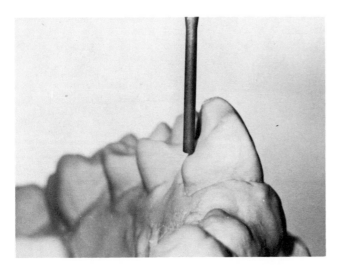

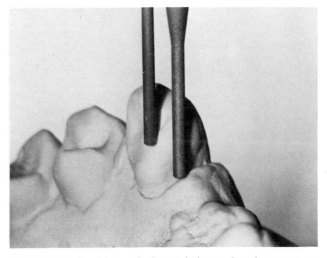

Fig. 9-28A The analyzing rod is used to determine whether access still exists for the rests to be seated.

Fig. 9-28B Double analyzing rod shows that the rest seat will be accessible together with the mesial surface of the canine.

B. SHAPE OF THE ARCH—CATEGORY I DESIGN.

1. May affect seating of a rotational prosthesis.

2. A square arch will have radii that are parallel, bilaterally passing through all abutments perpendicularly from the rotational axis. The amount and extent of blockout may be readily assessed.

3. A tapering arch will have shorter radii if they are extended perpendicularly from axis of rotation to a point on the proximal surface of the tooth. A shorter radius requires more blockout than a longer radius.

4. All blockout of interferences must be determined by radii that are extended at right angles from the axis of rotation. (Figs. 9–37A, B &C)

C. SHAPE OF THE ARCH—CATEGORY II DESIGN.

1. For the replacement of anterior teeth, the distance between the fulcrum line and the incisal edges of the teeth will influence the amount of retention necessary on the molar abutments.

81

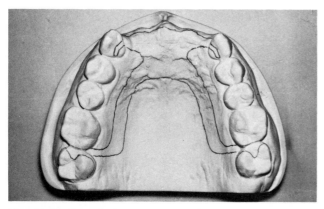

Fig. 9-29 A preliminary outline is drawn on the diagnostic cast indicating rest areas and any additional tooth modifications.

A tissueward force, when incising, exerts a displacing force on the posterior clasps which increases as the distance between the fulcrum line and the incisal edges increases. (Figs. 9–38 and Figs. 9–39A to D)

2. This factor may dictate the amount of undercut that must be engaged by the molar clasp.

3. As a general rule, the more posteriorly the retentive undercut is located, the more favorable is the leverage factor.

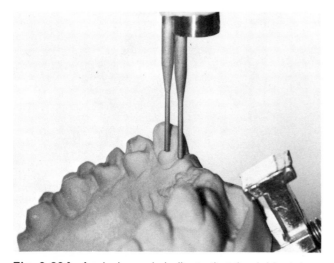

Fig. 9-30A Analyzing rods indicate that the rigid retainer can seat without interference.

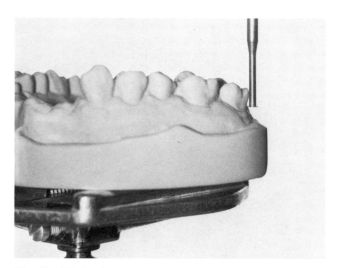

Fig. 9-30C Undercut gauge used to measure depth of undercut on the molar abutment.

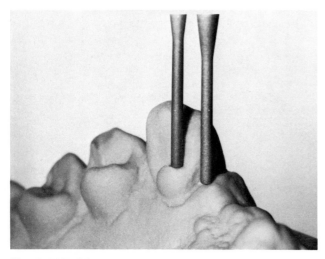

Fig. 9-30B Closeup view from Fig. 9-30A.

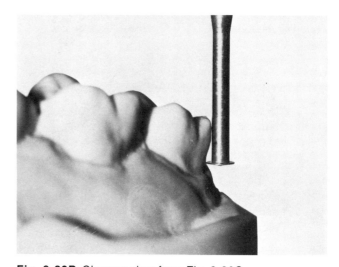

Fig. 9-30D Closeup view from Fig. 9-30C.

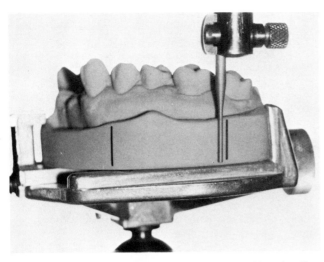

Fig. 9-31A Cast is tripodized for each position by first placing three widely spaced vertical lines are drawn on the sides of the cast at the zero degree tilt.

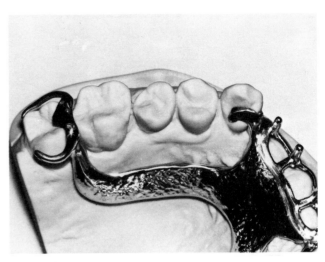

Fig. 9-32A Partial denture is seated anteriorly first.

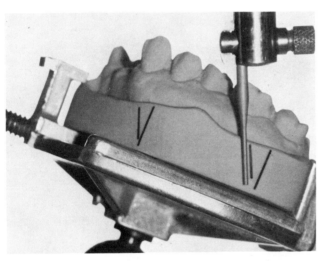

Fig. 9-31B Three additional lines are drawn on the sides of the cast at the tilt which will permit the initial seating (straight path of placement) without interferences.

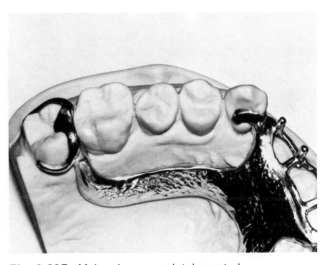

Fig. 9-32B Molar clasp completely seated.

D. LINGUALLY TILTED TEETH.

1. In the mandibular arch, when utilizing the rotational path, the major connector may require excessive relief to clear the teeth when being seated. This can create a food trap and become bothersome to the patient's tongue.

2. Problems associated with lingually tilted teeth become more acute with a tapered arch, as indicated above.

3. If modification of the involved teeth does not rectify the problem, the rotational path probably should not be used.

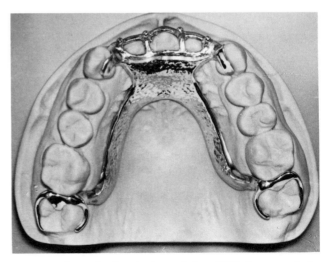

Fig. 9-32C Occlusal view of the RPD framework in place.

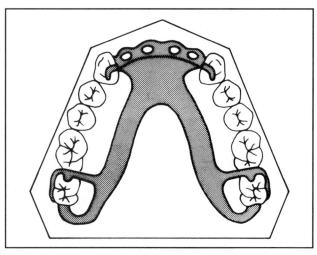

Fig. 9-33 Rigid proximal plates on the distal surfaces of the molars will diminish the possibility of anterior horizontal movement of the partial denture during function which increases the resistance to anterior vertical displacement.

E. MULTIPLE ROTATIONAL PATHS.

1. At times more than one rotational path may be used for a single partial denture.

2. A path of placement may be evaluated by fabricating a template in the form of the proposed design.

3. Carding wax strips or other suitable materials may be used to confine an autopolymerizing resin to the outline of the proposed design. (Fig. 9–40A) Interferences must be blocked out.

4. After the resin has polymerized, the wax is removed.

5. The resin template is analyzed to be certain that it covers only the area of the proposed design.

6. The template is then removed, taking care not to fracture the teeth on the stone cast, and finished for evaluation.

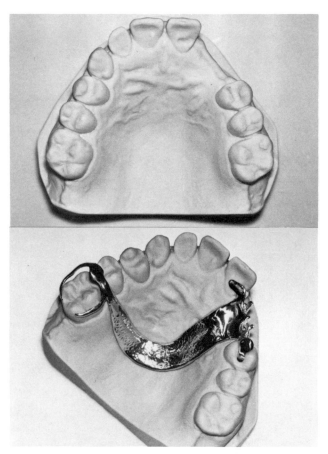

Fig. 9-34A Master cast of patient with lateral incisor and canine missing.
Fig. 9-34B Lateral path of placement.

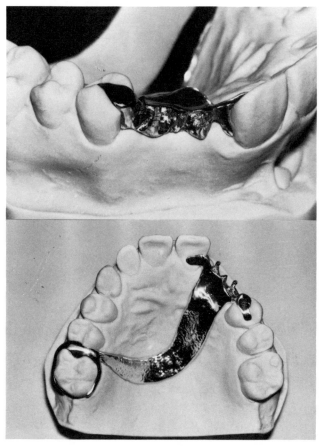

Fig. 9-34C Minor connector engaging mesiobuccal undercut on the premolar and a distal undercut on the central incisor.
Fig. 9-34D RPD framework completely seated on master cast.

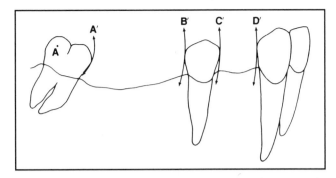

Fig. 9-35 The further the minor connector is from the axis of rotation the straighter the arc that it must follow. The closer the minor connector is from the axis of rotation, the greater the curvature that it must follow requiring more blockout.

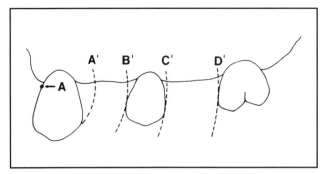

Fig. 9-36 Maxillary arch. The amount of blockout on the distal surface of the canine is much greater than that required on the mesial surface of the molar. This is due to the close proximity of the distal surface of the canine to the rotational center (A).

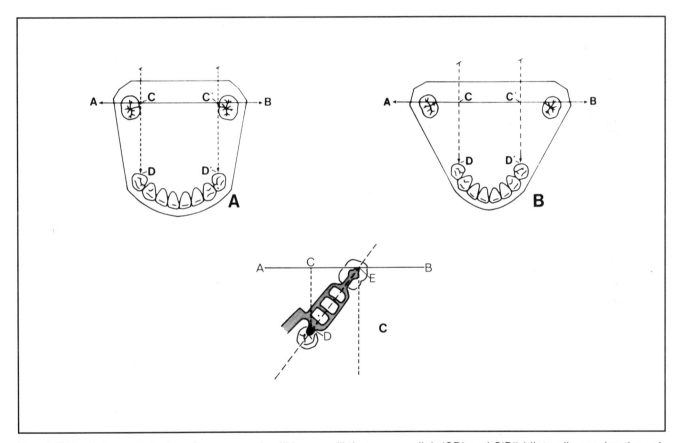

Fig. 9-37A Category I design. A square arch will have radii that are parallel, (CD) and C'D') bilaterally passing through all abutments perpendicularly from the rotational axis (AB).

Fig. 9-37B A tapering arch will have shorter radii (CD) and (C'D') if they are extended perpendicularly from the rotational axis (AB) to a point on the proximal surface of the tooth. A shorter radius requires more blockout than a longer one. All blockout of undercuts must be determined by radii that are extended at right angles from the rotational axis.

Fig. 9-37C Section of a tapering arch with framework in position. Line (CD) is shorter than (ED). Line (CD) is used to determine the blockout on the distal surface of the premolar.

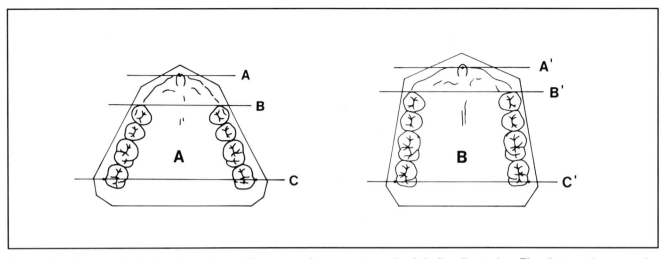

Fig. 9-38 Category II design. A tapering arch compared to a square arch of similar dimension. The distance between the mesial surface of the first premolars and distal surface of the second molars is identical. An anterior tissueward force exerted a displacing force on the posterior clasps which increases as the distance between line (A) and line (B) increases or the distance between line (B) and line (C) decreases. Note the difference in these proportions with the square arch. The distance between line (A') and line (B') is less than in the tapering arch and the difference between (B') and (C') is greater than in the tapering arch. As a general rule the more posteriorly the retentive undercut is located the more favorable the leverage.

7. A template that cannot be removed easily may indicate that the proposed design should not be used.

8. The template should be studied carefully, making certain that no elements will be added that would interfere with the placement of the casting.

9. The template may be sent to the laboratory as a guide in fabricating the framework.

F. DISTAL EXTENSION BASE PARTIAL DENTURES.

1. The rotational path of placement is not usually recommended for replacement of anterior teeth in combination with a distal extension base partial denture. Tissueward movement of the base may result in unfavorable torquing of the anterior abutments. (Fig. 9–41)

2. The use of a stress releasing attachment on the posterior abutments, however, may permit the use of the rotational path.

G. SPLAYED ANTERIOR TEETH.

1. The rotational path (dual path) of placement may be used when splayed anterior teeth cannot be clasped in a conventional manner.

2. A facial clasp arm is used on an anterior tooth, but, it may be placed at the cervical one third of the tooth. (Figs. 9–42A & B)

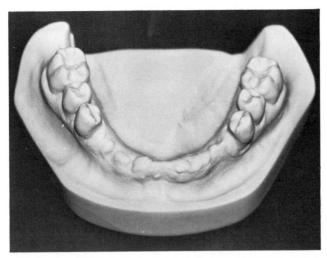

Fig. 9-39A Master cast for reception of an AP rotational path partial denture. The resistance arm of the partial denture is relatively short due to the absence of the second molars. A selective pressure impression of the anterior edentulous area is necessary to improve muco-osseous support.

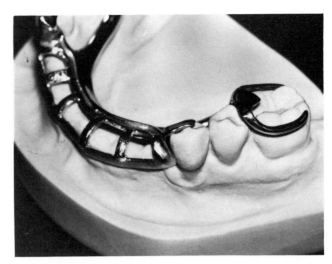

Fig. 9-39B Lateral view of the framework being seated.

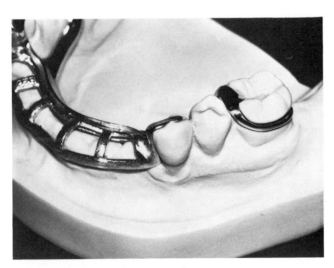

Fig. 9-39C Molar clasp seated.

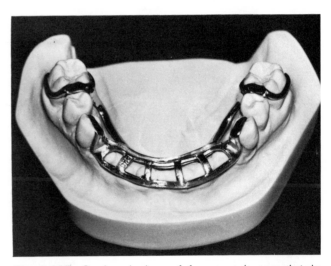

Fig. 9-39D Occlusal view of framework completely seated.

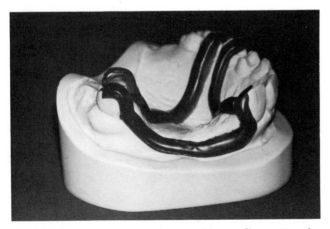

Fig. 9-40A Carding wax strips used to confine autopolymerizing resin in constructing a template.

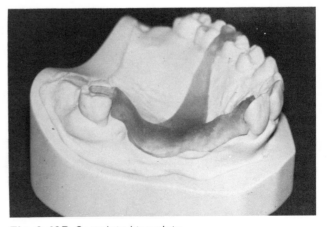

Fig. 9-40B Completed template.

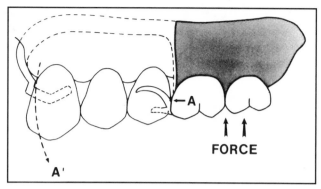

Fig. 9-41 A distal extension base partial denture with missing anterior teeth utilizing an AP rotational path. Force applied to the distal extension base results in torquing the anterior abutments. (A) is the center of rotation around which the anterior portion of the partial denture will tend to rotate following the arc (A'). The use of the rotational path of placement for extension base partial dentures is usually not recommended.

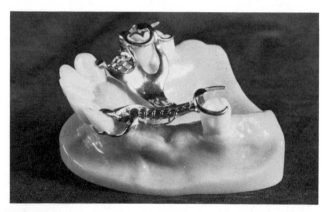

Fig. 9-42A Dual path of placement utilizing a clasp on the lateral incisor. Model shows splayed anterior teeth. The clasp designed for the lateral incisor is placed first followed by seating of the posterior clasps as the partial denture is rotated into position.

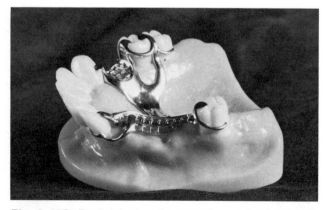

Fig. 9-42B Partial denture framework completely seated.

88

Chapter X

TOOTH-MUCOSA BORNE (EXTENSION BASE) PARTIAL DENTURE DESIGN

A tooth-mucosa borne partial denture derives support from the dento-alveolar and muco-osseous segments. The soft tissues of the muco-osseous segment demonstrate significantly greater displaceability upon loading than the dento-alveolar tissues. This variation allows rotational movements of the prosthesis to occur during loading of the denture base supported by the muco-osseous segment. The ability of the segments to bear the applied forces must be evaluated and designs which maximize muco-osseous support and which equitably distribute the forces between the segments are recommended. Movement of the prosthesis during function should not result in unfavorable forces directed to the dento-alveolar segment. Since the majority of tooth-mucosa borne partial dentures have distal extension bases, this chapter reviews designs for these situations.

FORCES ACTING ON DISTAL EXTENSION BASE PARTIAL DENTURES

A. VERTICAL SEATING FORCES—BILATERAL.

    1. Origin.

        a. Mastication (bilateral).

        b. Swallowing.

        c. Parafunction (clenching).

    2. Resultant movement. Tissueward movement of the extension bases bilaterally. Rotation around the fulcrum line axis. (Fig. 10–1)

    3. Counteracted by:

        a. Denture bases.

        b. Maxillary major connector.

        c. Rests.

        d. Non-stress releasing clasps.

B. VERTICAL SEATING FORCES— UNILATERAL.

    1. Origin.

        a. Mastication (unilateral).

        b. Parafunction.

    2. Resultant movement. Tissueward movement of the extension base on the loaded side. Rotation around a longitudinal axis formed by the ridge crest. Dislodging (lifting) of the base on the opposite side. (Fig. 10–2)

    3. Counteracted by:

        a. Denture base.

        b. Rigid major connectors.

        c. Clasps.

        d. Artificial tooth placement.

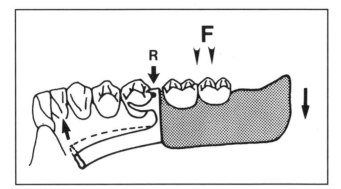

Fig. 10-1 Fulcrum line axis. Force (F) applied to the extension base causes tissueward movement. Rotation occurs around fulcrum line axis (R).

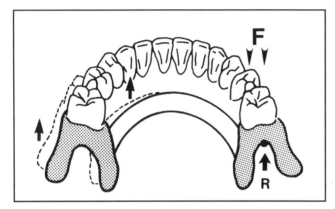

Fig. 10-2 Longitudinal axis. Force (F) applied to the extension base causes tissueward movement on loaded side. Rotation occurs around a longitudinal axis formed by the ridge crest (R). Base on opposite side dislodges (lifts).

C. HORIZONTAL (LATERAL) FORCES.

  1. Origin.

    a. Mastication. Loading forces may be applied obliquely and generate horizontal components of force.

    b. Parafunction (bruxing).

  2. Resultant movement. Buccolingual movement of the partial denture (fish tail effect). Rotation around a vertical axis near center of arch. (Fig. 10–3)

  3. Counteracted by:

    a. Denture base (primarily flange extensions).

    b. Maxillary major connector.

    c. Adequate bracing.

      i. Rigid major connectors.

      ii. Clasp bracing components.

D. VERTICAL DISLODGING FORCES.

  1. Origin.

    a. Mastication (sticky foods).

    b. Muscles of lips, tongue and cheeks.

    c. Gravity (maxillary).

  2. Resultant movement. Movement of extension base away from the ridge. (Fig. 10–4)

  3. Counteracted by:

    a. Direct retainers.

    b. Indirect retainers.

    c. Guiding planes & minor connectors.

    d. Gravity (mandibular).

MOVEMENTS OF A DISTAL EXTENSION BASE PARTIAL DENTURE DURING FUNCTION
(Figs. 10–1 to 10–5 and Chart 1)

A. ROTATION AROUND A FULCRUM LINE AXIS. The axis passes through the two rests closest to the edentulous area. (Fig. 10–1)

B. ROTATION AROUND A LONGITUDINAL AXIS. The axis passes along the edentulous ridge crest. (Fig. 10–2)

C. ROTATION AROUND A VERTICAL AXIS. The axis passes perpendicular to the occlusal plane and is located near the center of the arch. (Fig. 10–3)

D. ROTATION AROUND A HORIZONTAL AXIS. The axis passes through the two retentive clasp tips adjacent to the edentulous areas (when adequate indirect retention is absent). (Fig. 10–4)

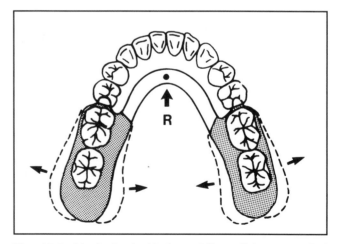

Fig. 10-3 Vertical axis. Horizontal (lateral) forces applied to the extension bases cause buccolingual movement of the partial denture. Rotation occurs around a vertical axis near the center or toward the anterior of the arch (R).

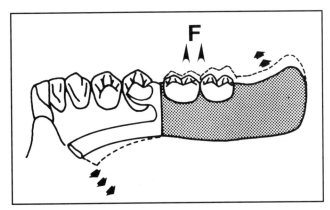

Fig. 10-4 Horizontal axis. Vertical dislodging forces applied to extension base causes dislodgement (lifting) of base when indirect retention is lacking.

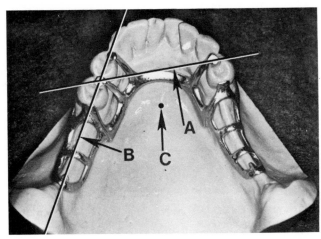

Fig. 10-5 Line (A) represents the fulcrum line axis, passing through the two rests closest to the edentulous areas. Line (B) represents the longitudinal axis, passing along the edentulous ridge crest. Point (C) represents a point on the vertical axis which is usually located near the center or toward the anterior of the arch.

EXAMINATION IMPORTANT CONSIDERATIONS

A. EVALUATE DENTO-ALVEOLAR SUPPORT POTENTIAL.

 1. Teeth.

 2. Periodontium.

 3. Alveolar bone.

B. EVALUATE MUCO-OSSEOUS SUPPORT POTENTIAL.

 1. Mucosa.

 2. Submucosa.

 3. Bone.

C. EVALUATE POTENTIAL OF APPLIED FORCES.

 1. Opposing occlusion.

 2. Muscular force potential.

 3. Parafunctional habits.

 4. Length of edentulous span.

 5. History of prosthesis failure.

 6. History of poor tissue tolerance.

DESIGN CONSIDERATIONS

A. OPTIMUM MUCO-OSSEOUS SUPPORT. Reduce potential for tissueward movement of the denture base.

 1. Pre-prosthodontic surgery.

  a. Removal of displaceable hyperplastic tissue to improve support.

  b. Removal of bony exostoses or tori to permit optimal extension of denture base.

 2. Maximum denture base coverage.

  a. Coverage of primary force bearing areas.

  b. Maximum extensions, as limited by movable soft tissues.

 3. Maxillary major connector coverage of horizontal hard palate.

 4. Impression procedures.

  a. Altered cast impression.

  b. Relining of extension base at delivery.

B. OPTIMUM DENTO-ALVEOLAR SUPPORT.

 1. Periodontal therapy.

  a. Professional maintenance and home care oral hygiene program instituted.

  b. Definitive treatment of existing periodontal disease.

  c. Reduction of excessive abutment tooth mobility.

  d. Develop an adequate zone of attached gingiva around abutment teeth.

 2. Restorative treatment. Establish structurally sound abutment teeth.

  a. Restore structurally compromised teeth.

  b. Splinting of abutment teeth to reduce hypermobility or to control abnormal forces.

CHART I

Description of rotational movements of a bilateral extension base partial
denture around various axes

FULCRUM LINE AXIS

FORCE	RESULTANT MOVEMENT	COUNTERACTED BY
Occlusal loading bilaterally	Tissueward movement of the extension bases bilaterally	1. Denture bases 2. Maxillary major connectors 3. Rests 4. Non-stress releasing clasps

LONGITUDINAL AXIS FORMED BY CREST OF RIDGE

FORCE	RESULTANT MOVEMENT	COUNTERACTED BY
Occlusal loading unilaterally	Tissueward movement of the extension base on the loaded side Lifting of the denture base on opposite side	1. Denture base 2. Rigid major connectors 3. Clasps 4. Tooth placement

VERTICAL AXIS NEAR CENTER OF ARCH

FORCE	RESULTANT MOVEMENT	COUNTERACTED BY

Lateral components of masticatory force during occlusal loading	Buccolingual movement of the extension base (fish tail effect)	1. Denture base
		2. Maxillary major connector
		3. Adequate bracing
		   a. Rigid major connector
		   b. Rigid bracing clasp arms

3. Modifications of abutment tooth contour.

    a. Guiding planes.

    b. Height of contour (survey line) adjustment.

    c. Retentive grooves.

    d. Rest seats.

C. EQUITABLE DISTRIBUTION OF FORCES TO THE DENTO-ALVEOLAR AND MUCO-OSSEOUS SEGMENTS. An equitable distribution of forces to the segments is required. The relative distribution is based upon the amount of force involved and the ability of the segments to withstand the applied forces.

1. **Designs to increase loading of the muco-osseous segments.** Utilize components that increase loading of the residual ridge (muco-osseous segment), and minimize lateral torquing forces directed to the abutment teeth (dento-alveolar segment) during function.

    a. Stress releasing clasps.

    b. Stress releasing attachments.

    c. Split major connectors.

2. **Designs to increase loading of the dento-alveolar segment.** Utilize components that increase loading of the abutment teeth (dento-alveolar segment), and minimize loading of the residual ridge (muco-osseous segment) during function.

    a. Non-stress releasing clasps.

    b. Non-stress releasing attachments.

D. REDUCTION OF FORCES APPLIED TO THE EXTENSION BASE.

1. Decrease the faciolingual width of the occlusal table.

2. Decrease the number of posterior teeth.

3. Space teeth with diastemas.

4. Maintain occlusal surface anatomy.

5. Plastic teeth may decrease the forces transmitted to the residual ridge.

FACTORS DETERMINING THE SELECTION OF MAJOR CONNECTORS

A. SUPPORT. The tooth-mucosa borne partial denture derives support from the dento-alveolar and muco-osseous segments.

1. Maxillary major connectors. Plate designs which derive support from the muco-osseous segment (horizontal hard plate) are usually required. Strap designs are usually not recommended.

2. Mandibular major connectors. Mandibular major connectors do not provide support since they do not contact the underlying mucosa. Relief is required since rotational movements are anticipated, and the underlying mucosa does not withstand mechanical forces.

B. LOCATION OF EDENTULOUS AREA(S). The major connector must connect the restored edentulous area(s).

C. ANTICIPATED LOSS OF NATURAL TEETH. Plating the lingual surfaces of natural teeth facilitates the addition of artificial teeth to the partial denture, however, it requires unfavorable coverage of teeth and gingival tissues.

D. FUNCTIONAL DEPTH OF THE LINGUAL VESTIBULE (FLOOR OF MOUTH). When an inadequate depth exists for a lingual bar (less than 7 mm) a sublingual bar or a lingual plate may be used. (See Chapter V)

E. INCLINATION OF THE REMAINING TEETH. In rare situations when mandibular teeth are severely lingually inclined a labial bar major connector may be required.

F. TISSUE RESTRICTIONS. The presence of certain hard or soft tissue structures may limit major connector selection.

G. PATIENT PREFERENCE. The major connector of patient's previous partial denture should be noted, and the patient's acceptance should be evaluated.

FACTORS DETERMINING THE SELECTION OF DENTURE BASES

A. SUPPORT. Maximum muco-osseous support should be maintained to minimize rotational movements of the prosthesis and to distribute the applied forces over the greatest mucosal supporting area. Resin bases which may be relined to compensate for resorptive changes, are indicated for the extension base areas.

B. ADJUSTMENTS. The rotational movements of the RPD during function may excessively displace underlying mucosal tissues. Resin bases are easily adjusted to eliminate tissue impingement.

FACTORS DETERMINING THE SELECTION OF CLASPS

A. DISTRIBUTION OF FORCES. The equitable distribution of forces to the muco-osseous and dento-alveolar segments is required. Stress releasing clasps minimize lateral torquing forces directed to abutment teeth, but may increase loading of the muco-osseous segment. Non-stress releasing clasps direct lateral torquing forces to the abutment teeth, but may minimize loading of the muco-osseous segment.

1. Non-stress releasing clasps.
    a. Circlet (Akers).
    b. Back action.
    c. Embrasure.
2. Stress releasing clasps.
    a. "RPI".
    b. "RPC".
    c. Cast circumferential and wrought wire circumferential (combination).
    d. Circumferential "C".
    e. Cast circumferential and cast bar (modified "T")—Distal rest.
    f. Cast circumferential and cast bar (modified "T")—Mesial rest.

B. LOCATION OF UNDERCUTS. The location of true undercuts on abutment teeth will influence the choice of retentive clasp arms.

C. MINIMAL TOOTH AND MINIMAL GINGIVAL COVERAGE. Clasps which minimize coverage of these tissues are preferred since they tend to reduce plaque accumulation.

D. ESTHETICS. The choice of a clasp arm may be influenced by its visibility during normal facial movements. Bar clasps contact less surface area and are usually confined to the gingival one third of the tooth. Since they approach the undercut from the gingival direction they are often less conspicuous than circumferential clasps.

E. CLASPS ON PREVIOUS REMOVABLE PARTIAL DENTURE.
    1. May indicate esthetic awareness and demands of the patient.
    2. May indicate amount of retention necessary.

COMPARATIVE MOVEMENTS OF CLASPS DURING FUNCTION

An analysis of the movement of clasp components during function demonstrates their potential for directing lateral torquing forces to abutment teeth.

A. CLASPS WITH MESIAL RESTS.
    1. Rotation occurs in area of mesial rest.

2. Clasp components located posterior to the fulcrum line axis move gingivally during occlusal loading. (Fig. 10–6A)

3. Clasp components located anterior to the fulcrum line axis move occlusally during occlusal loading. (Fig. 10–6A)

4. Mesial rest directs a mesial torquing and axial forces to the tooth. The tooth may be braced by an adjacent tooth. (Fig. 10–7A)

5. Mesial (remote) location of rest loads ridge more vertically than a distal rest. (Fig. 10–8)

B. CLASPS WITH DISTAL RESTS.
    1. Rotation occurs at area where minor connector breaks contact with the tooth.

    2. Clasp components located anterior to the fulcrum line axis move occlusally during occlusal loading. (Fig. 10–6B)

    3. Distal rest directs a distal torquing and axial forces to the tooth. With no adjacent tooth for bracing, more lateral movement may occur. (Fig. 10–7B)

    4. Distal (proximate) location of rest loads ridge more obliquely than a mesial rest. (Fig. 10–8)

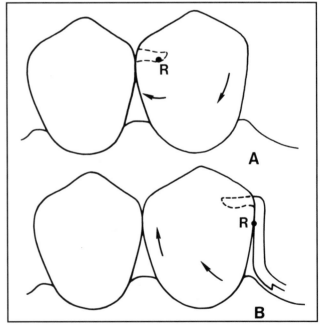

Figs. 10-6A & B (A) Clasp with mesial rest. Center of rotation (R). Arrows indicate movement of clasp components during occlusal loading. (B) Clasp with distal rest. Center of rotation (R). Arrows indicate movement of clasp components during occlusal loading.

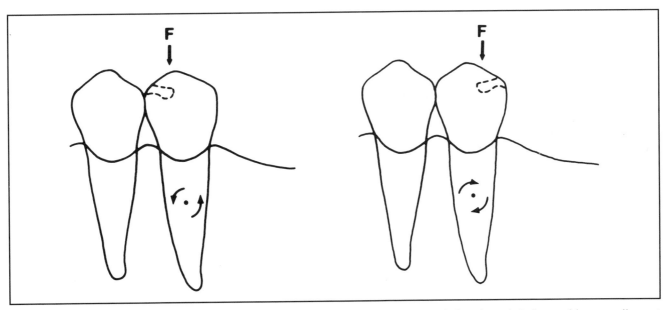

Fig. 10-7A Clasp with mesial rest. Force (F) on rest tends to tilt tooth mesially where it is braced by an adjacent tooth.

Fig. 10-7B Clasp with distal rest. Force (F) on rest tends to tilt tooth distally. The absence of a distally adjacent tooth for bracing, allows more lateral movement.

MECHANICS OF CLASPS THAT DO NOT PROVIDE STRESS RELEASE

A. CIRCLET CLASP. (Fig. 10–9)

1. Rotation occurs at area where minor connector breaks contact with tooth.

2. Cast retentive clasp arm tip moves occlusally during function and directs a distal torquing force to the tooth.

3. Apically inclined rest moves distally during function loading and directs a distal torquing force to the tooth.

B. BACK ACTION CLASP. (Fig. 10–10)

1. Rotation occurs in area of mesial rest.

2. Shoulder of cast retentive clasp arm moves gingivally during function and directs a facial torquing force to the tooth.

C. EMBRASURE CLASP.

1. Rotation occurs in area of occlusal rests.

2. Cast retentive clasp arm opposite the fulcrum line from the extension base moves occlusally during function and directs a lateral torquing force to the tooth.

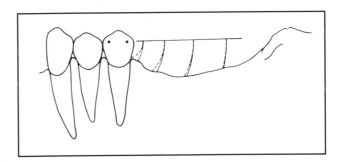

Fig. 10-8 Direction of force applied to residual ridge. Mesial rest tends to direct forces more vertically (solid line). Distal rest tends to direct forces more obliquely (dotted line).

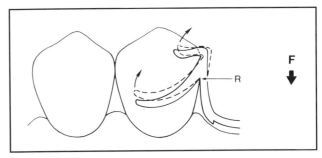

Fig. 10-9 Circlet clasp during function. Loading force (F) causes clasp to rotate at (R), where minor connector breaks contact with tooth. Retentive clasp arm tip moves occlusally during function and directs a distal torquing force to the tooth.

MECHANICS OF CLASPS THAT PROVIDE STRESS RELEASE

A. "RPI" CLASP. (Fig. 10–11)

1. Rotation occurs in area of mesial rest.

2. "I" bar and proximal plate disengage from the tooth during function.

3. During function, forces are transmitted through the RPD components to the mesial rest directing mesial torquing and axial forces to the tooth. The abutment tooth is usually braced by a mesially adjacent tooth.

B. "RPC" CLASP. (Fig. 10–12)

1. Rotation occurs in area of mesial rest.

2. Circumferential clasp arm and proximal plate disengage from the tooth during function.

3. During function, forces are transmitted through the RPD components to the mesial rest directing a mesial torquing and axial forces to the tooth. The abutment tooth is usually braced by a mesially adjacent tooth.

C. CAST CIRCUMFERENTIAL AND WROUGHT WIRE CIRCUMFERENTIAL CLASP (COMBINATION). (Fig. 10–13)

1. Rotation occurs at area where minor connector breaks contact with tooth.

2. Wrought wire retentive clasp arm tip moves occlusally during function and directs a distal torquing force to the tooth. Magnitude of torquing forces are influenced by the flexibility of wrought wire clasp arm.

3. Flat rest seat preparation allows rest to slip distally during function.

D. CIRCUMFERENTIAL "C" CLASP. (Fig. 10–14)

1. Rotation occurs at area where minor connector breaks contact with tooth.

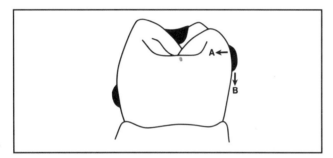

Fig. 10-10 Back action clasp on a premolar. Arrow (A) represents the buccal force exerted on the tooth when an occlusal force applied to the extension base tends to move the clasp gingivally. (B) The lingual portion of the clasp arm is above the height of contour and produces the buccal force.

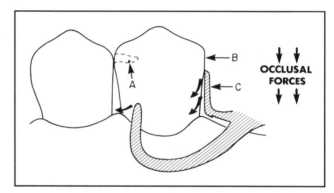

Fig. 10-11 "RPI" clasp during function. (A) Indicates the center of rotation. (B) Indicates the guiding plane. (C) Indicates the proximal plate. Note that the "I" bar clasp arm and the proximal plate move in a mesiogingival direction disengaging from the tooth.

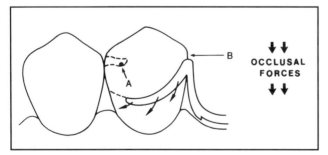

Fig. 10-12 "RPC" clasp during function. (A) Indicates the center of rotation. (B) Indicates the guiding plane. Note that the circumferential clasp arm and proximal plate move in a mesiogingival direction disengaging from the tooth.

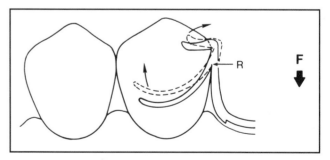

Fig. 10-13 Wrought wire (combination) clasp during function. Loading force (F) causes clasp to rotate at (R), where minor connector breaks contact with tooth. Wrought wire clasp arm tip moves occlusally and directs a distal torquing force to the tooth. Flexibility of wrought wire arm limits torquing.

2. Retentive "C" clasp moves mesio-occlusally during function and directs torquing forces to the tooth, which may be braced by a mesially adjacent tooth..

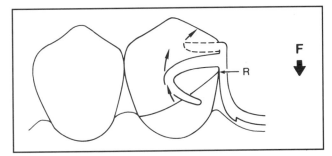

Fig. 10-14 Circumferential "C" clasp during function. Loading force (F) causes clasp to rotate at (R) where minor connector breaks contact with tooth. Retentive clasp tip moves mesio-occlusally, while rest rotates distally.

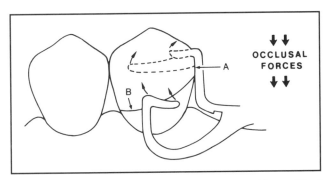

Fig. 10-15 Distal rest combination clasp with modified "T" bar during function. (A) Indicates center of rotation. (B) Indicates the height of contour (survey line). Only the retentive terminal of the buccal clasp arm engages the undercut, permitting the more rigid portion to disengage the tooth. The retentive terminal exerts a mesio-occlusal force on the tooth counteracting the distal force that may be exerted by the distal movement of the rest.

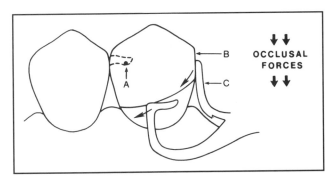

Fig. 10-16 Mesial rest combination clasp with modified "T" bar during function. (A) Indicates center of rotation. (B) Indicates the guiding plane. (C) Indicates the proximal plate. The retentive clasp moves mesiogingivally during function. It may disengage the tooth if the gingival convergence is pronounced.

3. Flat rest seat preparation allows rest to slip distally during function.

4. During function, forces are transmitted through the RPD components to the distal rest directing distal torquing and axial forces to the tooth.

E. CAST CIRCUMFERENTIAL AND CAST BAR (MODIFIED "T")—DISTAL REST. (Fig. 10–15)

1. Rotation occurs at area where minor connector breaks contact with tooth.

2. Modified "T" bar clasp tip moves mesio-occlusally during function and directs torquing forces to the tooth.

3. Flat rest seat preparation allows rest to slip distally during function.

4. During function, forces are transmitted through the RPD components to the distal rest directing distal torquing and axial forces to the tooth.

F. CAST CIRCUMFERENTIAL AND CAST BAR (MODIFIED "T")—MESIAL REST. (Fig. 10–16)

1. Rotation occurs in area of mesial rest.

2. Proximal plate disengages from the tooth during function.

3. Modified "T" bar clasp tip moves mesiogingivally during function.

DESIGN OF THE "RPI" CLASP
(Figs. 10–17, 10–18A to D, 10–19 A & B)

A. REST.

1. Rest is located on mesial of abutment tooth. Rest seat preparation should be smooth and rounded to facilitate rotation of rest. (Fig. 10–18D)

2. The minor connector is placed into the mesio-lingual embrasure but does not contact the adjacent tooth. (Figs. 10–17,10–18B, 10–19A, B & C)

3. A 2 to 3 mm guiding plane may be formed at the occlusal one third of the mesiolingual embrasure.

B. PROXIMAL PLATE.

1. A guiding plane is prepared on the distal surface of the abutment tooth in the occlusal one third.

2. The guiding plane is approximately 2 to 3 mm in height occlusogingivally. (Figs. 10–18A, C & D)

3. An undercut should exist below the guiding plane to permit movement of the proximal plate.

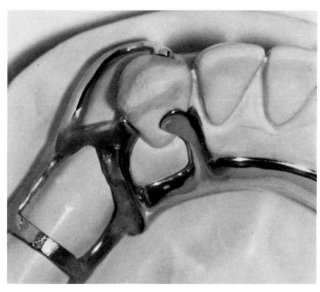

Fig. 10-17 Occlusal view of an "RPI" clasp on a mandibular canine.

4. The distal guiding plane should be parallel to the mesiolingual guiding plane in an occlusogingival direction.

5. The distal guiding plane extends lingually far enough to accept a proximal plate of proper faciolingual dimension. (Figs. 10–18B, 10–19A &B, 10–20A &B)

6. The proximal plate extends lingually just far enough so that together with the mesial rest it provides adequate encirclement to prevent potential lingual movement of the tooth.

7. The superior edge of the proximal plate contacts 1 mm of the gingival portion of the guiding plane. This should approximate the junction of the occlusal and middle one thirds of the clinical crown. (Fig. 10–18C)

8. The proximal plate is 1 to 1.5 mm thick.

9. The portion of the proximal plate adjacent to the gingival tissues is relieved (30 gauge) and highly polished. (Figs. 10–21 & 10–22)

10. The internal finish line should be located 3-4 mm from the natural tooth, and form a well defined butt joint with the denture base resin.

11. The base of the proximal plate should swing back to join the major connector in a rounded acute angle in order to increase gingival exposure. (Figs. 10–19A & B and 10–23)

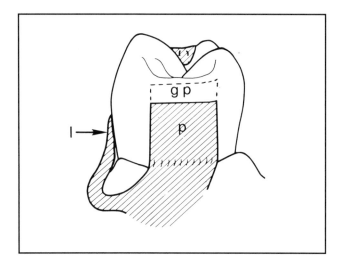

Fig. 10-18A   Distal view. The guiding plane (gp) is approximately 2 to 3 mm in height occlusogingivally. The faciolingual width of the guiding plane and proximal plate (p) is determined by the contour of the tooth (Fig.10-18B). The "I" bar (I) makes a 2 mm contact with the tooth in an occlusogingival direction. Note the slight relief over the gingival margin.

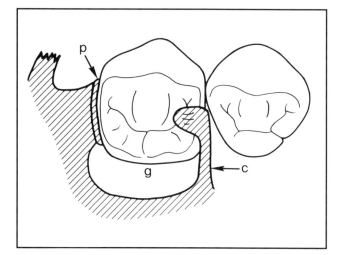

Fig. 10-18B   Occlusal view. The proximal plate (p) extends faciolingually far enough so that the distance between its lingual margin and the mesial minor connector is less than the width of the tooth. The mesial minor connector should not contact the adjacent tooth. The proximal plate should extend facially far enough to permit development of a normal embrasure with the adjacent artificial tooth. The major connector comprising a part of the clasp should be located at least 3 mm from the gingival margins (g) for mandibular partial dentures and at least 6 mm from the gingival margins for maxillary partial dentures.

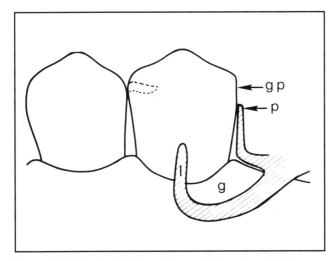

Fig. 10-18C Facial view. The guiding plane (gp) is approximately 2 to 3 mm in height occlusogingivally. The proximal plate (p) contacts approximately 1 mm of the gingival portion of the guiding plane. The proximal plate is 1 to 1.5 mm thick. The approach arm of the "I" bar is located at least 3 mm from the gingival margin (g) and may be designed to follow its contour. The "I" bar should cross the gingival margin at a 90 degree angle.

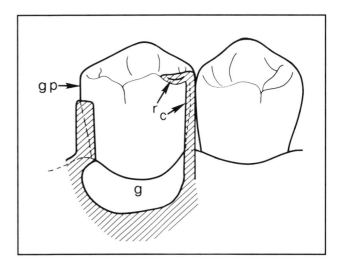

Fig. 10-18D Lingual view. The guiding plane (gp) is approximately 2 to 3 mm in height occlusogingivally. The rest seat preparation should be smooth and rounded to facilitate rotation of the rest (r). The proximal plate extends lingually far enough so that together with the mesial minor connector (c) they may prevent lingual movement of the tooth (Fig. 10-18B). The major connector comprising a part of the clasp should demonstrate adequate exposure of the gingival tissues (g).

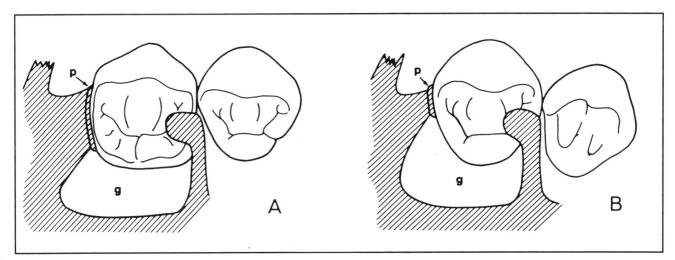

Fig. 10-19A & B Illustration showing comparative width of the proximal plates for teeth with different contours. (A) Proximal plate (p) relatively wide due to square contour of second premolar. (B) Proximal plate relatively narrow due to tapering contour of first premolar. The proximal plate should be as narrow as possible but still prevent potential lingual migration of the tooth. The base of the proximal plate should swing back to join the major connector to increase the exposure of gingival tissues (g).

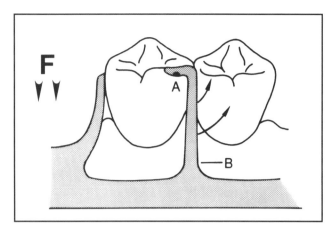

Fig. 10-19C Lingual view of "RPI" clasp during function. (A) Indicates center of rotation and (B) mesial minor connector. Minor connector rotates mesio-occlusally toward adjacent tooth requiring relief.

C. "I" BAR.

1. From an occlusal view, the "I" bar may be placed on the facial surface at the greatest prominence. It may be placed mesial to the greatest prominence, but not distal to it. Placement of the "I" bar to the mesial enhances the reciprocation from the proximal plate and increases the gingival exposure between the approach arm and the denture base. (Figs. 10–24 and 10–25)

2. Approximately 2 mm of the "I" bar contacts the tooth surface. The "I" bar contact should not extend above the height of contour. (Fig. 10–18A)

3. Inferior contact of the "I" bar is at 0.010 inch undercut.

4. The "I" bar tapers from the base to tip but does not come to a point. The terminal end is blunt.

5. From a facial view the "I" bar tip is usually placed in the gingival one third of the tooth.

6. When the undercut area of the clasp is located at or above the rotational (fulcrum line) axis occlusogingivally, the "I" bar should not engage an undercut anterior to the fulcrum line.

D. MODIFICATIONS OF THE "RPI" CLASP.

1. When two teeth are splinted the mesial rest may be placed on the anterior tooth and the proximal plate on the posterior tooth. The "I" bar is placed on the mesiofacial surface of the posterior tooth. (Fig. 10–26)

2. When fabricating an extension base partial denture where an isolated tooth is involved, the "RPI" clasp may be placed on the tooth anterior to the isolated tooth. Proximal plates may be placed on the mesial and distal surfaces of the isolated tooth without a rest. This design minimizes lateral forces directed to the isolated

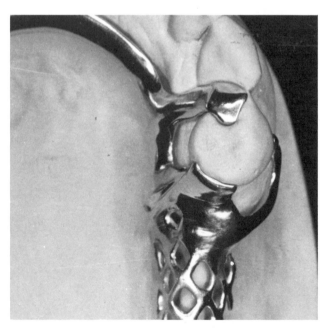

Fig. 10-20A Proximal plate too wide faciolingually for the contour of the tooth.

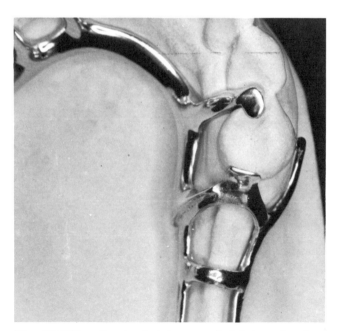

Fig. 10-20B Proximal plate properly fabricated makes minimal tooth contact and permits greater exposure of the gingival tissues.

tooth by promoting disengagement of the proximal plates during loading. The superior borders of the proximal plates on the isolated tooth should be located at, or gingival to the occlusogingival level of the rest of the "RPI" clasp to ensure stress release. (Fig. 10–27)

3. When a bar is used to splint mandibular canines the bar acts as the rest. The proximal plate is placed on the distal surface of the canine, and the "I" bar on the mesiofacial surface of the canine. The "I" bar should contact the tooth gingival to the height of the bar to allow the "I" bar to disengage. (Figs. 10–28A, B & C)

4. The amount of contact between the proximal plate and the guiding plane may be varied. While several designs have been proposed, there have been no published studies comparing the designs. Whichever design is selected, a functional adjustment of the framework should be performed to minimize potential torquing of the abutment teeth. (Figs. 10–29A, B & C)

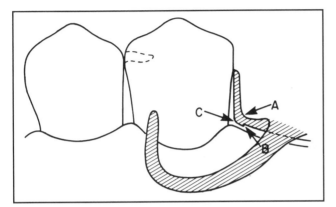

Fig. 10-21 Illustration showing proper design of the proximal plate. (A) Junction of proximal plate with framework. Too much thickness in this area may compromise placement of the artificial tooth. (B) Internal finish line is located 3 to 4 mm from the natural tooth and forms a well defined butt joint with the denture base resin. (C) Tissue surface of the proximal plate is relieved (30 gauge) and highly polished.

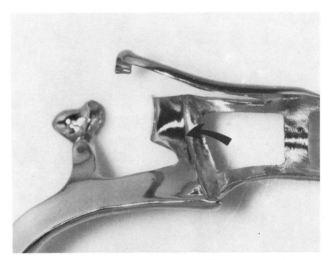

Fig. 10-22 Tissue surface of a mandibular partial denture framework. Arrow indicates internal finish line. Note highly polished proximal plate.

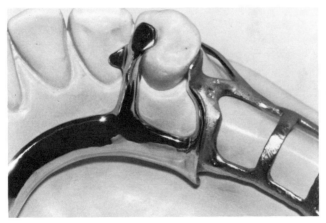

Fig. 10-23 Lingual view of "RPI" clasp. Base of proximal plate swings distally to join lingual bar increasing the exposure of gingival tissues.

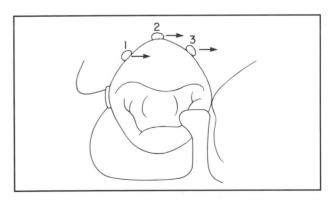

Fig. 10-24 Occlusal view of an "RPI" clasp. Placement of the "I" bar at the greatest prominence (2) or to the mesial (3) permits the "I" bar to disengage from the tooth during function. An "I" bar placed distal to the greatest prominence (1) does not disengage during function and torques the tooth.

E. CONTRAINDICATIONS FOR THE "RPI" CLASP.

1. Insufficient vestibular depth. The approach of the "I" bar should not interfere with movable tissues. The superior border of the arm should be located at least 3 mm from the gingival margin. (Figs. 10–30A & B)

2. Deep tissue undercut. The approach arm usually should not be located more than 2 mm from the soft tissue. Excessive relief may form a food trap, interfere with patient comfort or irritate the mucosa of the lip or cheek. (Fig. 10–31)

3. Lack of facial undercut. When mouth preparation (recontouring) or a restoration cannot create an adequate undercut for the "I" bar clasp. (Fig. 10–31)

4. Mesial inclination. When the tooth is tilted mesially, and no undercut is present gingival to the distal guiding plane, the proximal plate cannot disengage from the tooth during function.

5. Use of a lingual plate. When a lingual plate is required, its placement above the height of contour on the abutment tooth will produce a facial torquing during function (similar to a back action clasp). (Fig. 10–10)

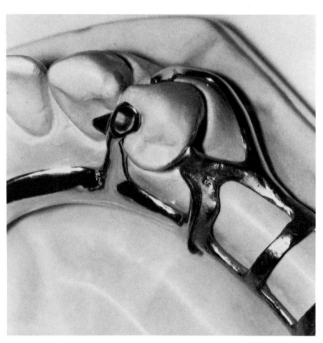

Fig. 10-25 Occlusal view of an "RPI" clasp on a mandibular first premolar. Placement of the "I" bar mesial to the greatest prominence enhances the reciprocation from the proximal plate, and increases the gingival exposure between the approach arm and the denture base.

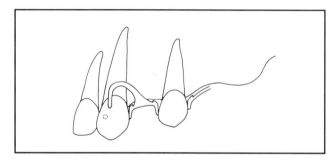

Fig. 10-27 Illustration of an "RPI" clasp on a maxillary canine with proximal plates on the isolated second premolar. Note that the proximal plates on the premolar are located gingival to the indicated position of the ball rest of the "RPI" clasp.

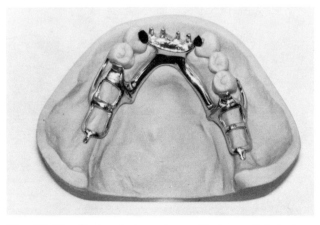

Fig. 10-26 Occlusal view of mandibular partial denture with "RPI" clasps bilaterally. On the left the two teeth are splinted, while on the right a fixed partial denture is present. The rests are placed on the mesial retainers, while the "I" bars and proximal plates are placed on the distal retainers.

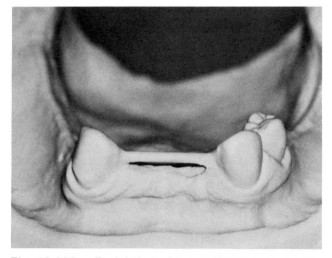

Fig. 10-28A Facial view of a mandibular cast with the canines splinted with a bar. Note that the left canine is also splinted to the first premolar.

DESIGN OF THE "RPC" CLASP

A. REST. As described for the "RPI" clasp.

B. PROXIMAL PLATE. As described for the "RPI" clasp.

C. CAST CIRCUMFERENTIAL RETENTIVE CLASP ARM. (Figs. 10–32A &B)

   1. The rigid portion of the circumferential clasp arm is fabricated so that only the superior border contacts the tooth at the height of contour.

Relief of the clasp arm is provided gingival to the contact to permit disengagement during function. (Figs. 10–32A &B and 10–12)

   2. The retentive tip of the clasp arm contacts the tooth without relief.

   3. A round cast clasp arm may be utilized. It should be placed at the height of contour except at the retentive tip to permit disengagement during function. (Fig. 10–33C)

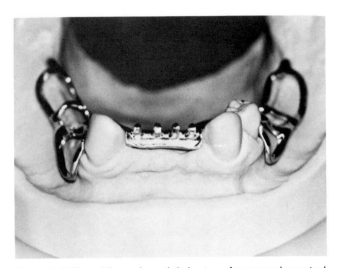

Fig. 10-28B View of partial denture framework seated on cast from Fig. 10-28A. The "I" bar contacts the right canine gingival to the superior border of the bar to permit disengagement during function.

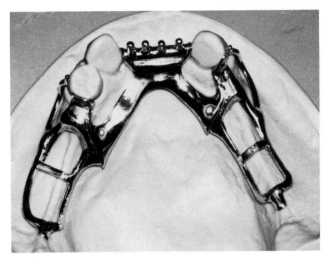

Fig. 10-28C Occlusal view of the partial denture framework from Fig. 10-28B.

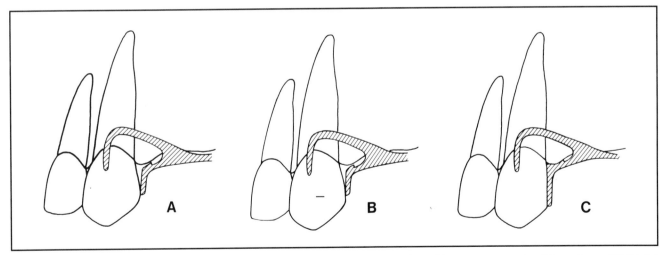

Fig. 10-29A, B & C (A) Proximal plate contacting distal surface of canine without a prepared guiding plane. (B) Distal guiding plane prepared in incisal one third of canine. The superior edge of the proximal plate contacts 1 mm of the gingival portion of the guiding plane. Note relief of proximal plate over gingival tissues. This design is described in detail in this syllabus. (C) Distal guiding plane prepared on entire distal surface of canine. Note absence of relief of proximal plate over gingival tissues.

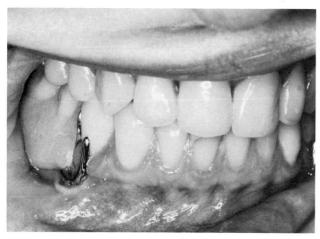

Fig. 10-30A Mucosal ulceration under approach arm of "I" bar due to insufficient depth of vestibule. The vestibular depth should be evaluated clinically by manually activating the associated soft tissue attachments.

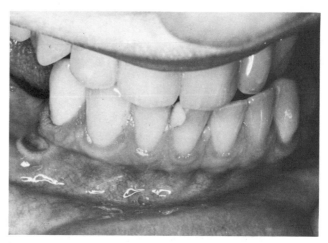

Fig. 10-30B Ulceration under "I" bar approach arm is apparent. A functional vestibular depth of 5 mm is required.

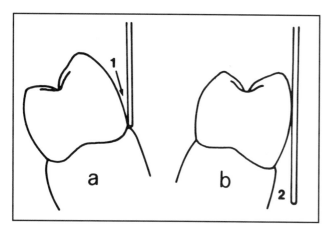

Fig. 10-31 Illustration of tilted premolars. (a) No facial undercut is present as indicated by number (1). (b) Deep tissue undercut is indicated by number (2).

DESIGN OF THE CAST CIRCUMFERENTIAL AND WROUGHT WIRE CIRCUMFERENTIAL CLASP (COMBINATION CLASP)

A. REST. Rest seat preparation is flat. Allows rest to slip distally during occlusal loading. (Fig. 10–13)

B. CAST CIRCUMFERENTIAL BRACING CLASP ARM.

C. WROUGHT WIRE CIRCUMFERENTIAL RETENTIVE CLASP ARM.

1. Flexibility of wrought wire retentive arm minimizes distal torquing of the abutment tooth.

2. The wrought wire gauge and composition should be selected to achieve the required flexibility.

3. The wrought wire should be attached to the framework at some distance from the retentive tip. This maintains the wire's flexibility. (Figs. 6–21A & B)

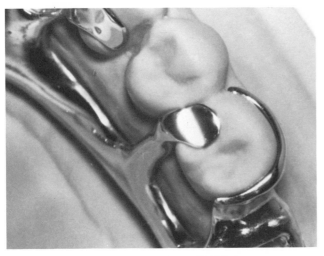

Fig. 10-32A Occlusal view of an "RPC" clasp on a mandibular second premolar. Note facial cast circumferential retentive clasp arm originating from the proximal plate.

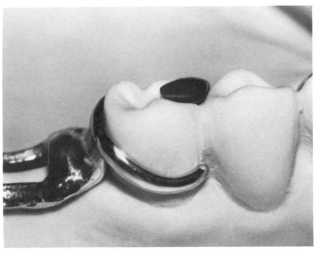

Fig. 10-32B Facial view of "RPC" clasp from Fig. 10-32A.

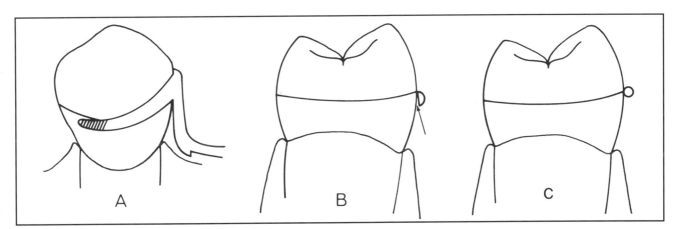

Fig. 10-33A, B & C (A) Illustration of the cast circumferential retentive clasp arm of an "RPC" clasp. The superior border of the shoulder portion contacts the tooth at the height of contour. The retentive tip of the clasp arm contacts the tooth without relief. (B) Cross-sectional view of the shoulder portion of the "RPC" clasp arm. Note the relief (arrow) gingival to the contact of the superior border with the tooth at the height of contour. (C) Cross-sectional view of a round cast clasp arm. Relief is present gingival to the contact of the arm at the height of contour.

Chapter XI

DENTURE BASE DESIGN

Proper base design incorporates coverage of muco-osseous supporting structures. This is most important for the tooth-mucosa borne partial denture where the base contributes to the support of the prosthesis. In the mandibular arch, the buccal shelf and the pear-shaped pad are the two areas most resistant to resorption. The most resistant areas in the maxillary arch are the horizontal hard palate and posterior residual ridges. When maximum support is required, designs that cover these areas are required.

DEFINITION

The denture base is that component of the partial denture which contacts the oral mucosa and to which the artificial teeth are attached.

REQUIREMENTS OF BASES

A. SHOULD BE EXTENDED TO COVER SUPPORTING AREAS.

B. SHOULD PROVIDE ADEQUATE RETENTION OF THE ARTIFICIAL TEETH.

C. SHOULD BE SUFFICIENTLY STRONG TO AVOID FRACTURE DURING FUNCTION.

D. MUST BE PROPERLY LOCATED IN RELATION TO GINGIVAL AND MOVABLE SOFT TISSUES.

E. MUST NOT IMPINGE ON OR DEPEND ON MARGINAL GINGIVA FOR SUPPORT.

TYPES OF BASES

A. DENTURE BASE RESIN ON METAL FRAMEWORK.

  1. Indications.

    a. For extension bases in tooth-mucosa borne partial dentures.

    b. For long span tooth borne bases.

    c. When denture base resin is needed to restore anatomic contour and esthetics.

    d. When the need to reline or adjust the base is anticipated.

  2. Structural details.

    a. Base should be optimally extended with respect to surrounding soft tissues.

    b. Sufficient metal thickness at the junction of the base and the minor connector is essential to prevent fracture.

    c. The external finish line is positioned just far enough lingual to the ridge crest to position the artificial teeth. (Figs. 11–1 & 11–3)

    d. The external finish line fades into minor connectors or proximal plates as it approaches the occlusal surfaces of the contacted teeth. (Fig. 11–2)

    e. The internal finish line should be located to allow resin to cover muco-osseous areas where resorptive changes are anticipated. This permits the base to be relined to reestablish muco-osseous support. (Fig.11–3) (See Chapter V)

    f. The internal finish line should be located 3-4 mm from the natural teeth. This allows a highly polished metal surface to be placed adjacent to the free gingival margins. (Figs. 11–4A & B)

    g. The internal finish line should form a well defined butt joint with the denture base resin. (Fig. 11–3)

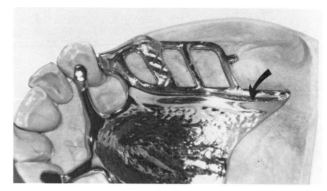

Fig. 11-1 Arrow indicates external finish line.

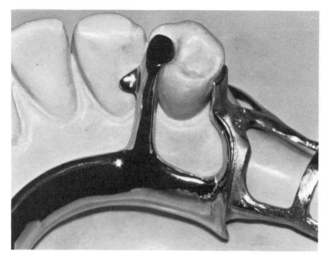

Fig. 11-2 External finish line fades into proximal plate on mandibular first premolar.

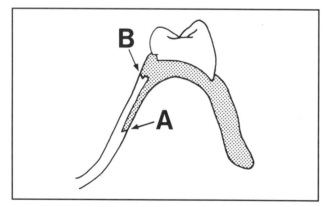

Fig. 11-3 Cross sectional view of a maxillary tooth-mucosa borne partial denture. The internal finish line indicated by arrow (A) is placed approximately at the junction of the vertical and horizontal planes of the palate to permit relining. Arrow (B) indicates the external finish line that is placed just far enough lingual to the ridge crest to position the artificial teeth.

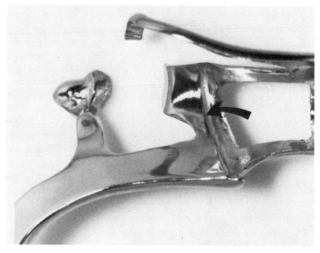

Fig. 11-4A Arrow indicates internal finish line.

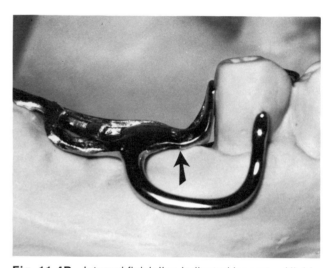

Fig. 11-4B Internal finish line indicated by arrow. Highly polished metal is placed adjacent to gingival margin, while resin is used over residual ridge.

  h. The internal line angle of the internal and external finish lines should be less than 90 degrees to provide mechanical retention for the denture base resin. (Fig. 11–3)

  i. The metal-resin interface exhibits a potential space which may enlarge during thermocycling and permit the entrance of microorganisms and fluids. This may lead to discoloration, plaque accumulation and resin deterioration at the interface. Recently developed denture base resins which bond to base metal alloys may reduce this microleakage.

j. The internal and external finish lines should not be superimposed. A staggered (offset) relationship maintains framework strength.

k. The open lattice design with large openings for the resin provides the greatest retentive strength for the resin. The longitudinal strut(s) should be placed facial and lingual to the crest of the ridge with connecting cross struts spaced to facilitate placement of artificial teeth. A longitudinal strut should not be positioned along the ridge crest as it may act as a wedge in the resin and may cause resin fracture. (Fig. 11–5)

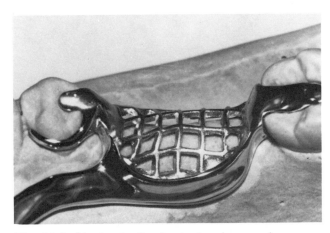
Fig. 11-6 Mesh retention for denture base resin.

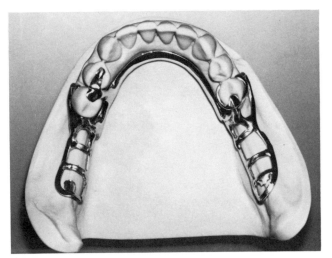
Fig. 11-5 Open lattice retention for denture base resin.

l. Retention mesh may be used, but it makes the mold packing procedures of painting the cast with a separating medium and packing with resin more difficult. Additionally, the attachment of the resin to the retention mesh is weaker because the smaller metal openings decrease the bulk of the resin. (Fig. 11–6)

m. Retentive posts, loops, or beads may be used to enhance the retention of the resin. This is especially critical when anterior teeth are involved. Posts provide the greatest reinforcement for artificial teeth. Proper post placement usually requires the fabrication of a matrix or template which indicates tooth position to the laboratory technician. (Figs. 11–7, 11–8A & B)

n. The resin retentive structure should extend posteriorly one half to two thirds the length of the residual ridge. Further extension of

the framework may interfere with base adjustment and may weaken the resin.

o. A metal stop should be used on the extension base framework for stabilization of the framework during mold packing with denture base resin. When an altered cast impression technique is utilized, the metal stop will require readaptation in order to restore contact with the cast prior to record base fabrication and processing. (See Chapter XVII) (Fig. 11–9)

3. Types of resin.

   a. Polymethylmethacrylate
      i. Most commonly used.
      ii. Wide variety of shades.

   b. Grafted polymethylmethacrylate.
      i. Resists impact fracture.
      ii. Resists flexure fatigue failure.

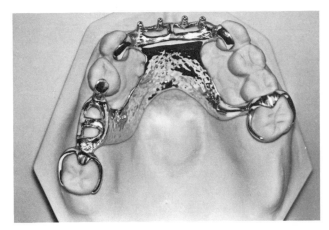
Fig. 11-7 Retentive posts used in anterior edentulous area.

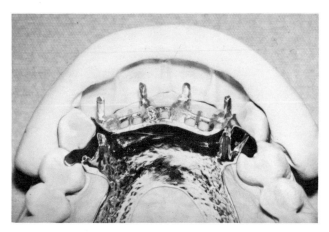

Fig. 11-8A Template on master cast with partial denture framework. Template facilitates precise placement of posts.

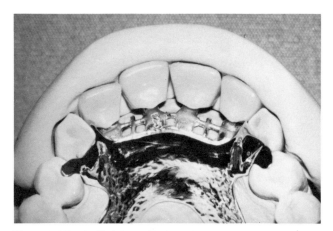

Fig. 11-8B Artificial teeth placed on posts.

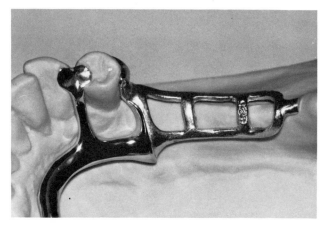

Fig. 11-9 Metal stop on extension base framework.

c. 4-META (4-methacryloxyethyl trimellitate anhydride).

   i. Potential to chemically bond to alloys capable of oxidation.

   ii. Increased bond strength of resin to metal.

   iii. Reduced microleakage at metal-resin interface.

d. Other.

   i. Polyvinyl.

   ii. Composite.

B. METAL BASE.

1. Indications.

   a. For short span tooth borne bases.

   b. When vertical height is limited, and insufficient space exists for use of denture base resin.

   c. When maximum strength is required and relining is not anticipated.

   d. When a significant vertical overlap of anterior teeth exists.

   e. When cast metal pontics or overlays are utilized.

2. Structural details.

   a. Base should be optimally extended with respect to surrounding movable soft tissues.

   b. Base may be thinner than resin-metal bases.

   c. To preserve contact with the underlying mucosa, the tissue surface should be electropolished only, without abrasive finishing.

   d. When a short span is to be restored in the posterior region, a cast metal pontic, with or without a resin facing, should be considered. (Fig. 11 – 10)

   e. Retentive posts, loops, or beads should be used to enhance the retention of the artificial teeth. (Fig. 11 –11)

IMPORTANT CONSIDERATIONS

A. SUPPORT SHOULD BE THE PRIMARY CONSIDERATION in selecting, designing and fabricating a denture base for an extension base denture.

B. THE EXTENSION BASE OF THE TOOTH-MUCOSA BORNE PARTIAL DENTURE OBTAINS ITS SUPPORT FROM THE ABUTMENT TEETH AND MUCO-OSSEOUS STRUCTURES AS LISTED.

1. The residual ridge.

2. The buccal shelf.

3. The pear-shaped pad.

4. The horizontal hard palate.

C. MAXIMUM SUPPORT FROM THE UNDERLYING STRUCTURES IS OBTAINED ONLY WHEN USING BROAD ACCURATE DENTURE BASES. Broad coverage furnishes the most favorable support with the least load per unit area. Close to the distal abutment tooth the base is supported primarily by the dento-alveolar segment. Further from the tooth, the base is supported primarily by the muco-osseous segment.

D. IN AN EXTENSION BASE PARTIAL DENTURE, THE BASE SHOULD COVER THE GREATEST SURFACE AREA POSSIBLE WITHOUT ENCROACHING ON MOVABLE TISSUES.

CRITERIA FOR SELECTION

A. THE NEED TO RELINE.

1. Tooth-mucosa borne partial dentures direct functional forces as pressure to the muco-osseous tissues. When resorptive changes occur, the base requires relining to maintain optimum support. Resin bases are easily relined.

2. In tooth borne partial dentures with long span bases, the base may require periodic relining to compensate for idiopathic or pressure induced resorptive changes.

B. THE NEED TO RESTORE MISSING TISSUES. A resin base may be contoured and shaded to restore proper form and esthetics.

C. LIMITED VERTICAL SPACE. When vertical space is limited, the minimal space may require a stronger base.

D. MAGNITUDE OF APPLIED FORCES. The anticipated occlusal forces may influence the choice of materials.

E. EASE OF ADJUSTMENT. Resin bases are more easily adjusted than metal bases.

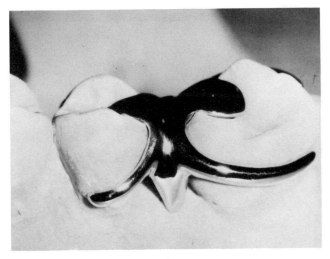

Fig. 11-10 Cast metal pontic.

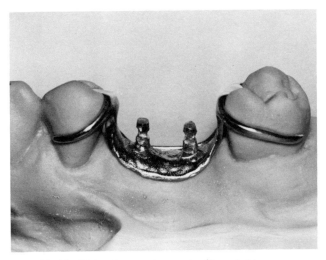

Fig. 11-11 Retentive posts used with metal base.

Chapter XII

PERIODONTAL CONSIDERATIONS IN REMOVABLE PARTIAL DENTURE DESIGN

Comprehensive prosthodontic therapy should contribute to the preservation of the remaining oral tissues. Since the primary etiologic factor contributing to the loss of teeth in adult patients is periodontitis, a preventive approach to removable partial denture design must incorporate periodontal considerations. Scientific investigations have implicated bacterial plaque as the primary etiologic factor in periodontal diseases.

Longitudinal clinical studies have demonstrated increased plaque accumulation on tissues covered by removable partial denture components and on the tissue surface of these components. This increased plaque accumulation is caused by reduced salivary flow and interference with the self-cleansing action of the lips, tongue, and cheeks. Increasing evidence of the adverse response of the periodontium to this increased plaque accumulation has been documented in the dental literature. Removable partial dentures should be designed to minimize plaque accumulation, particularly in the region of the gingival sulcus.

Mechanical force alone may cause pulpal hyperemia or increased tooth mobility but does not initiate periodontal diseases. It may, however, serve as an aggravating or accelerating factor in its progression. Since few patients are capable of maintaining a plaque free oral environment the control of mechanical forces directed to the dento-alveolar segment is important. However, some designs which may be effective in providing a broad distribution of force to the dento-alveolar segment may contribute to increased plaque accumulation. These designs often incorporate numerous framework components and undesirable coverage of gingival tissues.

Occasionally, the need for splinting of remaining natural teeth may dictate certain design features requiring additional components. Examples include the presence of hypermobile teeth which interfere with patient comfort and function, or the presence of excessive functional forces which may exceed the adaptive capacity of individually loaded abutment teeth.

This chapter presents guidelines for designing removable partial dentures with minimal tooth and gingival coverage. These design concepts may contribute to a more favorable response of the teeth and periodontium. Components of the removable partial denture framework should be eliminated whenever possible without compromising the biomechanical requirements of the prosthesis. Proper framework design and adequate mouth preparation also reduce the incidence of component failures and the resulting adverse effects on the periodontium.

MAJOR CONNECTORS

A. MAXILLARY MAJOR CONNECTORS.

1. The borders are placed at least 6 mm from the gingival margins. (Fig. 12–1)

2. Where a 6 mm distance from the gingival margins cannot be obtained, the metal may be extended onto the cingula of anterior teeth or the lingual surfaces of posterior teeth.

3. Usually, relief is not required on the tissue surface of the major connector, except where it crosses the gingival margins. In this area, the framework should be lightly relieved.

4. The metal should not be highly polished on the tissue surface to preserve intimate tissue contact, except where it crosses the gingival margins. In this area, the framework should be lightly relieved and highly polished.

5. The beading of the periphery of the maxillary major connector should fade within 6 mm of the gingival margins to prevent tissue impingement in this area.

B. MANDIBULAR MAJOR CONNECTORS.

1. The superior borders are placed at least 3 mm from the gingival margins. (Fig. 12–2)

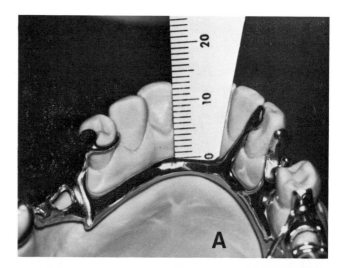

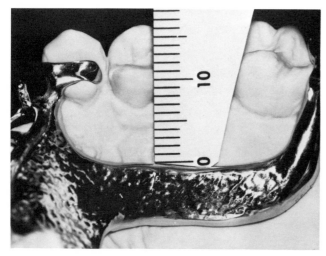

Fig. 12-1 The beaded borders of maxillary major connectors should be positioned at least 6 mm from the gingival margin.

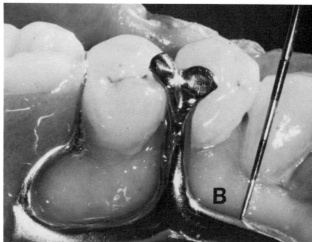

Fig. 12-2 (A) The superior border of the lingual or sublingual bar is positioned at least 3 mm from the gingival margin. (B) Intraoral view.

2. Where a 3 mm distance from the gingival margins cannot be obtained, the metal should extend onto the cingula of anterior teeth or the lingual surfaces of the posterior teeth. (Fig. 12–3)

3. The metal should be highly polished on the tissue side to minimize plaque accumulation.

4. Relief is required under the major connector to prevent tissue impingement at rest or during function. More relief is required with tooth-mucosa borne partial dentures. (See Chapter V)

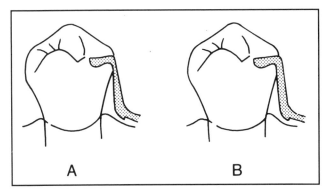

Fig. 12-4 Illustration of (A) inadequate and (B) adequate thickness at the junction of rest and minor connector.

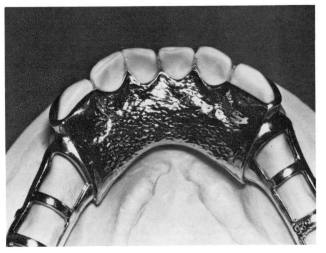

Fig. 12-3 Lingual plate design applied when insufficient vestibular depth is present.

MINOR CONNECTORS

A. THE JUNCTION OF THE REST WITH THE MINOR CONNECTOR REQUIRES A MINIMUM METAL THICKNESS OF 1.5 MM FOR BASE METAL ALLOYS (2 MM FOR GOLD ALLOYS). This minimizes the potential for fracture of the rest, which may result in a destructive settling of the partial denture into the peridental structures. (Fig. 12–4)

B. SHOULD BE LOCATED AT LEAST 5 MM FROM OTHER VERTICAL COMPONENTS THAT CROSS GINGIVAL MARGINS.

C. SHOULD EXHIBIT MINIMAL GINGIVAL COVERAGE.

1. Lingual minor connectors should cross the gingival tissues directly, joining the major connector at a right angle (90 degrees). (Fig. 12–5)

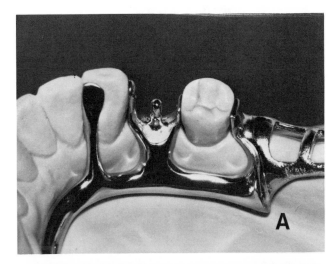

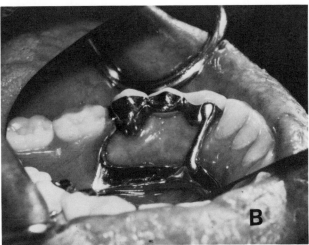

Fig. 12-5 (A) The lingual minor connector crosses the gingival tissue at 90°. Gingival exposure is increased by swinging back the base of proximal plates when joining the major connector. (B) A clinical view of increased gingival exposure by advancing the mesial rest and swinging back the proximal plate of the "RPI" clasp contacting a 3 unit fixed prosthesis.

2. The base of mesial and distal minor connectors and proximal plates adjacent to edentulous areas should swing back to join the major connectors in a rounded acute angle to increase gingival exposure. (Fig. 12–5)

3. Maximum gingival exposure may be provided for mesial and distal minor connectors and proximal plates by increasing the relief which exists gingival to their contact with the guiding plane. (Fig. 12–6)

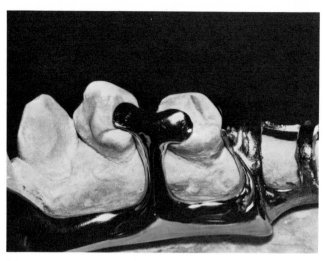

Fig. 12-7 Minor connector requires relief of the tissue surface opposing the first premolar and overlying the gingival tissues to prevent impingement during movement of the extension base.

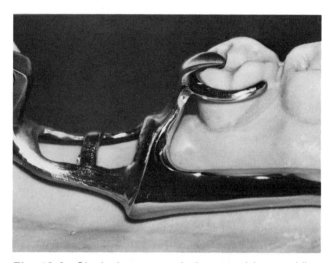

Fig. 12-6 Gingival exposure is increased by providing relief of the tissue surface of minor connectors and proximal plates increasing the angle of approach to the base area.

F. THE TISSUE SURFACES OF MINOR CONNECTORS THAT CROSS GINGIVAL TISSUES SHOULD BE HIGHLY POLISHED TO MINIMIZE PLAQUE ACCUMULATION. (Fig 12–8)

CLASPS

A. SHOULD EXHIBIT MINIMAL TOOTH AND GINGIVAL COVERAGE TO REDUCE PLAQUE ACCUMULATION.

D. RELIEF IS REQUIRED WHERE CROSSING GINGIVAL TISSUES.

1. Tooth-mucosa borne partial dentures. Relief (30 gauge) of minor connectors adjacent to extension base areas is required to prevent gingival impingement upon rotation of the partial denture during function. Other minor connectors require only minimal relief (32 gauge). (Fig. 12–7)

2. Tooth borne partial dentures. Minimal relief (32 gauge) is required.

E. RELIEF OF THE MINOR CONNECTOR WHERE CROSSING ADJACENT TEETH IS USUALLY REQUIRED WITH TOOTH-MUCOSA BORNE PARTIAL DENTURES IN ORDER TO ACCOMMODATE MOVEMENTS DURING FUNCTION. The minor connector should be slightly relieved (32 gauge). (Fig. 12–7)

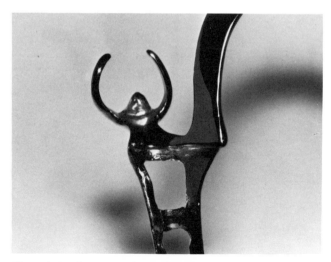

Fig. 12-8 Tissue surface of minor connector highly polished adjacent to gingival tissues.

B. BAR CLASP ARMS.

1. The approach arm must never impinge on soft tissue. The tissue surface of bar clasp arms should be smooth, polished, and lightly relieved (30 gauge).

2. The superior border of the approach arm should be located at least 3 mm from the free gingival margins. A minimum vestibular depth of 5 mm during function is required. (Fig. 12–9)

3. The approach arm should cross the free gingival margin at a right angle (90 degrees). (Fig. 12–9)

4. The vertical portion of the approach arm should be located at least 5 mm from other vertical components. (Fig. 12–9)

C. CIRCUMFERENTIAL CLASP ARMS.

1. Circumferential clasp arms should be placed at the junction of the middle and gingival one third of the tooth occlusogingivally, whenever possible. (Fig. 12–10)

2. Circumferential clasp arms located in the gingival one third of the tooth occlusogingivally may increase plaque accumulation apical to the clasp arm.

3. Circumferential clasp arms should not contact the free gingival margins.

4. Circumferential clasp arms located in the occlusal one third may increase forces transferred to the abutment teeth.

RESTS

A. THE JUNCTION OF THE REST WITH THE MINOR CONNECTOR REQUIRES A MINIMUM METAL THICKNESS OF 1.5 MM FOR BASE METAL ALLOYS (2 MM FOR GOLD ALLOYS). This minimizes the potential for fracture of the rest which may result in destructive settling of the partial denture into the peridental tissues. (Fig. 12–4).

B. SHOULD BE USED ONLY ON SURFACES THAT WILL DIRECT FORCES ALONG THE LONG AXES OF TEETH. A prepared rest seat is required to properly transmit the horizontal and vertical forces. Restorations may be required to achieve a positive rest seat. (Fig. 12–11)

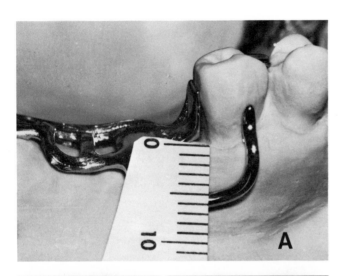

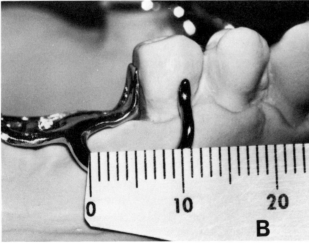

Fig. 12-9 (A) A properly designed "I" bar maintained at least 3 mm from the gingival margin during its approach and crossing it at 90°. (B) 5 mm is maintained between the vertical portion of the "I" bar and the base area.

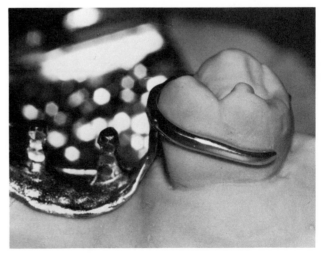

Fig. 12-10 Proper positioning of circumferential clasp arms promotes a favorable gingival response.

BASES

A. BASES FOR TOOTH-MUCOSA BORNE PARTIAL DENTURES SHOULD EXHIBIT OPTIMAL EXTENSION TO MAXIMIZE MUCO-OSSEOUS SUPPORT. This minimizes torquing of the abutment teeth and promotes equitable loading of the residual ridge.

B. WHERE THE BASE CROSSES GINGIVAL TISSUES, RELIEF IS REQUIRED TO PREVENT IMPINGEMENT.

C. ADJACENT TO ABUTMENT TEETH OR OTHER COMPONENTS THE BASE SHOULD BE CONTOURED TO EXPOSE AS MUCH GINGIVAL TISSUE AS POSSIBLE. (Fig 12-12)

D. THE INTERNAL FINISH LINE SHOULD BE LOCATED 3-4 MM FROM THE GINGIVAL MARGINS OF ABUTMENT TEETH. This allows highly polished metal to be adjacent to the gingival tissues. (Fig. 12-13)

IATROGENIC PERIODONTAL DESTRUCTION

A. LOSS OF DENTO-ALVEOLAR SUPPORT DUE TO FRAMEWORK FRACTURE OR ABUTMENT TOOTH MIGRATION.

   1. Inadequate metal thickness.

      a. Inadequate tooth preparation.

      b. Excessive finishing or polishing.

      c. Excessive occlusal adjustment of framework.

   2. Insufficient tooth modification without apical inclination of rest seats.

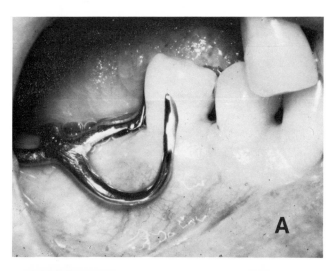

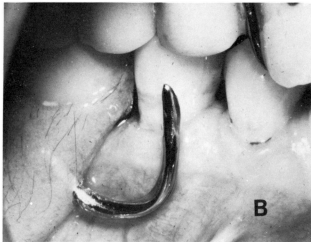

Fig. 12-12 (A) "I" bar correctly positioned in relationship to the gingival tissues. (B) Base resin contoured to promote gingival tissue exposure.

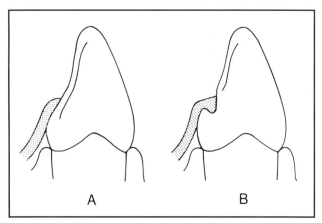

Fig. 12-11 Apically inclined rest seats are required to ensure axial force transmission. (A) Inadequate preparation. (B) Adequate preparation.

   3. Porosity within framework.

   4. Consequences. RPD usually settles into peridental tissues. (Fig. 12-14)

      a. Lingual bar or sublingual bar properly designed. Usually settles into floor of mouth without impingement on gingival tissues adjacent to abutment teeth. Adverse tissue response is usually acute and reversible. (Fig. 12-15)

      b. Lingual bar or sublingual bar improperly designed. Without adequate relief or distance from free gingival margins, the bar may settle into the gingival tissues adjacent to the teeth. The adverse tissue response is usually acute and irreversible. It may result in the loss of crestal alveolar bone. (Fig. 12-16)

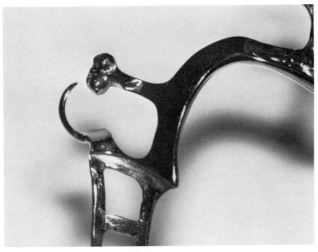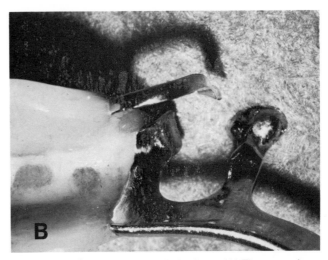

Fig. 12-13 Proper internal finish line location permits highly polished metal to overlie marginal gingivae. (A) Tissue surface of "RPC" clasp. (B) Tissue surface of "RPI" clasp after processing of the base resin.

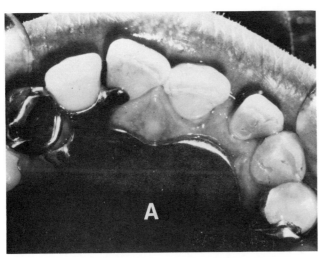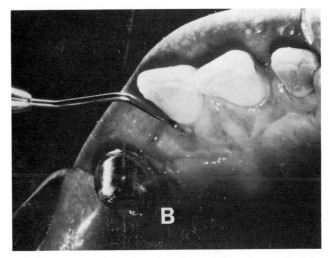

Fig. 12-14 (A) The absence of a rest seat permits the transmission of lateral forces to the abutment tooth resulting in migration of the central incisor. (B) Increased pocket depth is evident due to gingival coverage, increased plaque accumulation, and physical trauma in the area of the marginal gingiva.

c. Lingual plate. Usually settles slowly into the gingival tissues adjacent to the teeth. The adverse tissue response is usually chronic and irreversible. It may result in the loss of crestal alveolar bone. (Fig. 12–17)

B. INADEQUATE MUCO-OSSEOUS SUPPORT. Allows excessive tissueward movement of RPD during function. This increases the torquing forces on abutment teeth and may direct forces inequitably to the muco-osseous supporting areas.

1. Failure to incorporate corrected impression procedures (altered cast impression).

2. Underextension of denture base.

3. Inadequate palatal major connector coverage.

C. INSUFFICIENT RELIEF. Results in tissue impingement during functional loading. (Fig. 12–18)

1. Bar clasp approach arms.

2. Minor connectors and proximal plates where crossing marginal gingiva.

3. Mandibular major connectors.

D. INADEQUATE GINGIVAL EXPOSURE. Results in increased plaque accumulation and subsequent inflammation if not removed. (Fig. 12–19)

1. Lingual and sublingual bar.

2. Lingual plate.

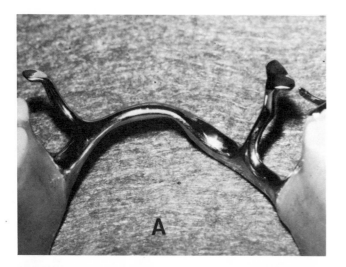

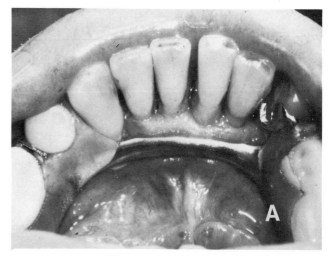

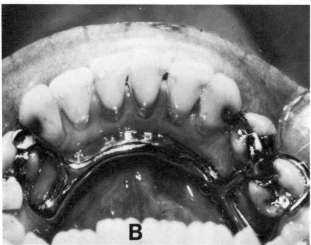

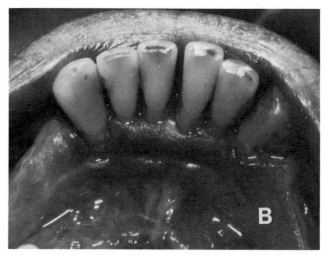

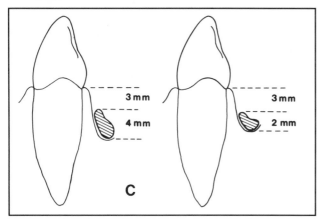

Fig. 12-15 (A) A sublingual bar opposite the central incisors gradually changing to a lingual bar further posteriorly. (B) Intraoral view demonstrates a sufficient 3 mm distance from the free gingival margins. Failure of a rest would not result in impingement of the gingival tissues. (C) Illustration of lingual bar (left) and sublingual bar (right). Note dimensions and relief.

Fig. 12-16 (A) Major connector demonstrates insufficient relief and distance from the free gingival margin expecially lingual to the canines. (B) Physical trauma contributes to the periodontal tissue destruction observed.

3. Vertical components. Minor connectors and proximal plates.

4. Bar clasp approach arms.

5. Denture base.

CAST RESTORATIONS FOR ABUTMENT TEETH

Permits optimal abutment tooth contours.

A. LEDGED CAST RESTORATIONS PERMIT CLASP ARMS TO BE CONTAINED WITHIN NORMAL ANATOMIC CONTOURS OF ABUTMENT TEETH. (Fig. 12–20)

B. FLAT GINGIVAL CONTOURS.

1. Rotational path designs. Bell-shaped contours enhance retention in the occlusal half of the abutment tooth but the gingival half is flattened. (Fig. 12–21)

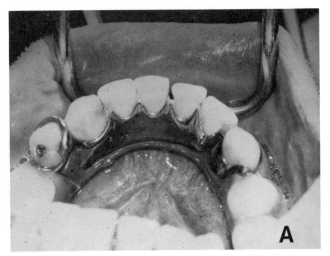
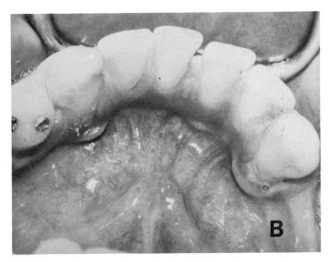

Fig. 12-17 (A) Lingual plate is settling into the gingival tissues following fracture of a rest. (B) Note the irreversible loss of lingual periodontal supporting tissues.

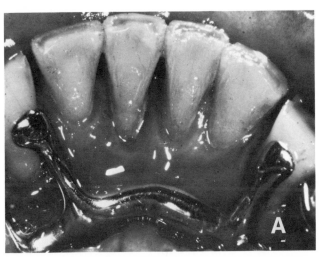
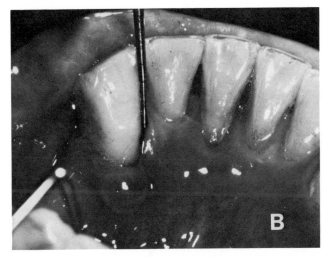

Fig. 12-18 (A) Demonstrates the results of inadequate relief of the tissue surface of the minor connectors and inadequate rest seat preparation for this extension base RPD. (B) Unfavorable periodontal tissue response.

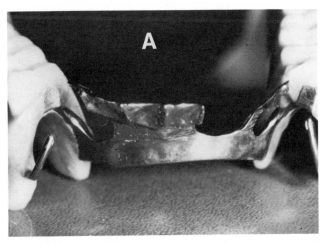
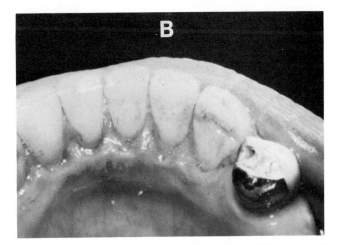

Fig. 12-19 Coverage of teeth and gingival tissues results in increased plaque accumulation on the covered tissues and on the fitting surface of the framework. (A) This framework was part of a clinical study. It was fabricated with a major connector one half lingual bar and one half lingual plate. (B) Note the increased plaque accumulation demonstrated with the application of disclosing solution on the side covered by the plate after a period of 20 hours following insertion.

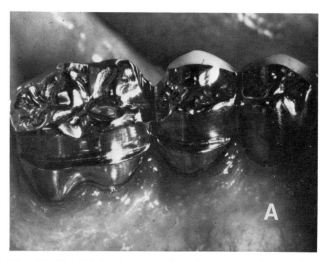 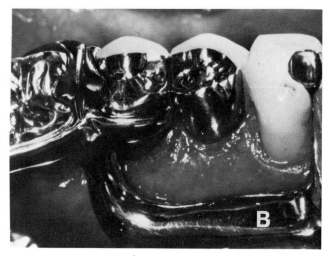

Fig. 12-20 (A) Cast restorations incorporate lingual ledges to accomodate the bracing clasp arms. Note also the rest seats and embrasures designed to permit minor connector placement. (B) Clasp components do not interfere with normal anatomic contours.

2. Furcation areas. Flat contours reduce plaque accumulation and facilitate oral hygiene procedures. (Fig. 12–22)

C. ADEQUATE TOOTH PREPARATION.

1. Rest seat areas. Promotes axial force direction, inhibits tooth movement and ensures adequate metal thickness at the junction of the rest with the minor connector.

2. Ledged casting areas—promotes normal axial tooth contours.

3. Intracoronal attachment areas. Permits matrix to be confined within normal abutment tooth contours. (Fig. 12–23)

D. EXTENDED OCCLUSAL RESTS MINIMIZE ABUTMENT TOOTH TIPPING AND ENHANCE BRACING. (Figs. 12–22 & 12–24)

SPLINTING

A. DEFINITION: The joining of two or more teeth into a rigid unit by means of fixed or removable restorations or devices to increase the resistance to lateral or horizontal forces in all directions (increases bracing).

B. ADVANTAGES.

1. Reduce hypermobility. Generally some degree of mobility may be acceptable in an otherwise healthy periodontium. Hypermobility may require treatment.

   a. When increasing in magnitude.

   b. When interfering with patient comfort or function.

2. Resist abnormal forces. The classification of a force as abnormal depends on both the magnitude of the force and the tooth's ability to resist force.

   a. Primary occlusal traumatism. Increased functional or parafunctional forces directed toward an otherwise healthy periodontium.

   b. Secondary occlusal traumatism. Normal functional forces directed toward a compromised periodontium.

Fig. 12-21 Cast restorations on anterior abutments demonstrate rounded contours occlusally but flattened contours in the gingival one half.

C. DISADVANTAGES.

1. Increased tooth and gingival coverage by additional or extended components may increase plaque accumulation.

2. Fixed splinting which involves rigid connectors between adjacent teeth may compromise embrasure form and complicate home care oral hygiene procedures.

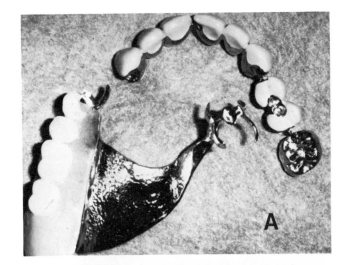

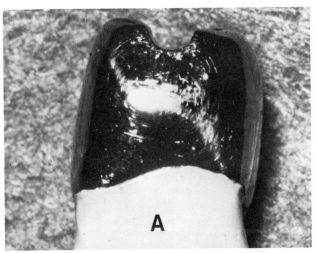

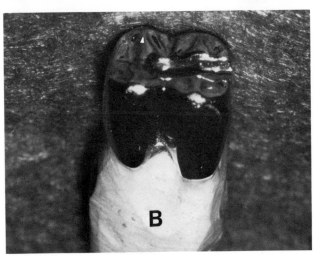

Fig. 12-22 (A) Cast restorations should demonstrate flattened contours in the gingival one half. (B) This is difficult to achieve in furcation areas.

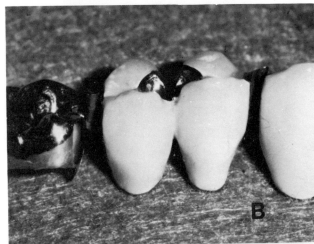

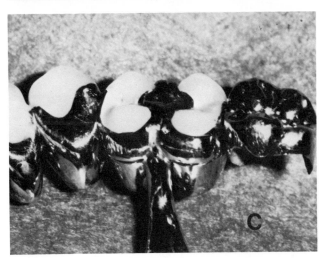

Fig. 12-23 To promote normal anatomic contours of restored abutments additional tooth modification was necessary to accomodate (A) an intracoronal attachment matrix, (B) an occlusal rest, and (C) lingual ledges.

D. DESIGNS THAT PROMOTE SPLINTING IN RPDs—Note that all RPDs contribute to cross arch splinting through the incorporation of a rigid major connector.

1. Multiple extended occlusal rests. (Figs. 12–24 and 12–25)

2. Continuous or multiple clasps.

3. Lingual plates. When used in conjunction with positive rest seats placed on the covered teeth. (Fig. 12–25)

4. Swing lock RPDs.

5. Multiple precision attachments.

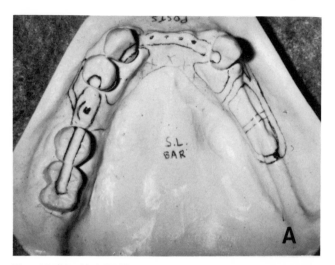 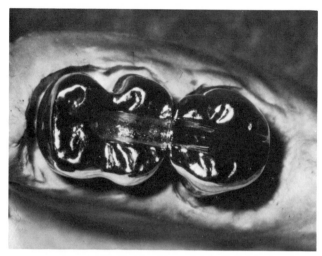

Fig. 12-24 (A & B) Extended occlusal rest assists in splinting the second molar and the distal half of the hemisected first molar without the need for a solder joint. Bracing and support are enhanced.

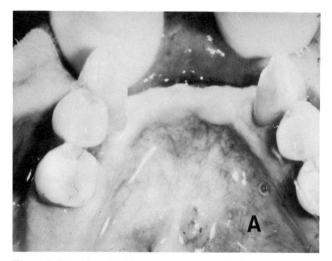 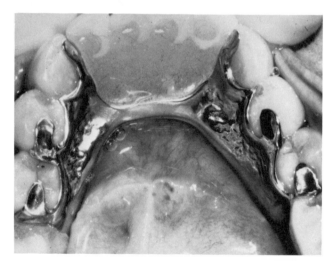

Fig. 12-25 (A & B) Lingual plate may promote splinting of the remaining teeth in conjunction with the rests provided on each abutment.

Chapter XIII

THE DESIGN PROCESS

The word "design" means to create according to a plan. A removable prosthesis should be designed only when the biomechanical and functional requirements of the patient and prosthesis are understood. The incorporation of engineering principles in the design of a prosthesis contributes to the preservation of the teeth and peridental tissues. The design process begins with the identification of a problem and ends with its resolution through the application of sound biomechanical concepts. In most instances, a variety of designs may be acceptable.

FACTORS INFLUENCING DESIGN

A. PRESERVATION OF TEETH AND PERIDENTAL STRUCTURES. A primary objective in design is to maintain healthy bone, teeth, and supporting soft tissue structures.

B. MINIMAL TOOTH AND MINIMAL GINGIVAL COVERAGE. Designs which minimize coverage of these tissues are preferred since they tend to reduce plaque accumulation.

C. THE NATURE OF THE PARTIAL DENTURE, TOOTH BORNE OR TOOTH-MUCOSA BORNE. In the tooth-mucosa borne partial denture, consideration must be given to equitable distribution of forces between the abutment teeth and the residual (edentulous) ridge. (See Chapter III)

D. ANATOMIC LIMITATIONS. The presence of certain congenital or acquired anatomic features such as bony exostoses, reduced vestibular depth, undercuts, or defects may influence the design.

E. TOOTH INCLINATION, POSITION, OR CONTOUR. May prevent a design feature from being utilized, dictating an alternative choice.

F. CONTINGENCY PLANNING. Possible future loss of teeth may require provision for modifications of the prosthesis.

G. POTENTIAL MAGNITUDE OF APPLIED FORCES. Increased functional forces or parafunctional forces, may increase the structural requirements of the framework or require splinting of abutment teeth.

H. EASE OF PLACEMENT AND REMOVAL. Handicapped individuals may be limited in their ability to place and remove the partial denture.

I. ESTHETICS. May be the most important factor from the viewpoint of the patient. May influence the type of clasps used.

J. DESIRES AND PREVIOUS EXPERIENCE OF THE PATIENT. The desires of the patient and the opinion of the dentist may not always be in accord. Whenever possible, acceptable options should be presented to the patient.

One or more of the above-mentioned factors may strongly influence the final design. They should never do so, however, to the detriment of the patient's health or function. A partial denture usually permits a variety of designs which are acceptable in meeting established criteria. It is within this range of acceptability that freedom in the design of a partial denture lies.

GENERAL PROCEDURAL SEQUENCE

A. EXAMINATION.

B. DIAGNOSIS.

C. TREATMENT PLAN AND DESIGN.

    1. Mount diagnostic casts.

    2. Survey diagnostic casts.

    3. Design diagnostic casts.

    4. Verify mouth preparation.

    5. Survey master cast.

    6. Design master cast.

THE DESIGN SEQUENCE

A. COMPLETE THE SURVEYING OF THE DIAGNOSTIC OR MASTER CAST AND REMOVE IT FROM THE SURVEYOR. Survey lines should be drawn and the cast should be tripodized. The exact location of undercut areas for retentive elements may be indicated with a red line 1-2 mm in length. (Fig. 13–1)

B. UTILIZING SHARP RED, BLUE, AND GREEN PENCILS, OUTLINE THE FRAMEWORK ON THE CAST.

C. THE PRIMARY DIFFERENCE BETWEEN THE DIAGNOSTIC CAST AND THE MASTER CAST IS THAT ALL MOUTH PREPARATION, INCLUDING TOOTH MODIFICATION, IS INDICATED ON THE DIAGNOSTIC CAST AND COMPLETED PRIOR TO OBTAINING THE MASTER CAST. Areas shaded in green may be used to indicate the need for tooth modification on the diagnostic cast.

D. OUTLINE THE RESTS IN BLUE CONFINED TO THE REST SEAT PREPARATIONS. (Fig. 13–2)

E. OUTLINE THE MINOR CONNECTORS AND PROXIMAL PLATES IN BLUE, INDICATING EXACT WIDTH, HEIGHT, AND RELATIONSHIP TO PREPARED GUIDING PLANES. (Fig. 13–3)

F. OUTLINE THE MAJOR CONNECTOR IN BLUE INCORPORATING MAXIMUM GINGIVAL TISSUE EXPOSURE IN THE AREAS JOINING THE MINOR CONNECTORS AND PROXIMAL PLATES. (Fig. 13–4)

G. OUTLINE ALL CLASP ARMS IN BLUE, INDICATING PRECISE WIDTH, TAPER, AND RELATIONSHIP TO SURVEY LINES AND THE FREE GINGIVAL MARGINS. (Fig. 13–5)

H. OUTLINE THE RETENTIVE MESH OR LATTICE OF THE RESIN BASE AREAS IN BLUE, INCLUDING A METAL STOP FOR EXTENSION BASES. LIMIT THE POSTERIOR EXTENSION TO ONE HALF TO TWO THIRDS THE LENGTH OF THE EDENTULOUS SPAN. The external finish lines may also be indicated in blue. (Fig. 13–6)

I. THE INTERNAL FINISH LINE MAY BE INDICATED USING A SHARP RED PENCIL. (Fig. 13–7)

J. HIGHLIGHT ANY ADDITIONAL FEATURES OF THE DESIGN SUCH AS POSTS, LOOPS, OR BEADS, UTILIZING A RED OR BLUE PENCIL. (Fig. 13–8)

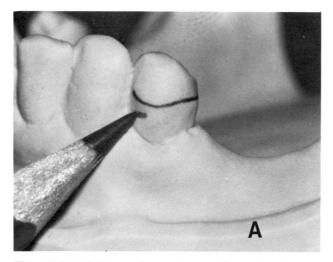 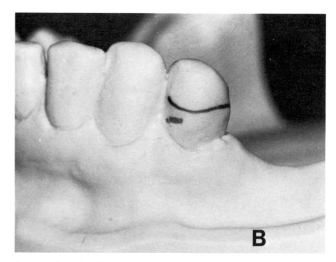

Fig. 13-1 (A & B) A sharp red pencil is used to demonstrate the precise depth of undercut required and its relationship to the survey line.

K. THE MEASURED DEPTH OF UNDERCUT MAY BE WRITTEN ON THE CAST TOGETHER WITH OTHER SPECIAL INSTRUCTIONS SUCH AS GAUGE OF RELIEF OR THE USE OF SPECIFIC MATERIAL SUCH AS 19 GAUGE WROUGHT WIRE. (Fig. 13-9)

Note: The final design should be drawn on the master cast or on a diagnostic cast which would accompany the master cast. A thin, clear, air dried cyanoacrylate coating may be applied to the abutment teeth of the master cast. This helps to protect the surface of the cast from abrasion and may improve casting adaptation.

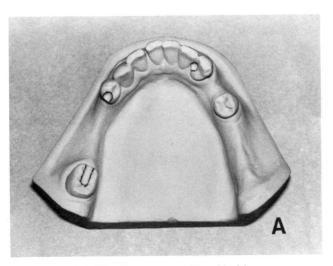
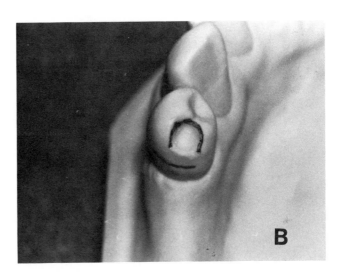

Fig. 13-2 (A & B)   Rests are outlined in blue.

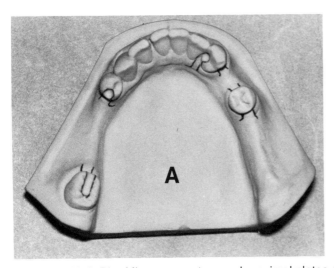
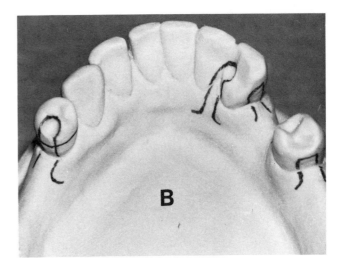

Fig. 13-3 (A & B)   Minor connectors and proximal plates are outlined in blue.

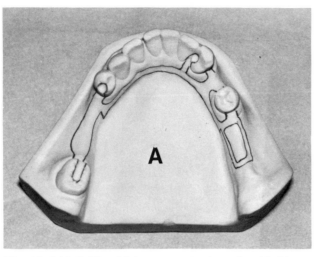
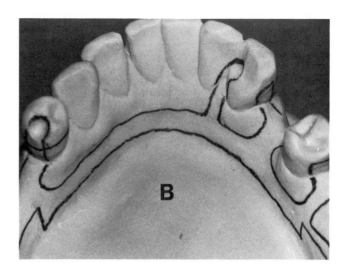

Fig. 13-4 (A & B)   Major connector is outlined in blue.

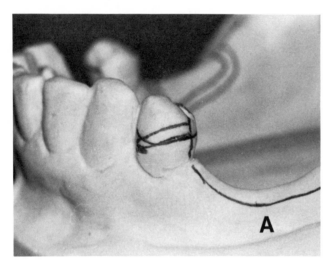
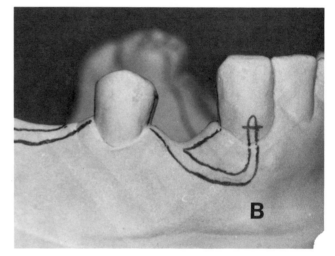

Fig. 13-5 (A & B)   Clasp arms are precisely outlined in blue, indicating the relationship of the clasp tip to the undercut area and survey line.

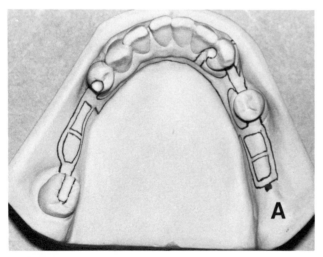
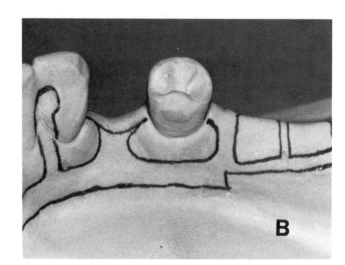

Fig. 13-6 (A & B)   The retentive mesh is outlined in blue.

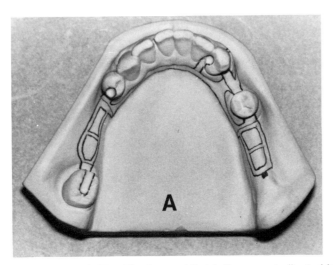
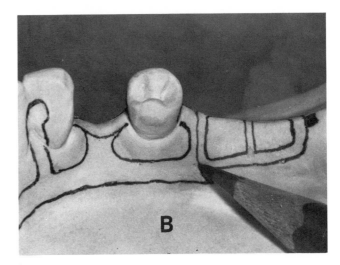

Fig. 13-7 (A & B) The internal finish lines are indicated in red.

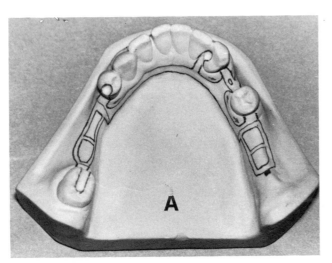
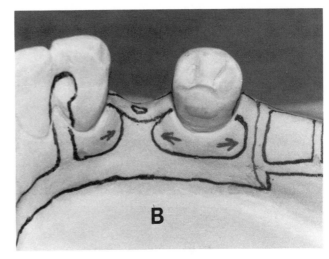

Fig. 13-8 (A & B) The post in the metal base area of tooth #28 is indicated.

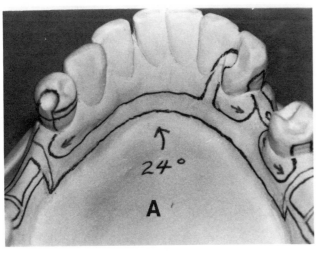
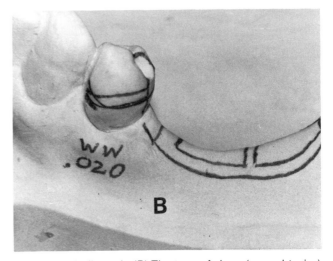

Fig. 13-9 (A & B) The relief of the tissue surface of the major connector is indicated. (B) The type of clasp (wrought wire) and depth of undercut (0.020) is written.

Chapter XIV

SELECTION OF TEETH FOR PARTIAL DENTURES

The selection of teeth for removable partial dentures depends upon the nature of the opposing dentition, strength required to prevent failure, abrasion resistance, available space, size of the remaining natural teeth and esthetic requirements of the patient. The occlusion and articulation required by the prosthesis will also influence the selection of posterior teeth. Plastic teeth are usually indicated for removable partial dentures.

ANTERIOR TEETH

A. PLASTIC TEETH.

   1. Advantages.

      a. Bond with denture base resins.

      b. Easily recontoured and polished.

      c. May be used effectively in combination with cast metal posts or loops to enhance the mechanical retention and strength.

      d. Teeth may be characterized.

      e. Lingual contour usually more closely approximates natural tooth contour.

   2. Disadvantages.

      a. Decreased abrasion resistance.

      b. Decreased stain resistance.

B. PORCELAIN TEETH.

   1. Advantages.

      a. Increased abrasion resistance.

      b. Increased stain resistance.

   2. Disadvantages.

      a. Increased abrasion of opposing natural teeth, plastic artificial teeth, or those restored with gold occlusal surfaces.

      b. May be used only when there is sufficient space for denture base resin to provide mechanical retention and ensure strength.

      c. Porcelain teeth are more susceptible to fracture.

      d. Mechanical bond required to denture base resins.

C. FACINGS.

   1. Advantages.

      a. Metal backing increases strength.

      b. May be used when there is insufficient space for denture base resin to provide mechanical retention and ensure strength.

   2. Disadvantages.

      a. May exhibit a flat appearance, lacking depth.

      b. Metal backing may affect shade and depth.

      c. Fabrication of a framework with a metal backing is more difficult due to occlusion and articulation.

FACTORS INFLUENCING THE SELECTION OF ANTERIOR TEETH

A. SIZE AND OUTLINE FORM OF REMAINING NATURAL TEETH. Artificial teeth should have size and outline forms that closely resemble the natural teeth.

B. SHADE OF REMAINING NATURAL TEETH. Artificial teeth should closely resemble adjacent natural teeth in shade.

Note: Numerous brands of artificial teeth are available. To achieve an acceptable esthetic result, several combinations of molds and shades may have to be evaluated. Selective recontouring may be required to improve the final appearance.

C. AMOUNT OF AVAILABLE SPACE. Artificial teeth must be placed within the available incisogingival and mesiodistal space.

D. MECHANICAL PROPERTIES. The selection of anterior teeth is influenced by the opposing occlusion, abrasion resistance, stain resistance, resistance to fracture, bond strength to denture base resin and ease of adjustment.

E. TEETH ON PREVIOUS PARTIAL DENTURE. May indicate patient's esthetic concerns.

POSTERIOR TEETH

A. PLASTIC TEETH.

1. Advantages.

   a. Bond with denture base resins.

   b. Easily recontoured and polished.

   c. Increased resistance to fracture.

   d. May be used where space is limited.

   e. Reduce wear of opposing restorations and natural teeth.

2. Disadvantages.

   a. Decreased abrasion resistance. The accelerated reduction in the occlusal vertical dimension can be minimized by using cast gold occlusal surfaces or by placing amalgam stops in the plastic teeth.

   b. Decreased stain resistance.

B. PORCELAIN TEETH.

1. Advantages.

   a. Increased abrasion resistance. This assists in maintaining the occlusal vertical dimension.

   b. Increased stain resistance.

2. Disadvantages.

   a. Increased abrasion of opposing gold restorations, plastic artificial teeth or natural teeth.

   b. May be used only where there is sufficient strength for denture base resin to provide mechanical retention and ensure strength.

   c. If porcelain teeth are modified to an extent which markedly alters the diatoric, the mechanical bond to the denture base resin may be compromised.

   d. Decreased resistance to fracture.

   e. Polishing of adjusted surfaces is time consuming and requires special instrumentation.

C. METAL TEETH.

1. Advantages.

   a. May be used where space is limited.

   b. Increased resistance to fracture and abrasion.

2. Disadvantages.

   a. May be unesthetic, however, the use of facial resin or composite veneers may be used to enhance esthetics.

   b. Difficult to adjust occlusion and articulation. Whenever metal occlusal surfaces are used, a suitable method must be utilized to develop an accurate occlusion and articulation during the framework fabrication. This minimizes the clinical adjustment required.

FACTORS INFLUENCING THE SELECTION OF POSTERIOR TEETH

A. SIZE OF REMAINING NATURAL TEETH. Artificial teeth should have occlusogingival, buccolingual and mesiodistal dimensions that are approximately the same as the natural teeth.

B. SHADE OF REMAINING NATURAL TEETH. Artificial teeth should closely resemble adjacent natural teeth in shade.

C. CUSP HEIGHT OF OPPOSING TEETH. Artificial teeth should have a cusp height that is equal to or slightly greater than the opposing teeth. This allows the teeth to be modified for proper articulation.

D. AMOUNT OF AVAILABLE SPACE. Artificial teeth must be placed within the available occlusogingival and mesiodistal space.

E. MECHANICAL PROPERTIES. The selection of posterior teeth is influenced by the opposing occlusion, abrasion resistance, stain resistance, resistance to fracture, bond strength to denture base resin, and ease of adjustment.

F. TEETH ON PREVIOUS PARTIAL DENTURE. May indicate the patient's preference for porcelain or plastic teeth.

G. CONDITION OF MUCO-OSSEOUS SUPPORTING TISSUES. An evaluation of the bone index and mucosal tissue tolerance should be made. When the patient exhibits a poor residual ridge bone index or a low tissue tolerance, the forces transmitted to the residual ridges should be decreased.

1. Decrease the faciolingual width of the occlusal table.

2. Decrease the number of posterior teeth.

3. Space teeth with diastemas.

4. Redefine the anatomy on occlusal surfaces after grinding to re-establish masticatory efficiency.

5. Plastic teeth may decrease the forces transmitted to the residual ridge.

Chapter XV

METAL ALLOYS USED IN PARTIAL DENTURE FABRICATION

The most commonly used metals for removable partial denture frameworks are the base metal alloys. Their popularity has been attributed to lighter weight, higher modulus of elasticity, lower material cost and greater tarnish resistance than that of gold alloys. When increased flexibility is required for retentive clasp arms, wrought metal alloys may be indicated.

ALLOYS USED FOR PARTIAL DENTURE FRAMEWORKS

A. BASE METAL ALLOYS. These alloys have either cobalt or nickel as their principal constituent. Chromium is the other major constituent. Minor amounts of other elements are also present.

　1. Cobalt-chromium alloys. These alloys contain approximately 60% cobalt and 25-30% chromium.

　2. Nickel-chromium alloys. These alloys contain approximately 65% nickel and 16% chromium.

B. GOLD ALLOYS. Gold alloys used for partial dentures are the Type IV (Extra-Hard) alloys.

　1. Yellow gold alloys (ADA Type IV). These alloys contain at least 75% gold and platinum group metals.

　2. Low gold alloys. These alloys contain less than 75% gold and platinum group metals, but exhibit similar physical and mechanical properties.

COMPARISON OF PHYSICAL AND MECHANICAL PROPERTIES

A. FUSION TEMPERATURE. Fusion temperatures for gold alloys are generally in the range of 875° - 1000° C, while for base metal alloys they are in the range of 1300° - 1500° C. The fusion temperature must be considered when the alloy is cast to a wrought wire clasp arm, when a wrought wire clasp arm is soldered to the framework or when the framework is soldered during a repair procedure.

B. DENSITY. Gold alloys have approximately twice the density of base metal alloys.

C. YIELD STRENGTH. Base metal alloys and hardened gold alloys have comparable yield strengths.

D. TENSILE STRENGTH. Base metal alloys and hardened gold alloys have comparable tensile strengths.

E. ELONGATION. Gold alloys have approximately twice the percentage of elongation as base metal alloys.

F. HARDNESS. Base metal alloys have a hardness approximately one third greater than gold alloys.

G. MODULUS OF ELASTICITY. Base metal alloys have a modulus of elasticity that is twice that of hardened gold alloys.

SELECTION OF METAL ALLOYS USED FOR PARTIAL DENTURE FRAMEWORKS

A. CRITERIA FOR SELECTION. Each alloy has advantages under certain conditions. The choice of alloy should be based on several factors:

1. Biocompatability.
2. Physical properties.
3. Dimensional accuracy.
4. Reproduction of surface detail.
5. Cost.
6. Versatility.

B. GOLD AND BASE METAL ALLOYS—COMPARABLE CHARACTERISTICS.

1. Biocompatability.
2. Wrought wire components may be attached to either alloy.
3. Dimensional accuracy.
4. Either alloy may be soldered for repairs.

C. ADVANTAGES OF BASE METAL ALLOYS.

1. Less thickness is required for adequate strength and rigidity. Greater clasp arm rigidity is desirable when the undercut on an abutment tooth is less than 0.010 inch.
2. The weight of base metal alloys is about one half that of gold alloys. Larger maxillary frameworks benefit from the reduced weight by minimizing the effects of gravity.
3. Base metal alloys do not tarnish as readily as gold alloys.

D. ADVANTAGES OF GOLD ALLOYS.

1. Gold alloys are approximately twice as flexible as base metal alloys.
2. The greater flexibility of gold alloys usually permits location of retentive clasp arm terminals in the gingival third of the abutment tooth, since a greater depth of undercut may be engaged.
3. Adjustments may be more easily made than with base metal alloys.
4. Gold alloys are more easily soldered during a repair procedure.

5. A gold casting is able to reproduce increased surface detail and may provide more intimate adaptation of the tissue surface of the framework.

ALLOYS USED FOR RETENTIVE CLASP ARMS

A. CAST ALLOYS. Retentive clasp arms are most commonly cast as part of the framework. The mechanical properties of the clasp arm are determined by the chosen alloy and structural design. (See Chapter VI)

1. Base metal alloys. Clasp arms of base metal alloys are approximately one half as flexible as gold alloys, given the same clasp shape, length, taper, and cross-sectional size (diameter).
2. Gold alloys. Clasp arms of gold alloys are approximately twice as flexible as base metal alloys, given the same clasp shape, length, taper, and cross-sectional size (diameter).

B. WROUGHT WIRE ALLOYS. Wrought metal alloys are occasionally used as retentive clasp arms.

1. Wrought gold alloys. These alloys generally contain a high percentage of gold and platinum group metals.
2. Wrought base metal alloys. These alloys contain no precious metals.
3. General considerations for wrought wire clasp arms.

   a. The wrought wire clasp arm is usually soldered to the framework.

   b. Excessive heating of the wrought wire should be avoided during casting or soldering procedures. This can induce a recrystallization, compromising the wire's mechanical properties. A recent report has demonstrated that wrought wire clasps exhibit reduced flexibility when base metal alloys are cast to them.

   c. The wrought wire should be attached to the framework at some distance from the retentive tip. This maintains the wire's flexibility and may reduce the potential for fracture. (Figs. 6–21A & B)

   d. Wrought wire for clasp arms is generally available in 18 to 20 gauge thicknesses. Gauge and flexibility are not directly correlated. The flexibility of the wrought wire is determined by its gauge and composition. Generally, 19 gauge wrought wire provides adequate flexibility for most tooth-mucosa borne RPDs. Many 18 gauge wrought wire clasps do not demonstrate adequate flexibility to ensure stress release in tooth-mucosa borne RPDs, while most 20 gauge wrought wires lack adequate strength for practical clinical application.

e. The gauge of the clasp arm may be confirmed by a wire thickness gauge.

Chapter XVI

MOUTH PREPARATION

Following the development of a comprehensive treatment plan, including the design for a removable partial denture, an appropriate sequence of mouth preparation procedures should be completed. This may include surgical, periodontal, endodontic, or orthodontic therapy in addition to restorative treatment and abutment tooth modification. This chapter primarily emphasizes those modifications of abutment tooth contours which promote the ease of placement, esthetics, retention, stability, support, and comfort of the partial denture. Abutment tooth contours are modified through preparation of the enamel or placement of restorations.

SURGICAL

A. PERIODONTALLY COMPROMISED OR SEVERELY MALPOSED TEETH. May require extraction.

B. EXTRUDED TEETH. May require extraction or dentoalveolar segmental osteotomy.

C. ENLARGED TUBEROSITIES. May require vertical or horizontal, soft tissue or bony reduction.

   1. Compromised interridge distance (less than 3 mm).

   2. Interference with the path of placement.

   3. Presence of loose, movable, redundant soft tissue.

D. BONY EXOSTOSES AND TORI. May require modification or removal.

   1. Interference with path of placement.

   2. Presence of thin mucosa overlying most tori may compromise force-bearing potential of the muco-osseous segment.

   3. May compromise optimum extension of RPD components.

E. HYPERPLASTIC DISPLACEABLE SOFT TISSUES. May require removal.

PERIODONTAL

A. PERIODONTAL DISEASE AND PLAQUE CONTROL.

   1. Home care instruction and professional hygiene recall should be implemented.

   2. Definitive treatment of disease including surgical treatment, if necessary.

B. INSUFFICIENT ATTACHED GINGIVA. The development of an adequate zone of attached gingiva may increase the resistance of the periodontium to mechanical forces. This is particularly true when subgingival restorations are planned or when physical trauma to the gingival tissues is anticipated.

C. SUPRABONY GINGIVAL POCKETS. Hyperplastic tissue may require surgical reduction in order to expose more of the clinical crown and improve abutment tooth contour.

ENDODONTIC

A. NON-VITAL TEETH SHOULD BE ENDODONTICALLY TREATED.

B. ENDODONTICALLY TREATED ABUTMENT TEETH.

1. Placement of conservative intraradicular posts with minimal removal of tooth structure may increase resistance to structural failure.

2. May require restoration with crowns to resist fracture.

ORTHODONTIC

A. ABUTMENT TEETH.

1. Axial inclination may require correction.

2. Infraeruption or supraeruption may compromise contours requiring correction.

B. OCCLUSAL PLANE. Irregularities may be corrected by orthodontic therapy.

C. ASYMMETRICAL OR UNDERSIZED EDENTULOUS SPANS. Areas which are not conducive to the artificial replacement of missing teeth may require modification.

RESTORATIVE

A. REMOVAL OF CARIES.

B. REPLACEMENT OF DEFECTIVE RESTORATIONS.

C. RESTORE STRUCTURALLY COMPROMISED TEETH.

D. OCCLUSAL PLANE MODIFICATION.

E. CORRECTION OF MALOCCLUSION.

F. SPLINTING OF NATURAL TEETH.

G. CORRECTION OF UNACCEPTABLE ABUTMENT TOOTH CONTOURS NOT CORRECTABLE THROUGH ENAMEL MODIFICATION.

H. EXPOSURE OF DENTIN DURING ABUTMENT TOOTH MODIFICATION.

1. Sensitivity.

2. Caries susceptibility.

MODIFICATIONS OF ABUTMENT TOOTH CONTOUR

A. OBJECTIVE.

1. Develop an acceptable path of placement.

2. Improve esthetics.

3. Enhance comfort.

4. Promote favorable biomechanical properties.

   a. Retention.

   b. Stability.

   c. Support.

B. ARMAMENTARIUM. All prepared tooth surfaces should be smooth, rounded and highly polished. (Fig. 16–1)

1. Assorted diamonds.

   a. Cylindrical.

   b. Round.

   c. Elliptical.

2. Assorted Burs.

   a. Round (#4,6,8).

   b. Multi-fluted finishing.

3. Polishing instruments.

   a. Points.

   b. Cups.

   c. Polish.

SEQUENCE OF TREATMENT

TOOTH MODIFICATION IS INITIATED FOLLOWING DETERMINATION OF DESIGN AND PRECEDING FINAL IMPRESSIONS.

A. GUIDING PLANES.

1. Prepared on certain proximal surfaces against which minor connectors or proximal plates will be placed. Guiding planes are not required for rotational path RPDs and may be of questionable value for tooth borne RPDs.

2. Dimensions.

   a. Occlusogingival. (Fig. 16–2)

      i. Confined to occlusal one third.

      ii. Two to three millimeters in length.

      iii. Flat occlusogingivally.

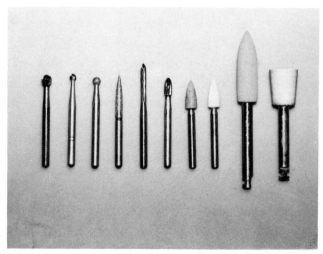

Fig. 16-1 An assortment of burs, diamonds, and polishing points provide the necessary armamentarium.

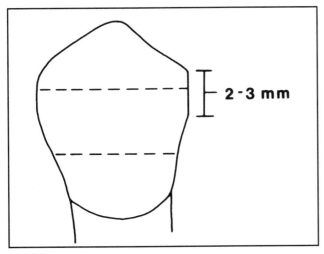

Fig. 16-2 Illustration of occlusogingival dimensions of a guiding plane prepared in the occlusal one third.

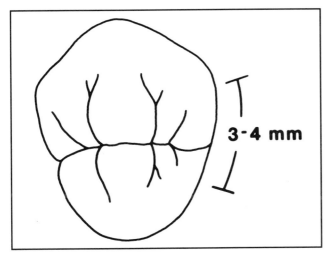

Fig. 16-3 Illustration of faciolingual dimensions of a guiding plane demonstrating rounded contour.

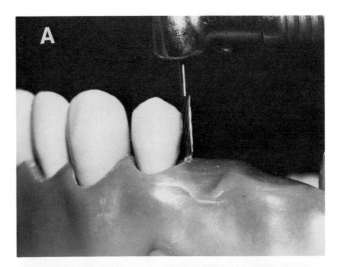

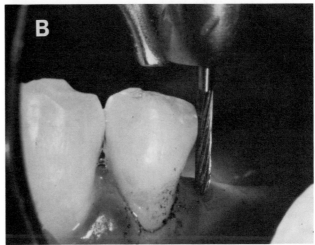

Fig. 16-4 A parallel-sided cylindrical bur prepares the guiding plane flat occlusogingivally. (A) On a model. (B) In the mouth.

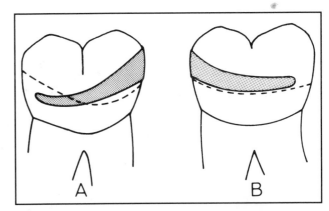

Fig. 16-5 Representation of proper circumferential clasp arm location. (A) Facial view. (B) Lingual view.

b. Faciolingual dimensions. (Fig. 16–3)

    i. Confined to proximal surface.

    ii. Three to four millimeters in width.

    iii. Rounded faciolingually in harmony with existing tooth contour.

c. Prepared with cylindrical diamonds or burs. Discs are not recommended since they tend to flatten the tooth surface in all directions. (Fig. 16–4)

B. HEIGHT OF CONTOUR ADJUSTMENT (SURVEY LINE).

1. Permits circumferential clasp arm location at the junction of the middle and gingival one third of the tooth occlusogingivally (Fig. 16–5). Circumferential clasp arms placed in the occlusal one third may create unfavorable le- verage. Circumferential clasp arms placed in the gingival one third may facilitate plaque accumulation in the area of the tooth apical to the clasp arm.

141

2. Reduces excessive relief required for minor connectors or lingual plates.

3. Eliminates sharp termination of guiding planes at facioproximal and linguoproximal line angles.

4. Establishes retentive undercuts at the junction of gingival and middle one third occlusogingivally.

5. Prepared with a cylindrical diamond or bur angled to the long axis of the tooth above the survey line. (Fig. 16–6)

C. RETENTIVE GROOVES.

1. Increases depth of undercut. (Fig. 16–7)

2. Dimensions.

   a. Proportional to retention required.

   b. Prepared with an elliptical or cylindrical diamond.

3. Gradual transition occlusogingivally (Gently sloping contour).

D. REST SEATS.

1. Tooth support is provided through rests requiring prepared rest seats to ensure axial force direction.

2. Tooth modification must be completed to permit a minimum thickness of base metal alloy of 1.5 mm at the junction of any rest with its minor connector.

3. Rests **require** the preparation of rest seats.

REST SEAT PREPARATIONS

A. OCCLUSAL RESTS.

1. Conventional.

   a. Indications. Posterior teeth.

   b. Dimensions.

      i. Apically inclined (spoon-shaped), except for distal rests for distal extension partial dentures. (Fig. 16–8)

      ii. From the occlusal view, the outline form resembles a rounded triangle whose base is at the marginal ridge.

      iii. One third of the faciolingual width of tooth. (Fig. 16–9)

      iv. One half of the width between the facial and lingual cusp tips.

      v. 1.5 mm marginal ridge reduction required for base metal alloys (2 mm for gold alloys).

      vi. The rest seat may be prepared with a #6 or #8 round bur, depending on the size of the tooth. (Fig. 16–10)

      vii. Embrasure rests require adequate tooth reduction to permit a sufficient thickness for the rests, minor connector and clasp arms. (Fig. 16–11)

2. Extended.

   a. Indications. Posterior teeth.

      i. Rotational path designs.

      ii. Splinting. (Fig. 16–12)

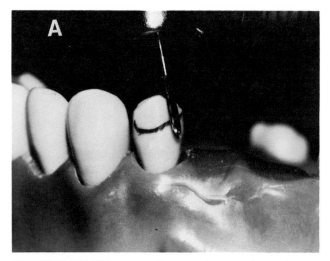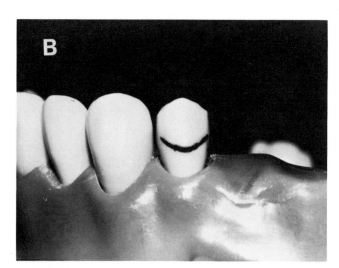

Fig. 16-6 (A) This survey line may be repositioned to a more gingival location through modification of the abutment tooth contour. (B) Survey line may be redrawn following modification.

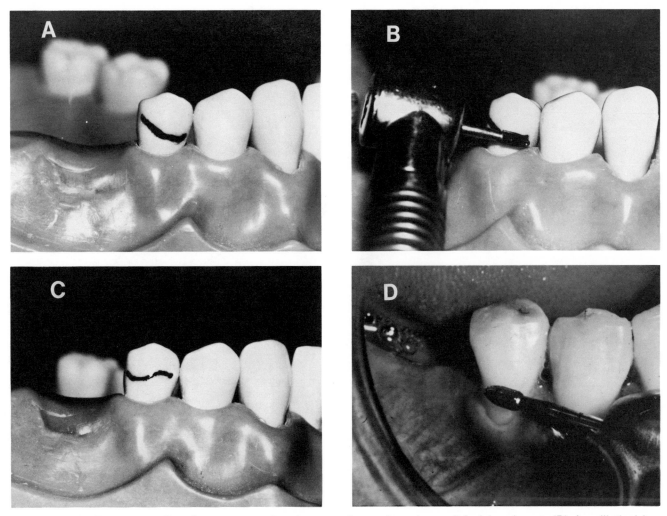

Fig. 16-7 (A) This survey line demonstrates the absence of an adequate mesiofacial undercut. (B) An elliptical bur enhances the depth of undercut. (C) The redrawn survey line demonstrates an increased undercut which should be confirmed on the surveyor. (D) A clinical example.

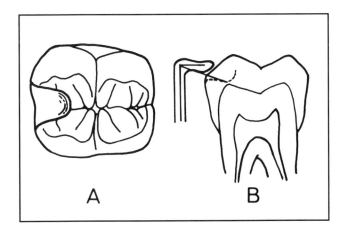

Fig. 16-8 Diagram demonstrates spoon shaped rest seat preparation. (A) Occlusal view. (B) Facial view.

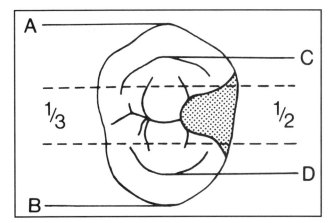

Fig. 16-9 Diagram demonstrates faciolingual dimensions of occlusal rest.

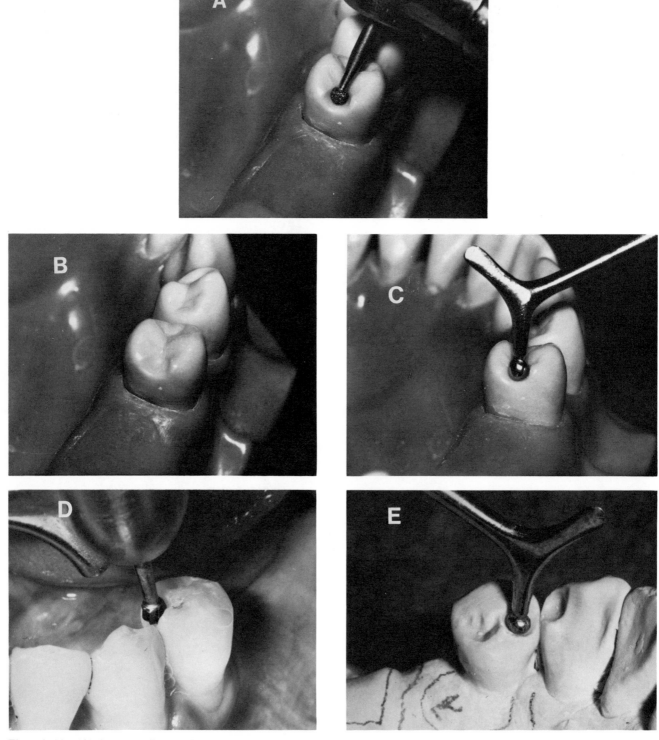

Fig. 16-10 (A) A round diamond prepares the occlusal rest seat primarily at the expense of the marginal ridge. (B) Completed rest seat. (C) Apical inclination is ensured as shown. (D) Clinical procedure. (E) Master cast.

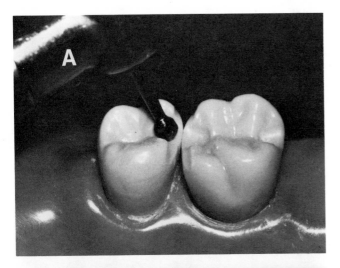

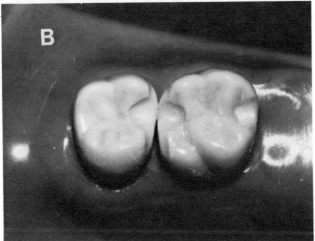

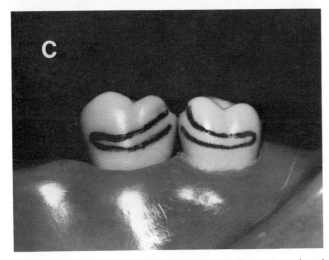

Fig. 16-11 (A) A round bur prepares adjacent occlusal rest seats. The completed rest seats and occlusal embrasure preparations. (B) Note that the contact area is not compromised by tooth modification. (C) Facial and lingual occlusal embrasures are prepared to permit clasp arms to extend from the rests without compromising thickness.

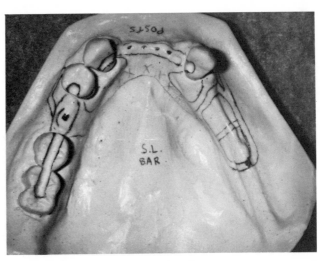

Fig. 16-12 An extended occlusal rest crosses crowned teeth #18 and 19 (mesial root resected) providing splinting without a solder joint when the partial denture is in place.

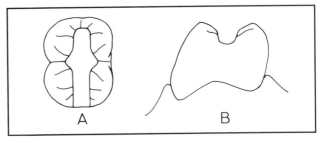

Fig. 16-13 Diagram of extended occlusal rest seat preparation. (A) Occlusal view. (B) Proximal view.

    iii. Tipped abutments. Assists in preventing further tipping.

    iv. Increased support and bracing.

  b. Dimensions. (Fig. 16–13)

    i. Slight apical inclination.

    ii. Greater than one half the mesiodistal width of the tooth.

    iii. 1.5 to 2.0 mm in depth.

    iv. From the occlusal view, an asymmetric outline form may be required for rotational path designs.

    v. Prepared with a #6 or #8 round bur. (Fig. 16–14)

 3. Overlay.

  a. Indications.

    i. Tipped teeth.

    ii. Undererupted teeth.

    iii. Increase in occlusal vertical dimension.

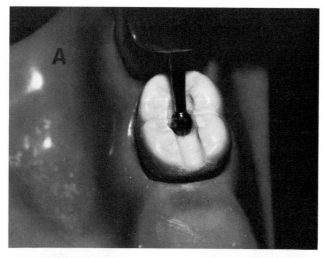

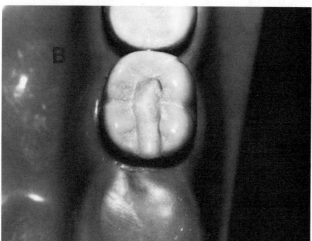

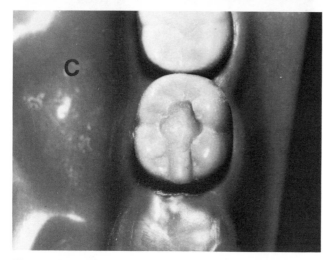

Fig. 16-14 (A) A round bur prepares the extended occlusal rest seat. (B) The completed rest seat. (C) Asymmetrical outline form or dovetails are important when extended occlusal rests are used in rotational path designs.

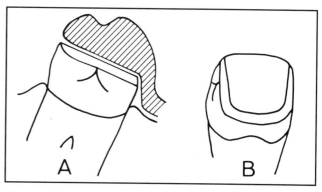

Fig. 16-15 (A) Illustration of an overlay rest. (B) The rest seat is bevelled and may include a flattened occlusal surface.

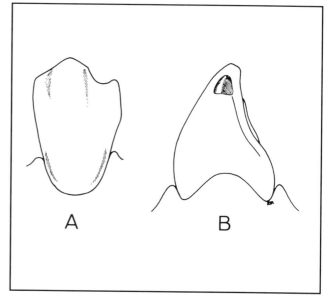

Fig. 16-16 Illustration of properly designed incisal rest seat preparation. (A) Facial view. (B) Proximal view.

     b. Dimensions. (Fig. 16–15)

        i. Bevel of occlusoproximal surfaces to prevent further tipping.

        ii. Occlusal contacts with opposing dentition.

B. INCISAL REST.

    1. Indications. Anterior teeth.

    2. Advantage. Does not require a prominent cingulum.

    3. Disadvantages.

      a. Unfavorable esthetics.

      b. Unfavorable mechanical leverage.

    4. Dimensions. (Fig. 16–16)

a. From the facial and proximal view, the outline form is saddle-shaped.

b. Faciolingually—convex.

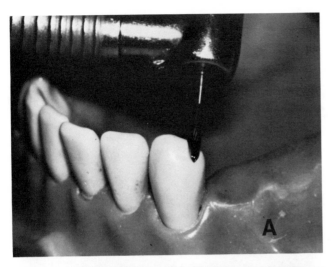

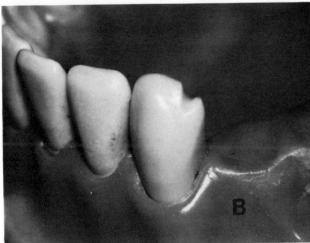

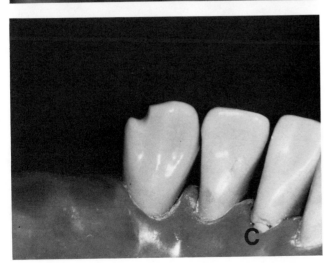

Fig. 16-17 (A) A cylindrical bur prepares the incisal rest seat. (B & C) The completed rest seat demonstrates apical inclination and saddle shape.

c. Mesiodistally—concave.

d. Prepared with elliptical or cylindrical burs or diamonds. (Fig. 16–17)

C. LINGUAL RESTS.

1. Cingulum rest.

   a. Indications. Anterior teeth.

   b. Advantages.

      i. Favorable mechanical leverage.

      ii. Favorable esthetics.

   c. Disadvantages.

      i. Requires prominent cingulum to minimize tooth modification.

      ii. Sharp internal line angles may compromise rest contact and axial force transmission in frameworks made from base metal alloys. This is due to the loss of surface detail of the casting associated with coarse refractory investment materials. Preparations which provide rounded internal line angles require deeper preparation but ensure more accurate adaptation of casting.

   d. Dimensions. (Fig. 16–18)

      i. Faciolingually—concave "V" or "U".

      ii. Mesiodistally—inverted "V" or "U".

      iii. Prepared with a cylindrical bur. Internal line angles should be rounded with corresponding round finishing burs and polishing points. (Fig. 16–19)

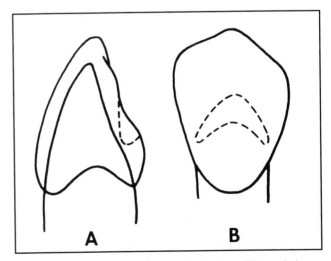

Fig. 16-18 Illustration of properly designed lingual cingulum rest seat. (A) Proximal view. (B) Lingual view.

2. Lingual ball rest.
   a. Indications. Anterior teeth.

b. Advantages.
   i. Favorable leverage.

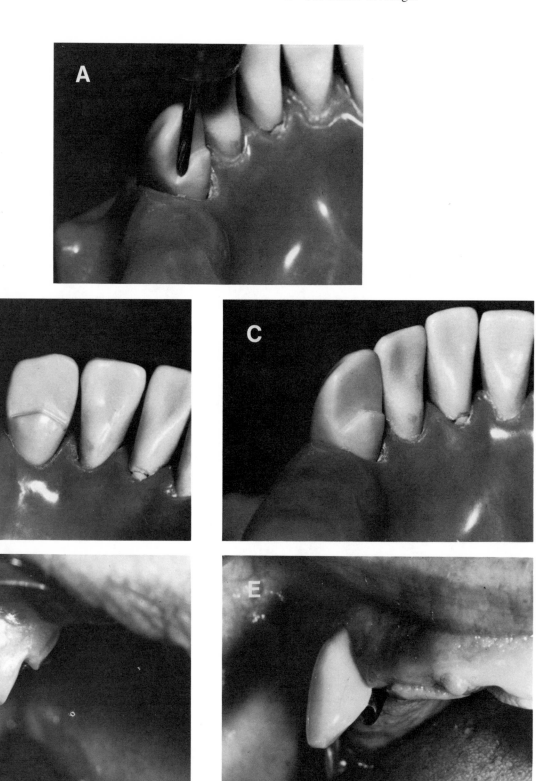

Fig. 16-19 (A) A cylindrical bur prepares the lingual cingulum rest seat. (B & C) Lingual and proximal views demonstrate apical inclination, rounded internal line angles, and the preservation of the lingual wall of the rest seat. (D) Prepared in enamel. (E) Ceramometal crown.

ii. Favorable esthetics.

iii. Does not require prominent cingulum.

c. Disadvantages. Tooth preparation may extend through dentinoenamel junction which may necessitate restoration.

d. Dimensions (Resembles occlusal rest seat). (Fig. 16–20)

i. Apically inclined.

ii. Marginal ridge reduction required.

iii. Rounded internal form.

iv. Prepared with #4 or #6 round bur. (Fig. 16–21)

RESTORATIONS ON ABUTMENT TEETH

A. CORRECTION OF UNACCEPTABLE ABUTMENT TOOTH CONTOURS.

1. Composite resin. Composite resin may be used to improve tooth contours but should not be used in force bearing areas.

a. May be used to establish the lingual wall of a rest seat. The floor of the rest seat should be prepared in tooth structure to minimize transmission of vertical seating forces to the composite resin. (Fig. 16–22)

b. May be used to increase depth of undercut.

i. Conventional clasps.

ii. Rotational path designs (see Chapter IX).

c. Some investigators suggest that the application of light cured microfilled composite resin to the internal area of a rest seat following framework fabrication may improve the seating of the rest providing improved contact of the central portion of the rest.

Long term clinical implications of this procedure are unknown.

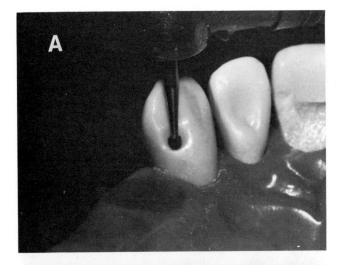

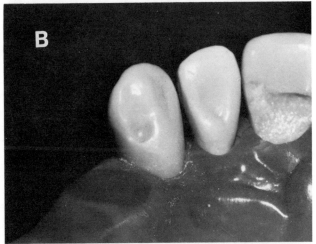

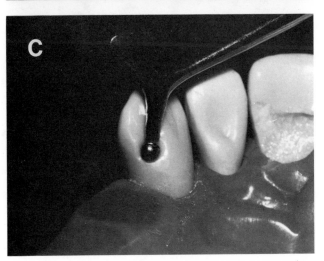

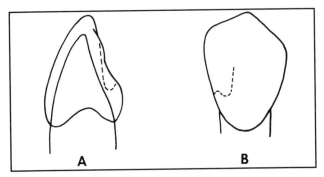

Fig. 16-20 Representation of a properly prepared ball rest seat. (A) Proximal view. (B) Lingual view.

Fig. 16-21 (A) A round bur prepares the lingual ball rest including reduction of the marginal ridge. (B) The completed rest seat. (C) A ball burnisher confirms apical inclination of rest seat.

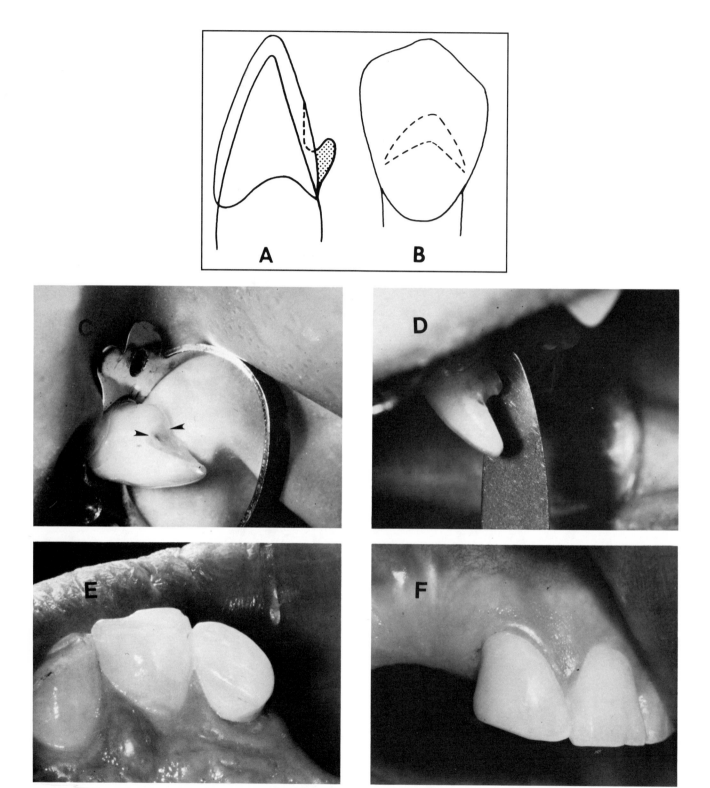

Fig. 16-22 The lingual wall of the rest seat may be developed by bonding composite resin to the enamel. The floor of the rest seat should be prepared in enamel to avoid directing vertical occlusal forces toward the restoration. Dotted line represents resin. (A) Proximal view. (B) Lingual view. (C) Placement of composite resin on an isolated tooth is shown. Arrows indicate junction of resin and enamel. (D) Completed rest seat demonstrating lingual wall of composite. Figures (E & F) demonstrate completed composite resin additions to (E) provide the lingual wall of the rest seat and (F) increase the proximal undercut for a rotational path RPD.

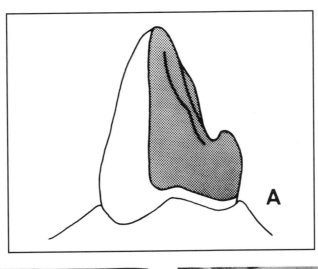

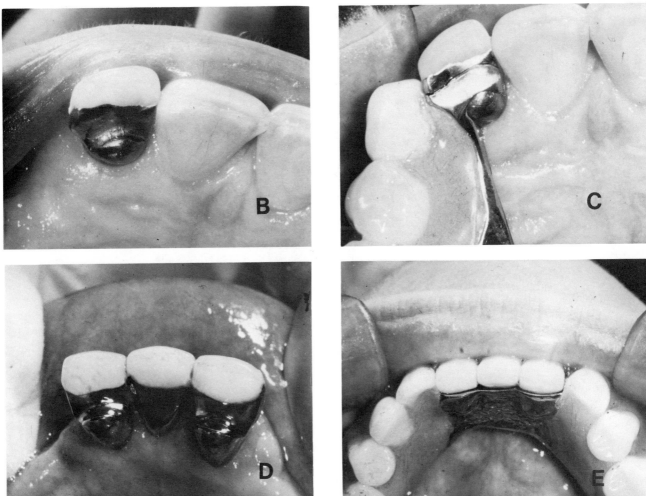

Fig. 16-23 (A) An inlay or 3/4 crown provided on an anterior tooth may be used to develop a cingulum rest seat when anatomic contours restrict tooth modification without restoration. (B) A cemented inlay. (C) RPD in place. (D & E) These splinted ceramometal crowns demonstrate lingual cingulum rests ideally contoured.

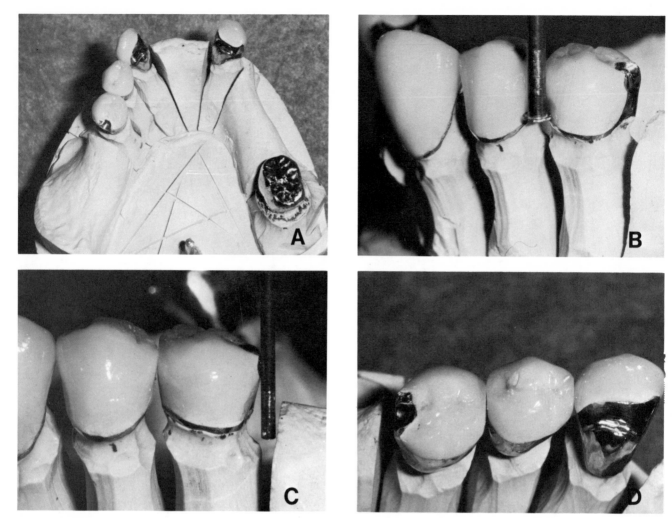

Fig. 16-24 (A) These restorations (B) demonstrate ideal undercuts, (C) guiding planes, and (D) rest seats as determined during the design phase.

2. Crowns.

    a. May provide ideal contours in all aspects of tooth modification. (Figs. 16–23 & 16–24)

    b. Metal preferred in force bearing areas such as rest seats. (Fig. 16–25)

    c. Ledged cast restorations. (Fig. 16–26)

       i. Axial wall of ledge parallel to path of placement.

      ii. Slightly rounded internal line angles preferred for base metal alloy to improve castability.

     iii. Requires additional abutment tooth preparation.

      iv. Improves stability.

      v. May improve support.

    d. Rotational path designs (see Chapter IX).

    e. Intracoronal or extracoronal attachments. (See Chapter XXII).

3. Pre-cast metal rest seats.

    a. Metal rest seats may be prefabricated or cast to fit abutment teeth. They may be bonded to etched enamel with composite resin.

    b. Metal rest seats may offer an alternative approach when optimal contours are difficult to achieve through abutment tooth modification (e.g. anterior teeth).

    c. Longitudinal *in vivo* studies are required to support these techniques for routine clinical use. The maintenance of a long term bond in a clinical environment when functional forces are involved, may be questionable.

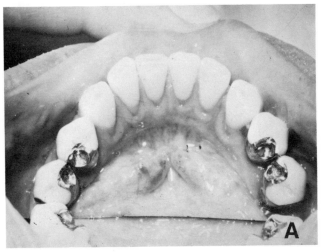 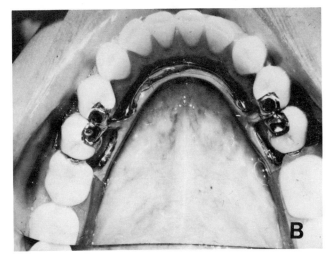

Fig. 16-25 (A & B) Occlusal rests are outlined in metal in these ceramometal crowns.

B. DENTIN EXPOSURE DURING TOOTH MODIFICATION.

1. Indications for restoring exposed dentin.
   a. Sensitivity.
   b. Caries susceptibility.

2. Restorations.
   a. Amalgam.
   b. Composite resin.
   c. Cast metal.

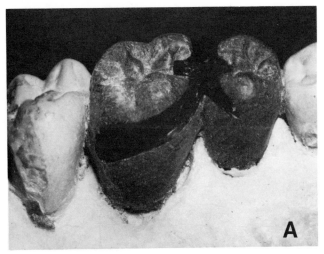 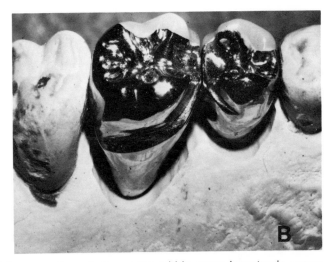

Fig. 16-26 Ledged cast restorations are provided to permit incorporation of clasp arms within normal anatomic crown contours. Adequate tooth reduction is required to permit the development of the ledges without overcontouring the gingival one third of the casting. (A) Wax contours. (B) Finished restorations.

Chapter XVII

IMPRESSION PROCEDURES

Support for tooth borne partial dentures is provided almost entirely by the dento-alveolar segment. Impressions for tooth borne partial dentures should accurately record the anatomic form of the teeth and surrounding tissues. This may usually be accomplished by a single stage impression procedure. For tooth-mucosa borne partial dentures, additional support is derived from the muco-osseous segment. Important factors in providing this support include maxillary major connector design, the extent of denture base coverage, and the selective pressure recording of primary and secondary force bearing anatomic regions. Such impression procedures are especially important for mandibular partial dentures where the quality and extent of muco-osseous tissues available for support is limited. Accurate recording of muco-osseous supporting areas requires that the mucosa is normal and that, if a prosthesis has been worn, tissue recovery has been achieved. Tissue recovery may usually be accomplished by removing the prosthesis for 24 to 72 hours or through the application of tissue conditioners.

TOOTH BORNE PARTIAL DENTURES

A. SINGLE STAGE ANATOMIC IMPRESSION—STOCK TRAY—IRREVERSIBLE HYDROCOLLOID. The purpose is to accurately record the anatomic form of the teeth and pertinent surrounding tissues.

1. Select a stock tray which allows for an adequate thickness of impression material without development of thin areas or pressure spots and which permits activation of muscle and frenal attachments without impingement. (Fig. 17–1)

2. Perforated stock trays usually demonstrate greater accuracy than rim lock trays due to the increased mechanical retention of the irreversible hydrocolloid. If necessary, adhesive may be applied to the tray to further increase the retention of the impression material.

3. Mix the irreversible hydrocolloid impression material following the manufacturer's instructions and load the tray.

4. Place the impression material into critical areas manually or with an impression syringe (e.g. rest seats, palatal vault and areas of framework contact). (Fig. 17–2)

5. Seat the tray in the mouth, being careful to center it accurately.

6. Prior to the initial set, continue to manually or functionally activate all pertinent muscle and frenal attachments. For mandibular impressions, the patient should be instructed to lightly place the tip of the tongue against the palate. (Fig. 17–3)

7. To achieve optimum strength, hold the tray in position for several minutes after the impression material reaches its final set.

8. Remove the set impression with a quick "snap."

9. Inspect the impression and remove the excess saliva. A water rinse, or application of a loose slurry mix followed by a water rinse, may be used to remove the saliva. The impression may be placed in a potassium sulfate bath to increase the surface hardness of the stone cast.

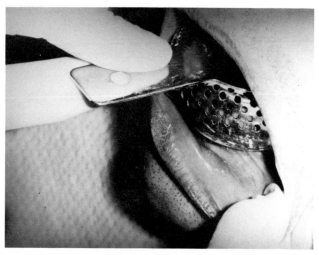

Fig. 17-1 A stock tray should be selected which provides adequate thickness of impression material to avoid thin areas which may pull away, resulting in distortion. Impingement of the vestibular tissues should be minimized as much as possible.

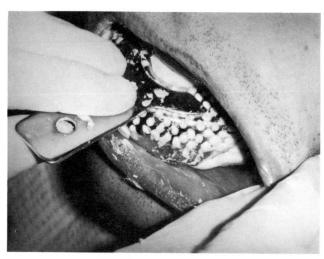

Fig. 17-3 Vestibular depth and contour is developed through manipulation and activation of the adjacent soft tissues while the tray is held in a stable position. The impression should only be removed following the final set of the impression material.

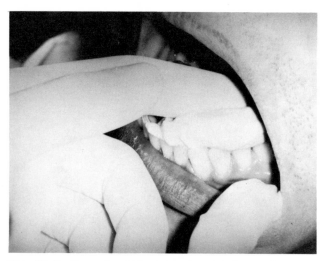

Fig. 17-2 Care should be taken to minimize the incorporation of air within the impression material during mixing. Irreversible hydrocolloid is manually placed in important areas where the framework is to be located.

B. SINGLE STAGE ANATOMIC IMPRESSION—CUSTOM TRAY—IRREVERSIBLE HYDROCOLLOID. The purpose is to accurately record the anatomic form of the teeth and pertinent surrounding tissues.

1. Fabricate a custom tray utilizing acrylic resin molded over the diagnostic cast. This procedure should be completed at least 1 hour before the impression is made to ensure complete polymerization of the tray resin.

2. Place baseplate wax as relief over the previously obtained diagnostic cast. Place one to two thicknesses of baseplate wax over the soft tissue areas and three to four thicknesses over the teeth. Place tissue stops in non-critical areas if desired. Tin foil may be placed over the cast and over the relief wax to facilitate wax removal from the cast and tray. Perforate the tray using a #8 round bur at 1/8 - 1/4 inch spacing. (Fig. 17–4)

3. Trim and adjust the tray clinically, allowing 3-5 mm of relief around the periphery to avoid impingement on soft tissue reflections. Manually or functionally activate all pertinent muscle and frenal attachments to ensure freedom of movement. (Fig. 17–5)

4. Follow steps 3 through 11 as previously described in Section A.

10. Pour the impression immediately, using an improved dental stone to register occlusal surfaces and critical areas. It should be poured in a non-inverted fashion or utilizing a double pour technique. Liquids to improve surface hardness may be used as a substitute for water.

11. If the impression cannot be poured immediately, it must be stored in an environment of 100% humidity.

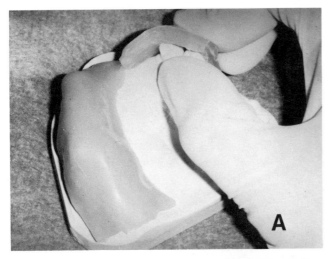

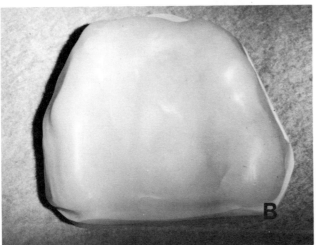

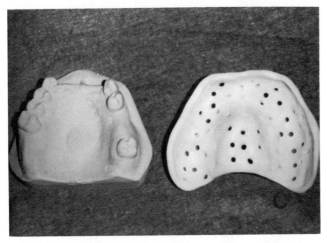

Fig. 17-4 (A) Wax spacer is placed over the teeth to a depth equivalent to 3 to 4 sheets of baseplate wax and (B) over the mucosal areas to a depth of 1 to 2 sheets. (C) Tray acrylic resin is adapted over the wax relief and perforated prior to initial set. The tray is removed, perforations completed, and extensions modified as required.

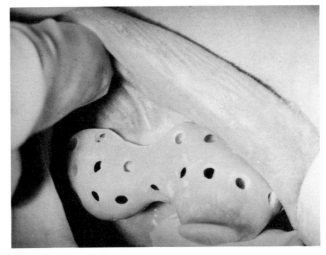

Fig. 17-5 The tray is adjusted clinically to ensure freedom of movement

C. RATIONALE FOR A STOCK TRAY.

  1. Advantages.

    a. Less laboratory time required.

    b. Fewer materials involved.

  2. Disadvantages.

    a. Usually less accurate tray adaptation.

    b. Less predictable thickness of impression material. This increases the possibility of thin areas which may lead to distortion. When an increased thickness of impression material is present in the palatal area, especially when using reversible hydrocolloid, slumping may result, causing distortion. This may be prevented by using a heavy bodied hydrocolloid or by building up the palatal area with wax, being certain that the wax does not come through the impression material.

    c. May interfere with the accurate recording of functional vestibular depth or soft tissue reflections, including muscle and frenal attachments which may result in overextended denture periphery.

  3. Indications.

    a. Tooth borne situations when accurate recording of soft tissue reflections is not critical.

    b. Tooth-mucosa borne situations when accurate recording of soft tissue reflections is not critical and a dual stage selective pressure impression is planned.

D. RATIONALE FOR A CUSTOM TRAY.

1. Advantages.

   a. Usually more accurate tray adaptation.

   b. Provides a more even thickness of impression material. This minimizes the tendency to develop thin areas which lead to distortions.

   c. Facilitates the adjustments of tray extensions, border molding procedures, and accurate recording of functional vestibular depth.

2. Disadvantages.

   a. More laboratory time required.

   b. More materials involved.

3. Indication. When a stock tray will not produce an acceptable impression.

E. COMPARISON OF IMPRESSION MATERIALS.

1. Irreversible hydrocolloid.

   a. Advantages.

      i. Permits use of custom tray.

      ii. Adequate accuracy and reproduction of surface detail, given the limitations of the refractory cast investment material.

      iii. Low tear strength may facilitate impression removal without distortion when severe undercuts are present (e.g. large open gingival embrasures).

      iv. Viscosity may be adjusted by varying the water to powder ratio.

      v. Setting time may be controlled by varying the water temperature.

      iv. Simple and expeditious.

      v. Inexpensive.

   b. Disadvantages.

      i. Incompatibility with dental stone may affect cast surface hardness.

      ii. Dimensional instability requires immediate pour.

      iii. More difficult to use with a syringe to minimize bubbles in critical areas.

2. Reversible hydrocolloid.

   a. Advantages.

      i. May demonstrate an improved reproduction of surface detail. This accuracy is negated by the coarseness of the refractory cast investment material.

      ii. Use of injectable syringe material may reduce bubble frequency.

   b. Disadvantages.

      i. Incompatibility with dental stone may affect cast surface hardness.

      ii. Lack of adequate viscosity may lead to slumping of material during setting— cooler areas against the mucosa and tray may set before the central body of the impression (e.g. when deep palatal vault is present).

      iii. Dimensional instability requires immediate pour.

      iv. Increased expense.

      v. Requires the use of a stock tray.

3. Elastomeric materials.

   a. Advantages.

      i. Permits use of custom tray.

      ii. May demonstrate an improved reproduction of surface detail. This accuracy is negated by coarseness of the refractory cast.

      iii. Increased dimensional stability.

      iv. Use of injectable syringe material reduces bubble frequency.

   b. Disadvantages.

      i. Increased rigidity of set material may create technical problems during retrieval of cast (e.g. fracture of teeth especially when long clinical crowns are present).

      ii. Increased tear strength may lead to impression distortion on removal when severe undercuts are present (e.g. severe overlapping of anterior teeth or open gingival embrasures).

      iii. Increased expense.

      iv. May require a longer setting time.

      v. Hydrophobic nature of most materials precludes presence of excessive moisture.

      vi. Remaking of impressions is more complex.

TOOTH-MUCOSA BORNE PARTIAL DENTURES

A. GENERAL CONSIDERATIONS.

1. Impression procedures for tooth-mucosa borne partial dentures should be designed to record

teeth and mucosal tissues in a manner that maximizes support.

2. Muco-osseous tissues have been described as being approximately 25 times more displaceable than the dento-alveolar tissues. This discrepancy and the variability in the displaceability of soft tissues overlying the different regions of the muco-osseous segment usually makes it impossible to obtain optimum support when utilizing a single stage impression procedure.

3. Within the area covered by a denture base are primary, secondary, and non-supporting mucosal tissues. (Fig. 17–6)

4. Resilient soft tissues of the primary supporting areas must be mildly displaced to promote their contribution to support. When primary supporting areas are loaded, long term resorptive changes are minimized. (Fig. 17–7)

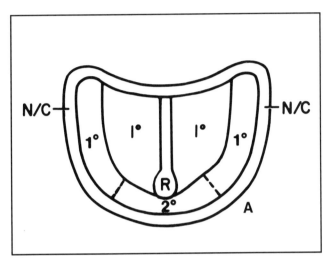
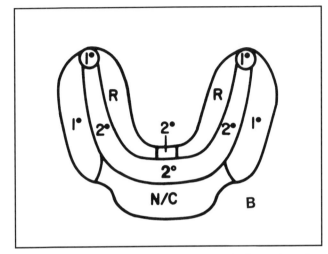

Fig. 17-6 (A) As described in Chapter III, primary (1°) supporting areas of the maxillary arch include the horizontal portion of the hard palate and the posterior ridge crest. (B) Primary (1°) supporting areas of the mandibular arch include the buccal shelf and the pear-shaped pad.

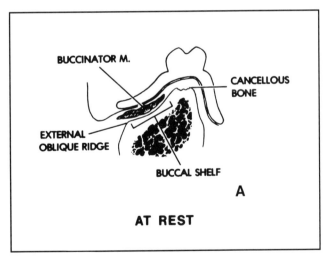
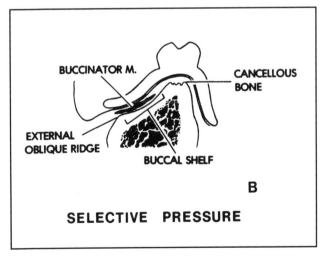

Fig. 17-7 (A) An anatomic impression which records the muco-osseous tissues at rest results in a prosthesis which directs functional forces to the more unyielding tissues overlying the ridge crest. These areas are not primary supporting areas. They are comprised of cancellous bone and demonstrate more rapid pressure-induced resorption. (B) A selective pressure impression which records the muco-osseous tissue with varying amounts of pressure, results in a prosthesis which directs functional forces toward the more displaceable tissues overlying the buccal shelf. These areas are primary supporting areas comprised of cortical bone, and demonstrate increased resistance to pressure-induced resorption. Note the increased tissue placement by the denture base overlying the buccal shelf following the use of a selective pressure impression.

5. Secondary and non-supporting areas should be recorded at rest to minimize the forces directed to these areas which are more susceptible to pressure-induced resorption or unable to tolerate functional forces.

6. Impression techniques for selectively recording muco-osseous tissues under varying degrees of pressure include:

    a. Varying the viscosity of impression material.

    b. Selective venting of the tray (escape holes).

    c. Selective relief of the tray.

7. Due to the limited quality and quantity of muco-osseous tissues available for support in the mandibular arch, a dual stage selective pressure impression (altered cast) is routinely recommended.

8. Due to the increased support achieved by major connector coverage of the hard palate in maxillary tooth-mucosa borne partial dentures, it is often not necessary to obtain a dual stage selective pressure impression. In addition, technical difficulties are often encountered in applying this procedure to the maxillary arch. These difficulties relate to the overflow of impression material beyond the internal finish line, the cutting of the cast at a position coincident with the internal finish line, etc.

9. The development of optimum soft tissue support for the maxillary major connector may require the use of a more viscous impression material when attempting a single stage selective pressure impression that promotes mild displacement of the mucosa overlying palatal supporting areas. This may be accomplished by decreasing the water : powder ratio of the irreversible hydrocolloid. Muco-osseous support may also be enhanced by using a reline procedure at or subsequent to delivery.

10. The patient should be instructed to remove the prosthesis 24-72 hours preceding the altered cast impression in order to promote mucosal tissue recovery.

B. DUAL STAGE SELECTIVE PRESSURE IMPRESSION (ALTERED CAST IMPRESSION)—CUSTOM TRAY—ELASTOMERIC MATERIAL. The purpose is to accurately record the anatomic form of the teeth and the form of the soft supporting tissues under selective pressures. Selective pressure refers to the recording of the tissues with varying degrees of displacement. This requires an altered or modified cast impression.

1. First stage anatomic impression (completed as outlined under tooth borne partial dentures).

2. Design framework on master cast incorporating a third point of reference. This facilitates an accurate, repeatable orientation of the framework on the teeth.

    a. Third rest. (Fig. 17–8)

    b. Incisal stop to be removed at delivery. (Fig. 17–9)

    c. Acrylic resin index. (Fig. 17–10)

3. Fabricate custom trays on the framework over muco-osseous denture supporting areas. Be certain that the primary supporting areas are covered (e.g. buccal shelf, pear-shaped pad). (Fig. 17–11)

4. Relief is provided over secondary and non-supporting areas to permit free flow of impression material (e.g. mandibular ridge crest, mylohyoid ridge, etc.).

    a. Grinding relief after tray fabrication is the preferred technique. (Fig. 17–12)

    b. Wax relief on cast prior to tray fabrication may interfere with complete reseating of framework on cast and subsequent tray fabrication.

5. Following adjustment of the framework, trim tray areas and adjust clinically to provide 3-5 mm of relief around periphery without impinging on mucosal reflections. Manually or functionally activate all pertinent muscle and frenal attachments to ensure freedom of movement.

6. Border mold the impression tray, following the principles of complete denture fabrication. (Fig. 17–13)

7. Remove the border molding material from within the tray except in areas where additional tissue displacement is required (e.g. buccal shelf).

8. Vent the tray overlying secondary and non-supporting areas where hydraulic pressures could develop (e.g. mandibular ridge crest) to minimize tissue displacement. (Fig. 17–14)

9. Dry the mucosal tissues and place gauze, as required, to minimize accumulation of saliva.

10. Select an elastomeric impression material based upon the required viscosity. More viscous materials will result in more mucosal displacement and, thereby, more functional forces directed toward those areas which are displaced.

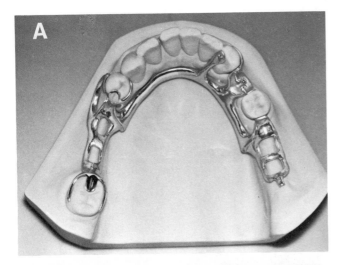

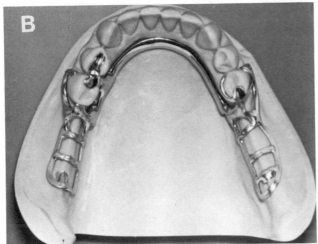

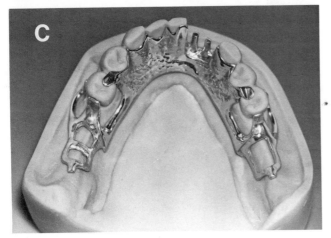

11. Mix the impression material and load the tray, pulling the material over the periphery and pre-shaping the impression.

12. Remove the gauze and insert the impression tray.

13. Ensure complete seating of all rests and third point of reference. Hold the framework in this position.

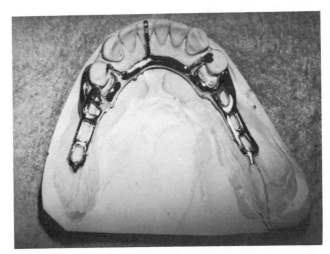

Fig. 17-9 When frameworks are fabricated without a third point of reference within the design, an incisal stop may be added which is removed later.

Fig. 17-8 (A) Frameworks for tooth-mucosa supported RPDs should routinely be designed to have a third point of reference by incorporating three rests. (B) To minimize placement of additional minor connectors, the third point of reference may be an extended occlusal rest, as on the first premolar. (C) Lingual plates require one or more rests designed on the covered teeth to provide an effective third point reference. Although not depicted in these illustrations note that the presence of two inverted "U" rests or long occlusal rests usually provide adequate framework orientation without the addition of a third reference point.

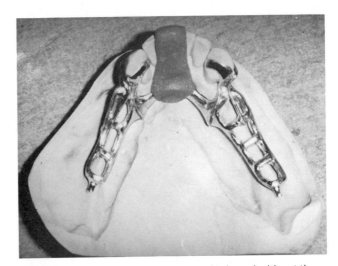

Fig. 17-10 When frameworks are designed without three rests a third point of reference in the form of an incisal stop may be fabricated utilizing acrylic resin. This index may be used during the altered cast impression procedure and then maintained as part of the patient's record for future reference. Note however that the use of two lingual inverted "U" or long occlusal rests may substitute for third reference points, due to their extended tooth contacts.

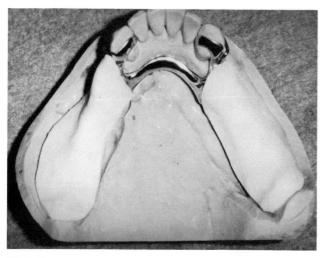

Fig. 17-11 Tray material is applied to the base areas prior to the frame try-in and altered cast impression appointment.

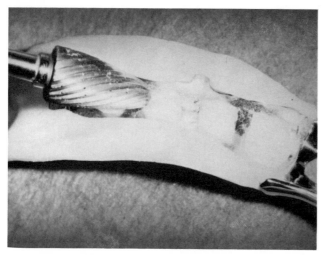

Fig. 17-12 Grinding the resin overlying the ridge crest provides relief.

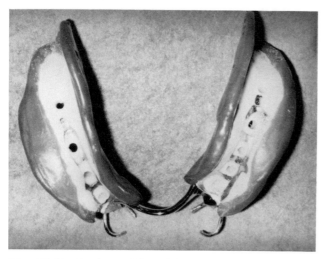

Fig. 17-13 Border molding of the base area is completed.

14. DO NOT DIRECT SEATING PRESSURE TO EXTENSION BASE TRAY AREAS!

15. During the setting of the impression material, continually activate all pertinent muscle and frenal attachments. (Fig. 17–15)

16. Remove the set impression.

17. Trim the excess impression material from the periphery. Cut away the impression material from the framework, precisely at the internal finish line. (Fig. 17–16)

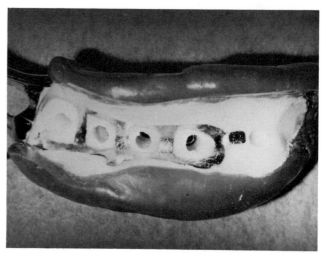

Fig. 17-14 The ridge crest area is vented. Positive pressure directed toward the buccal shelf may be ensured by permitting viscous border molding material to remain in this area.

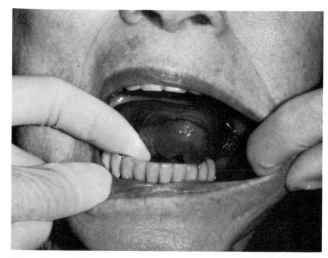

Fig. 17-15 During seating, pressure is placed only on the rests and any components serving as a third point of reference. Pressure is not directed on the base areas. The framework is held in position against the teeth while border molding manipulations are completed.

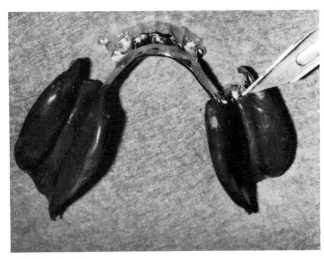

Fig. 17-16 Excess impression material is removed, including a cut at the internal finish line.

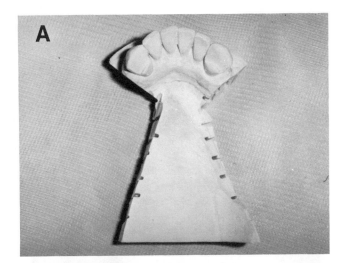

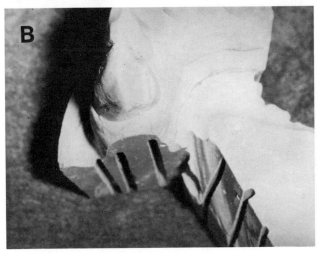

Fig. 17-17 (A) The master cast is cut along the area corresponding to the internal finish line. (B) Grooves or slots are cut into the cast to retain the stone.

18. Cut the cast in correspondence with the internal finish line of the framework or slightly closer to the abutment teeth to avoid contact of the impression material with the cast. Cut and remove the muco-osseous supporting areas of the initial cast which have been re-recorded by the second stage impression. (Fig. 17–17)

19. Seat the framework with the impression onto the sectioned cast, being certain that rests and third point of reference are fully seated. (Fig. 17–18)

20. Lute the framework into position. Check again to ensure that the impression material is not contacting the remaining stone cast, preventing complete seating. (Fig. 17–19)

21. Box the impression, soak in slurry water and pour the altered cast. (Fig. 17–20)

22. Contact between the metal stop and cast should be re-established on the corrected master cast using autopolymerizing acrylic resin prior to fabricating the record base and flasking. (Fig. 17–21)

23. Fabricate record bases and occlusion rims. (Fig. 17–22)

C. COMPARISON TO RELINE PROCEDURE AT DELIVERY. (See Chapter XX)

  1. Advantages.

    a. Accuracy of maxillomandibular records. Since the cast is altered prior to fabrication of record bases, the record bases will be more stable and the records more accurate.

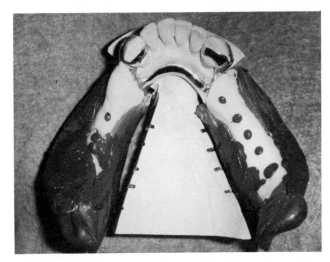

Fig. 17-18 The framework is seated on the cast, ensuring that all rests are completely seated.

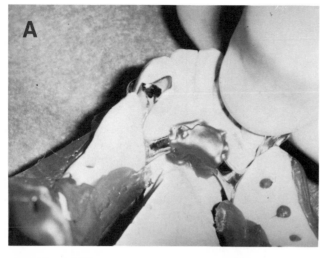

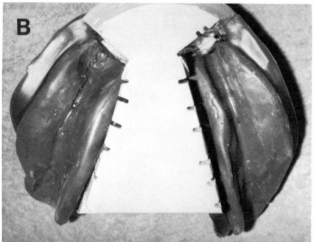

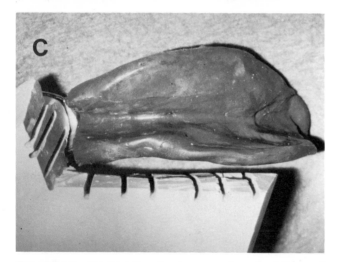

Fig. 17-19 (A) Stabilize the framework against the cast with sticky wax, continuing to observe seated rests. (B & C) Check to be certain that all tray and impression material is relieved of contact with the cast.

b. Less occlusal discrepancy apparent at clinical remount.

c. Use of dense heat polymerized resin on tissue surface may be more hygienic and color stable.

2. Disadvantages.

a. The technique is more demanding and the potential for errors may be increased.

b. Dimensional changes associated with the heat polymerized resin may make tissue adaption of the denture base less accurate than a denture base relined with autopolymerizing resin.

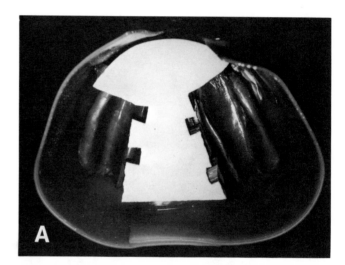

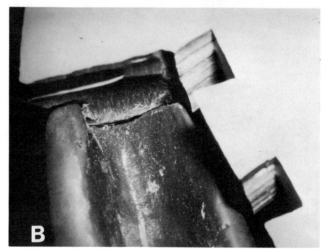

Fig. 17-20 The impression material may be boxed using several techniques. (A) Wax is the traditional material used in boxing. Note again the absence of contact between impression and cast. (B) Large undercut notches are an alternative to the grooves used for retention of the stone.

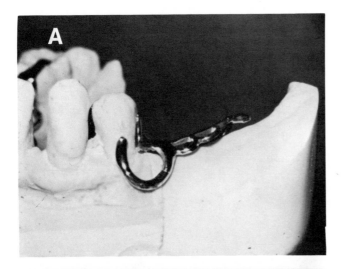

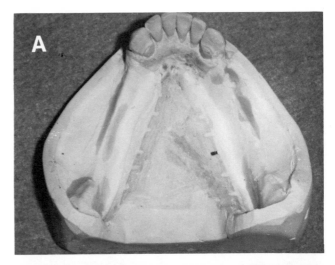

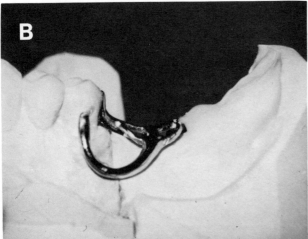

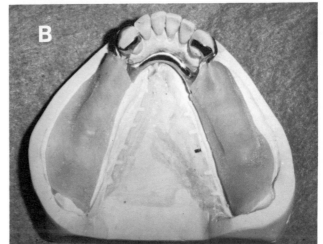

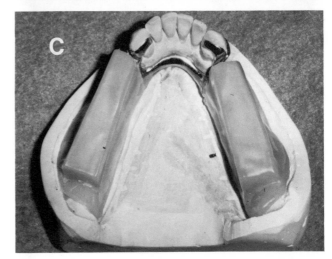

Fig. 17-21 (A & B) The tissue displacement achieved during the altered cast impression procedure requires that metal stop contacts be re-established utilizing autopolymerizing acrylic resin prior to record base fabrication and flasking.

Fig. 17-22 (A) Completed altered master cast. (B) Record base. (C) Occlusion rim. Stable occlusion rims adapted to the corrected master cast improve the accuracy of maxillomandibular records.

Chapter XVIII

FRAMEWORK EVALUATION

Evaluation of the framework is an essential procedure in the fabrication of a removable partial denture. The framework should be examined extraorally and intraorally for its conformation to the established design. Forces applied to the artificial teeth are transmitted by the framework to the abutment teeth. Accurate adaptation of the framework enhances the support, stability, and retention provided by the dento-alveolar segment. Frameworks for tooth-mucosa borne removable partial dentures should be functionally adjusted to minimize torquing of those teeth contacting the framework.

EXTRAORAL EVALUATION

A. EXAMINATION OF THE FRAMEWORK REMOVED FROM THE MASTER CAST.

1. Presence of defects. The framework should be evaluated for defects that might compromise its adaptation or strength.

   a. Positive bubbles or blebs. These may inhibit complete seating of the framework on abutment teeth or traumatize soft tissue.

   b. Voids or porosities. These may weaken the framework and lead to fracture. (Fig. 18–1)

2. Thickness of the components. The dimensions of the framework components should be evaluated to ensure that they are appropriate for the required mechanical properties.

   a. Major connectors. The major connector should demonstrate dimensions which provide rigidity and strength.

   b. Rest—minor connector junction. A minimum metal thickness of 1.5 mm at the junction of the rest with the minor connector is required for base metal alloys (2 mm for gold alloys). (Fig. 18–2)

   c. Clasp arm taper. Retentive clasp arms should taper uniformly in thickness and width. Bracing clasp arms should possess dimensions which provide rigidity and need not be tapered.

3. Finish lines.

   a. Staggered (offset) finish lines. In order to maintain framework strength, the internal and external finish lines should not be superimosed.

   b. Internal line angles. The internal line angles of external and internal finish lines should be less than 90 degrees to provide mechanical retention for the denture base resin.

4. Polish.

   a. Except where they cross gingival margins, maxillary major connectors should not be highly polished on the tissue surface in an attempt to preserve intimate tissue contact. Where crossing gingival margins the tissue surface of the framework should be highly polished and lightly relieved.

   b. Mandibular major connectors should be highly polished on their tissue surface.

   c. The tissue surface of other components which contact abutment teeth (rests, clasps, minor connectors and proximal plates) should not be highly polished as a means of preserving contact.

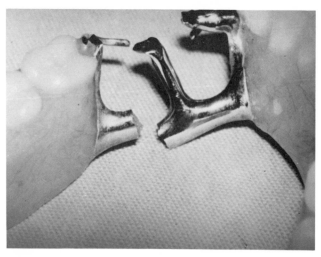

Fig. 18-1 Fracture of lingual bar major connector due to porosity.

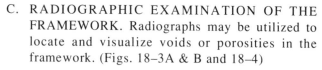

C. RADIOGRAPHIC EXAMINATION OF THE FRAMEWORK. Radiographs may be utilized to locate and visualize voids or porosities in the framework. (Figs. 18–3A & B and 18–4)

1. Porosity not visually detectable. Radiographs may demonstrate internal porosity.

2. Porosity visually detectable. Radiographs may indicate the size of a porosity which is only partially visible.

3. Technique.

   a. 10 MA - 100 KVP - $^{15}/_{60}$ seconds.

   b. 15 MA - 70 KVP - $^{15}/_{60}$ seconds.

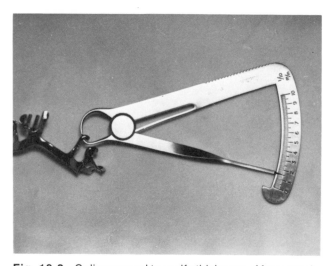

Fig. 18-2 Calipers used to verify thickness of framework. Rest-minor connector junction for base metal alloys should be at least 1.5 mm thick.

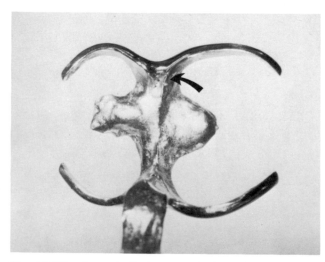

Fig. 18-3A Arrow indicates porosity in embrasure clasp.

B. EXAMINATION OF THE FRAMEWORK ON THE MASTER CAST.

1. Location of the components. The position of the framework components should correspond to the design indicated on the master cast.

2. Fit of the framework on the master cast.

   a. Complete and stable seating. The framework should demonstrate accurate adaptation of the rests to their rest seats without rebound.

   b. Adaptation. Confirm intimate adaptation of the framework to the master cast, where indicated.

   c. Relief. Confirm areas of relief between the framework and master cast, where indicated.

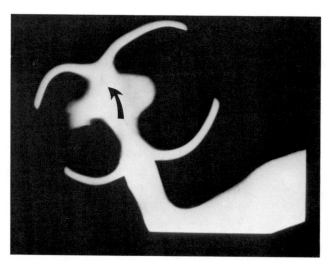

Fig. 18-3B Radiograph of clasp from Fig. 18-3A. Arrow indicates area of porosity.

INTRAORAL EVALUATION

A. COMPLETE AND STABLE SEATING. Excessive seating force should not be required and the framework should not rebound from the abutment teeth.

  1. Locating interferences. Contact between the framework and abutment teeth that prevents complete seating may be located by using rouge and chloroform, disclosing waxes, or other disclosing materials.

  2. Common interference areas. The most common areas of interference are above the survey line. They frequently occur under rests, in the shoulder region of circumferential clasps, on minor connectors and in the interproximal extensions of lingual plates.

  3. Framework modification. The areas of the framework that interfere with seating may be adjusted with carbide burs or abrasive stones using high speed instrumentation. Several adjustments may be required to obtain a complete and stable seating of the framework. All adjusted areas should be polished.

B. ADAPTATION. Confirm the intimate adaptation of the framework components to the underlying tissues where indicated.

  1. Abutment teeth. The contact of framework components with abutment teeth may be evaluated with rouge and chloroform, disclosing waxes or other disclosing materials.

  2. Mucosal surfaces. The contact of framework components with mucosal surfaces may be evaluated with disclosing waxes or pressure indicating pastes.

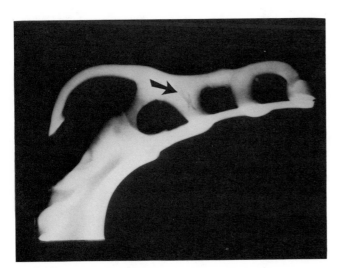

Fig. 18-4 Internal porosity in resin retention lattice.

C. RELIEF. Confirm areas of relief between the framework components and the underlying tissues where indicated. If visual verification is not adequate disclosing waxes or pressure indicating pastes may be used.

D. FUNCTIONAL ADJUSTMENT OF THE FRAMEWORK. Tooth-mucosa borne RPDs can be expected to rotate during function. To minimize the potential torquing of teeth contacted by the framework, optimum muco-osseous support should be provided. Proper framework design and fabrication is also important in decreasing the torquing forces applied to the abutment teeth. The framework should be adjusted to allow rotational movements to occur with minimal interferences from the teeth.

  1. Locating interferences.

    a. Seating forces. Vertical and lateral forces should be applied to the extension base areas. Impression trays or record bases should not be attached to the framework since they may restrict the movement.

    b. Disclosing materials. Rouge and chloroform, disclosing waxes or other disclosing materials are required to detect interfering areas.

  2. Framework modification. The areas of the framework that interfere with rotational movements may be adjusted with a carbide bur or abrasive stones in a high speed handpiece. Several adjustments are usually required to remove interfering areas. All adjusted areas should be polished.

E. OCCLUSAL EVALUATION. The framework should be examined for interferences with the occlusion and articulation.

  1. Vertical dimension. Except where indicated, the framework should not alter the occlusal vertical dimension.

    a. Locating interferences. Articulating paper, plastic strips or waxes may be used to visualize interferences. A matte finish of the occluding framework surfaces facilitates the marking with articulating paper.

    b. Adjustment. The framework is usually adjusted to remove interferences. Where the framework thickness is minimal for its required strength, the opposing dentition or restorations should be adjusted. If this adjustment is anticipated the patient should be informed prior to framework fabrication.

The adjusted and matte finished surfaces should be polished.

2. Articulation. The framework should not interfere with the articulation.

F. RETENTION. The resistance by the framework to vertical dislodging forces should be evaluated. The retentive components may require adjustment to provide optimum retention.

Chapter XIX

DELIVERY AND MAINTENANCE

At the delivery appointment, the adaptation of the removable partial denture to its supporting tissues must be evaluated and adjusted as required. Analysis of the occlusion and articulation should follow the confirmation of complete and stable seating of the partial denture. The patient should be given specific instructions on the care of the partial denture and oral tissues as well as on the need for periodic evaluation.

DELIVERY

A. SOFT TISSUE ADAPTATION.

1. Evaluate the relationship of the components to the underlying soft tissues.

   a. Components which should contact the soft tissues.

      i. Denture base.

      ii. Maxillary major connector, except where crossing the gingival margins.

   b. Components that require relief from the soft tissues.

      i. Mandibular major connectors.

      ii. Minor connectors and proximal plates.

      iii. Bar clasp approach arms.

2. Procedure for tissue surface adjustment.

   a. Visually and digitally inspect the finished partial denture. Examine closely for rough or sharp areas.

   b. Apply a pressure indicating paste to the tissue surface.

   c. Place the partial denture into the mouth and verify complete seating of the partial denture framework. Remove the partial denture and inspect the tissue surface for regions of paste displacement.

   d. Relieve the pressure areas where the paste has been displaced, using an appropriate bur. Repeat the process until the areas of unfavorable pressure have been removed.

   e. The denture base areas of tooth-mucosa borne partial dentures should also be examined while simulating occlusal loading forces under finger pressure.

   f. The tooth-mucosa borne partial denture should demonstrate the required muco-osseous support. Simulated loading forces applied to the extension base area usually should not cause the third point of reference to be elevated from its tooth contact. When movement of the third point of reference is noted, a relining of the base is usually indicated.

3. Evaluate the relationship of the components to the adjacent movable soft tissues. The partial denture should not impinge on movable soft tissues.

   a. Denture base.

   b. Major connectors.

   c. Bar clasp approach arms.

4. Procedure for periphery adjustment.

    a. Visually inspect the peripheral components of the seated partial denture in the mouth. Evaluate the extension.

    b. Manually activate or instruct the patient to move the lips, tongue, cheeks and jaw through simulated functional movements. Evaluate the extension.

    c. Where the periphery cannot be adequately observed and a question of peripheral extension exists, a disclosing wax may be utilized. The wax may show over extension or under extension.

    d. Modify the periphery as indicated by the visual or disclosing wax evaluation.

B. ABUTMENT TOOTH ADAPTATION. The framework components should be properly related to the abutment teeth.

1. The rests should demonstrate a complete and stable seating in their rest seats.

2. The clasp arms, minor connectors, and proximal plates should demonstrate the required contact with the abutment teeth.

C. RETENTION. The resistance to vertical dislodging forces should be evaluated. The retentive components may require adjustment to provide optimum retention. The amount of retention required is a subjective opinion determined by the dentist and patient.

D. OCCLUSION AND ARTICULATION.

1. Centric occlusion. Posterior teeth should demonstrate bilateral, even, simultaneous contact. Anterior teeth should demonstrate the appropriate relationship to opposing teeth.

2. Occlusal vertical dimension. The partial denture should demonstrate occlusal contacts at the correct occlusal vertical dimension. A visual inspection is required to verify that the RPD is not increasing the vertical dimension.

3. Articulation. The partial denture components should demonstrate appropriate occlusal contacts with the opposing dentition or restorations during excursive mandibular movements.

4. Adjustments.

    a. Tooth borne partial dentures. The occlusion and articulation may usually be evaluated and adjusted intraorally.

    b. Tooth-mucosa borne partial dentures. The evaluation and adjustment of the occlusion and articulation usually require a clinical remount procedure. The displaceability of the muco-osseous segment allows the extension base to move tissue-ward during occlusal loading forces. Deflective occlusal contacts usually cannot be evaluated intraorally.

    c. Opposing partial dentures. Initially, assess and adjust the occlusion and articulation of each partial denture independently. Then, repeat the process with both partial dentures in place.

    d. Evaluate patient response. The patient should be unaware of any change in the occlusion after the partial denture(s) have been adjusted. This does not apply to an intentional change in the occlusion, articulation or occlusal vertical dimension.

5. Clinical remount procedure. (See Chapter XXI)

PATIENT INSTRUCTIONS

A. CARE OF THE PARTIAL DENTURE. Describe and demonstrate proper maintenance procedures. Written instructions may augment the verbal communication.

1. Brushing technique.

    a. Use of a proper brush for the RPD.

    b. Brush over a sink with water or a towel in it. This minimizes the potential for damage if the RPD is dropped.

    c. Do not squeeze or bend RPD while brushing.

2. Cleaning agents.

    a. Hand soap. Patients should be advised not to use toothpastes or abrasive cleaners.

    b. Denture pastes or creams.

    c. Soak cleaners. May be used where stain accumulation is not controlled by brushing alone. Advise the patient to brush the RPD before and after soaking to maximize plaque and stain removal. Patients should be cautioned not to soak the RPD in a bleach solution.

    d. Ultrasonic baths. May be useful for patients who have difficulty brushing or as an adjunct cleaning procedure.

3. Adjustments. The patient should be advised not to adjust their RPD. If any difficulties with the fit or retention develop, they should contact their dentist.

B. CARE OF THE ORAL TISSUES.

1. Toothbrushing technique. Demonstrate the proper technique of sulcular brushing with a soft toothbrush.

2. Flossing technique. Demonstrate the proper flossing technique.

3. Adjunct devices. Where indicated, other devices may be recommended to improve plaque control.

   a. Floss holders.

   b. Tooth picks.

   c. Interproximal brushes.

4. Brushing of mucosal tissues adjacent to or covered by the RPD with a soft toothbrush.

5. Plaque reducing rinses. Over-the-counter or prescription solutions may be beneficial for patients who demonstrate less than optimal plaque control.

6. Fluoride. May be useful for patients who demonstrate an increased risk for caries.

   a. Rinses.

   b. Gels.

   c. Stents. Where patients demonstrate a high caries activity, stents may be used to carry a fluoride gel to the tooth surfaces.

   d. Fluoride on RPD. RPD framework may be used to carry a fluoride gel to the tooth surfaces.

C. PLACEMENT AND REMOVAL OF THE PARTIAL DENTURE. The proper placement and removal of the RPD should be demonstrated. The patient should be able to accomplish these procedures before leaving the office.

1. Finger pressure should be used to completely seat the RPD.

2. The patient should be cautioned not to seat the RPD with occlusal force (not "bite" into place).

3. Devices or modifications in the RPD may be required for patients who have difficulty removing the RPD with their fingers.

   a. Devices. Small smooth hooks placed in a toothbrush handle or modified dental hand instruments may aid the patient in removing the RPD.

   b. Modifications. Grooves or slots placed in the denture base or artificial teeth may improve the patient's ability to engage the partial denture.

D. WEARING THE PARTIAL DENTURE.

1. Initial accommodation period. Patients should be given specific instructions to help them adapt to their new prosthesis.

   a. Bulk of the RPD. It may take several days to several weeks before the patient accepts the presence of the partial denture, especially for the inexperienced patient.

   b. Speech. If the RPD alters enunciation, the patient should be instructed to practice reading aloud.

   c. Mastication. The patient should initially masticate smaller portions of softer foods.

   d. Saliva. A transient increase in salivary flow may be noticed initially.

2. Leave RPD out at night. Permits mucosa under RPD to receive normal stimulation. Several exceptions may be noted:

   a. RPD that splints hypermobile teeth. Teeth with mobility where patient experiences difficulty or discomfort in placement of RPD in morning.

   b. RPD that maintains the occlusal vertical dimension. When RPD prevents trauma to remaining natural teeth or mucosa. A splint may be used at night as a substitute for the RPD.

   c. When the RPD is worn at night, the patient should clean the oral tissues and prosthesis before retiring and again in the morning.

MAINTENANCE

A. PERIODONTAL TREATMENT.

1. Recall intervals appropriate for each patient.

   a. Shorter intervals for patients with active periodontal disease.

   b. Longer intervals for patients without active periodontal disease.

   c. Consider shorter intervals initially after RPD delivery.

2. Reinforce plaque control instructions at each appointment.

   a. Intraoral hygiene procedures.

   b. RPD maintenance procedures.

3. Evaluate periodontal health, especially RPD abutments.

4. Periodontal treatment as required.

B. RESTORATIVE EVALUATION. Usually performed at periodontal treatment appointments.

   1. Tooth examination.

      a. Caries.

      b. Defective restorations.

   2. Soft tissue examination. Examine all oral soft tissues, especially those adjacent to or supporting the RPD.

   3. RPD examination.

      a. Extraoral.

         i. Fracture of components.

        ii. Abrasion of teeth.

      b. Intraoral.

         i. Lack of muco-osseous support. Apply pressure to extension base areas of tooth-mucosa borne RPDs. Examine for movement of third point of reference indicating a need to reline the base.

        ii. Retention.

       iii. Stability.

       iv. Occlusion and articulation.

Chapter XX

RELINE PROCEDURES

The reline procedure offers an alternative to the altered cast procedure. At the time of delivery, a selective pressure impression of the muco-osseous segments is completed using the denture base as a tray. This technique is also applied to tooth-mucosa borne partial dentures at various intervals to re-establish muco-osseous support by compensating for the normal tissue remodelling. Such changes are primarily the result of pressure induced resorption associated with partial denture function. Generally speaking, tooth borne partial dentures do not require reline procedures unless they are fabricated after recent extractions and before the residual ridge has completely healed, or other factors are present causing muco-osseous changes. Note, however, that this simple reline procedure may be applied to any removable prosthesis containing resin bases.

RELINE PROCEDURE—CLINICAL PHASE

The purpose is to accurately record or re-record the functional (selective pressure) form of the muco-osseous supporting tissues while maintaining the proper relationship of the framework to the abutment teeth.

1. Remove the undercuts from the denture base. (Fig. 20–1)

2. Evaluate and correct the border extensions as required.

3. Provide relief and venting of the secondary and non-supporting muco–osseous tissues as required by selectively grinding the tissue surface and placing escape holes. (Fig. 20–2)

4. Select and mix the tissue conditioner or impression material according to the required viscosity and manufacturer's instructions.

5. Dry the mouth with gauze.

6. Load the denture base as a tray.

7. Seat the framework, being certain that the rests and the third point of reference are completely seated. (Fig. 20–3)

8. Do not direct seating pressure on the extension base areas.

9. During setting of the impression material, continually activate all pertinent muscle and frenal attachments. (Fig. 20–4)

10. The partial denture may be removed following the initial set of five to ten minutes. Inspect the impression. Additional material may be added to borders as required. The setting time of some tissue conditioners will be accelerated by spraying the impression surface lightly with tissue conditioner powder after the initial set. The excess powder should be removed by an air syringe before reinserting the partial denture. Reseat the impression for 10 to 15 minutes. (Fig. 20–5)

11. Remove the impression when set. Many tissue conditioners benefit from a total setting time of 20 to 30 minutes in the mouth.

RELINE PROCEDURE—LABORATORY PHASE

1. Pour the reline impression of the mucosal supporting areas in stone. (Fig. 20–6)

2. For mandibular partial dentures the area between the bases may be filled in with suitable block out material (e.g. modeling clay) to facilitate the fabrication of the cast.

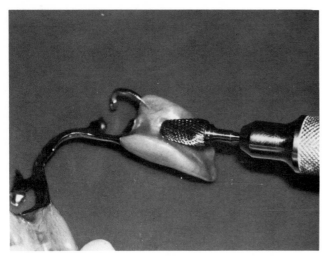

Fig. 20-1 Remove undercuts from the tissue surface of the denture base.

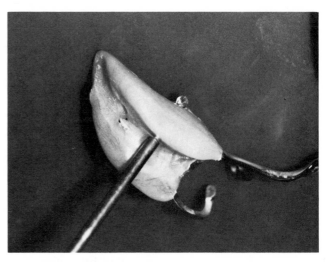

Fig. 20-2 Relieve the ridge crest and prepare vents directed from the ridge crest through the lingual flange with a round bur.

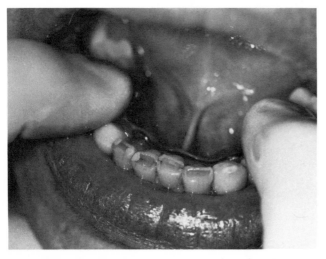

Fig. 20-3 The prosthesis is positioned so that the rests are completely seated. DO NOT PLACE PRESSURE ON THE BASE AREA.

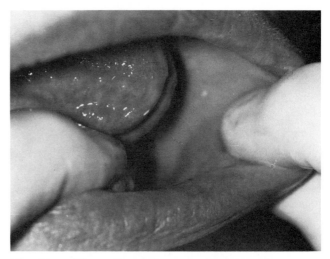

Fig. 20-4 The patient is instructed to move the tongue laterally and against the palate. The modiolus is manually directed superiorly, inferiorly, and forward to activate associated facial musculature.

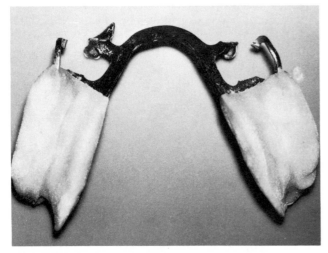

Fig. 20-5 The impression surface may be lightly sprayed with powder and reseated until final set.

3. After the cast has set, another mix of stone is used to make an index on the lower member of the reline device. (Fig. 20–7)

4. The upper member of the reline device is attached with mounting plaster. (Fig 20–8)

5. When the mounting plaster is set open the device, remove the partial denture from the cast, and clean away all of the impression material. Do not remove the prosthesis from the cast prior to this stage. (Fig. 20–9)

6. The resin should be ground slightly to yield a clean surface.

7. If a posterior palatal seal is to be carved on a maxillary cast, a clinical inspection should be

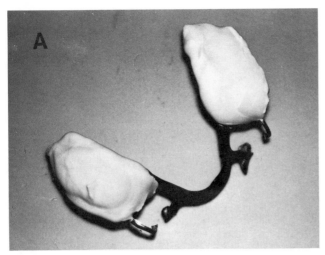
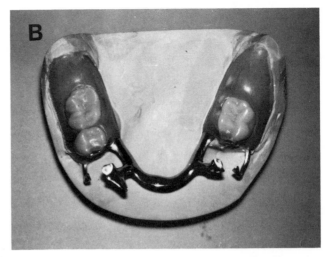

Fig. 20-6 (A) The impression of the base area is poured in stone. (B) A second pour is used to complete the cast fabrication. Stone should contact the framework to stabilize the prosthesis.

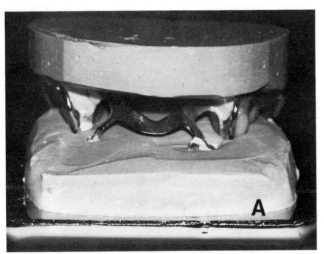
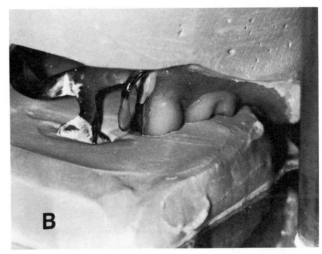

Fig. 20-7 (A & B) A viscous mix of stone is placed in the lower member of the reline device. The cast in inverted to form an index of the occlusal surfaces and rests in the stone.

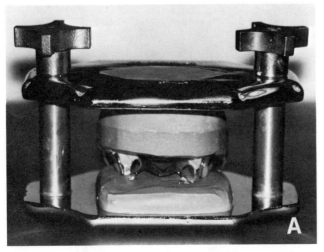
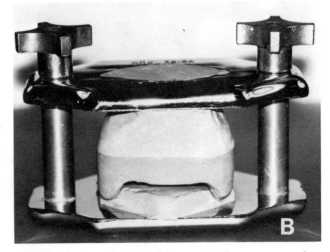

Fig. 20-8 (A) Anterior and (B) posterior views of the reline device following attachment of the cast to the upper member and tightening of the wing nuts. Note the space providing access to the lingual flange in the posterior view.

made of the junction of movable and immovable soft palate to determine the exact location and tissue resiliency. This will aid in establishing the position and depth of the seal to be carved in the cast.

8. Flush hot water over the cast and then paint a coat of separator on the warm cast and allow it to cool to room temperature. (Fig. 20–10)

9. Prepare a sufficient amount of an autopolymerizing resin and let it stand in a covered glass container until it appears to have a frosting-like consistency (following manufacturer's instructions).

10. Paint monomer on the denture base to ensure a positive bond with the new resin. (Fig. 20–10)

11. Use a small spatula to apply the resin in and around the peripheral margins on the cast. Avoid trapping air while spreading resin in the peripheral margins. Spread the resin over the inner surface of the denture base. (Fig. 20–11)

12. Place the denture back into the occlusal index and tighten the wing nuts until they secure the shoulder on the studs. Use a moistened gloved finger or cotton tipped applicator moistened with monomer to adapt the resin against the periphery and to remove the excess. (Fig. 20–12)

13. Place the assembly in a pressure container with just enough warm water (100°F) to cover the partial denture. Close the lid and apply 20 lbs. of

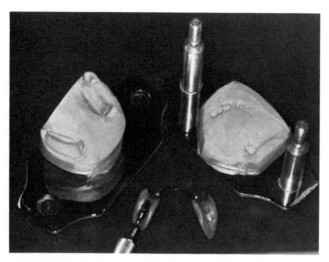

Fig. 20-9 The prosthesis is removed and cleaned of impression material. The denture base is roughened.

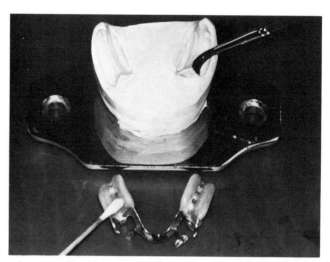

Fig. 20-10 Monomer is applied to the acrylic resin base area and a separating medium applied to the remount cast.

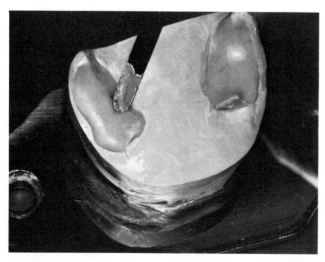

Fig. 20-11 Apply the resin to the impression surface of the cast and denture base.

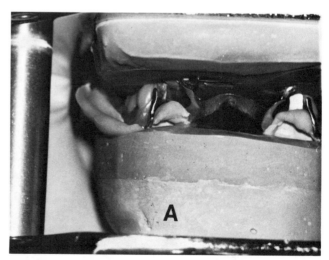

Fig. 20-12A The reline device is reassembled.

air pressure. The container may be opened after 20 minutes of processing time has elapsed. No heat is applied. The use of a timer is recommended to prevent premature disassembly.

14. After the assembly is removed from the pressure container, unscrew the wing nuts on the reline device. Remove the partial denture from the index and separate it from the cast. Finish and polish the partial denture in the usual manner. (Fig. 20–13)

15. A clinical remount procedure may be required to establish proper occlusion and articulation, especially if the partial denture is tooth-mucosa borne.

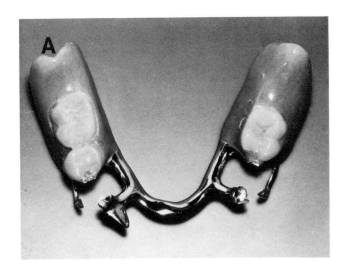

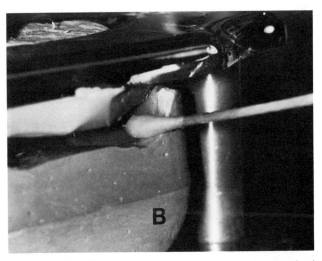

Fig. 20-12B Excess resin is removed and smoothed against the denture base using a cotton-tipped applicator or gloved finger moistened with monomer.

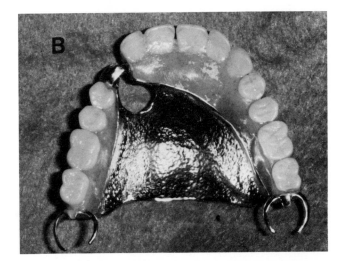

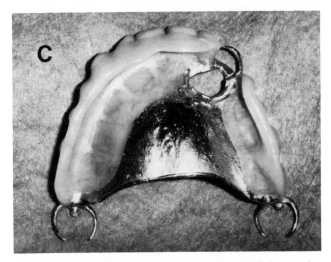

Fig. 20-13 (A) The prosthesis is polished, refining occlusal anatomy, and exposing the internal finish lines on the tissue surface. (B) A long span tooth and mucosa supported mesial extension prosthesis which required a reline procedure to re-establish muco-osseous support. (C) Note the finish line positions of the tooth borne segment as compared to the tooth mucosa-borne supported segment.

179

Chapter XXI

CLINICAL REMOUNT PROCEDURE

A clinical remount procedure is usually required when it is necessary to accurately evaluate or adjust the occlusion or articulation of tooth-mucosa borne removable partial dentures. The displaceability of the supporting tissues of the muco-osseous segment limits the ability of the clinician to evaluate occlusal contacts intraorally. Premature or deflective occlusal contacts result in denture base displacement upon mandibular closure which may prevent accurate assessment of the occlusion. The presence of such contacts may contribute to inequitable loading of the supporting tissues, increased frequency of pressure induced irritation of the mucosa, and accelerated resorption of the bone of the muco-osseous supporting tissues. Laboratory remount procedures are inadequate due to the release of strains developed in the processed denture base resin which occurs following retrieval from the master cast and the need to relate the processed base to the supporting tissues.

INDICATIONS

A. Delivery of tooth-mucosa borne prostheses usually requires a clinical remount procedure to compensate for malocclusion induced by dimensional changes associated with heat processed acrylic resin.

B. Reline of tooth-mucosa borne RPDs requires a clinical remount procedure to compensate for malocclusion induced by vertical changes resulting from the increased support provided by the muco-osseous segment.

C. Evaluation or adjustment of occlusion or articulation of tooth-mucosa borne RPDs.

PROCEDURE

A. Ensure appropriate tissue recovery prior to the procedure by instructing the patient not to wear tooth-mucosa borne prostheses 24 to 72 hours prior to the remount procedure.

B. Mount the maxillary cast utilizing a facebow. (Fig. 21–1)

 1. New facebow record.

 2. Preservation of previous facebow record.

C. Adjust the tissue surface of the prosthesis utilizing pressure indicating paste. (Fig. 21–2). To ensure complete seating and proper relationship of the prosthesis to the mucosa, the patient may be directed to occlude on cotton rolls placed in the posterior/molar region, one on each side positioned horizontally.

D. Make an impression of the seated RPD manually placing impression material in critical areas.

E. Block out undercuts in the impression with wax or appropriate material and pour the impression to form the remount cast. (Fig. 21–3)

F. Remove the prosthesis from the remount cast.

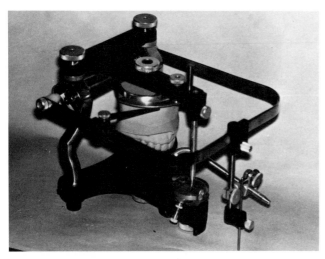

Fig. 21-1 The maxillary opposing cast is mounted with a new facebow record or through preservation of a previous facebow record.

G. Record centric relation with a pressure-free interocclusal record at a vertical dimension slightly beyond (1-2 mm) the occlusal vertical dimension. (Fig. 21–4)

H. Secure the prosthesis to the remount cast and lengthen the incisal pin to compensate for the thickness of the interocclusal record. Secure the remount cast to the maxillary cast, and mount it to the lower member of the articulator. (Fig. 21–5)

I. The occlusal surfaces of the casts may be coated with cyanoacrylate to improve surface hardness and reduce abrasion.

J. Complete the occlusal adjustment, refine the occlusal anatomy, and polish the prosthesis.

K. The remount cast, opposing cast and articulator number may be preserved as a permanent record for future reference.

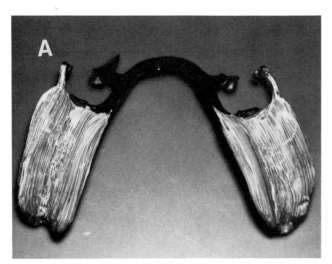
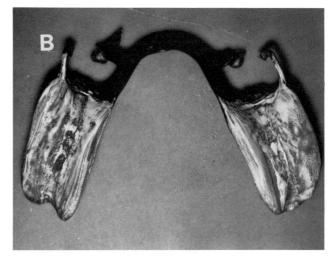

Fig. 21-2 (A) Pressure indicating paste is applied using a brush to provide clear, even markings on the denture base. (B) Adjustments of unfavorable pressure areas are completed as required.

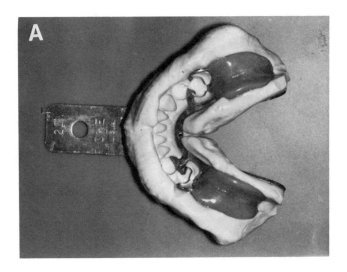

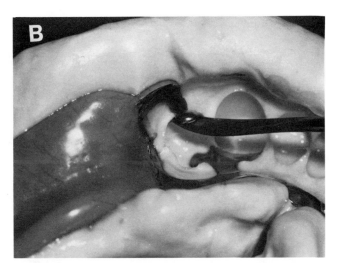
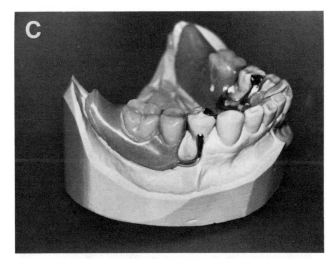

Fig. 21-3 (A) Irreversible hydrocolloid in a stock tray large enough to avoid interference with the prosthesis is used to form the remount impression. (B) Wax is used to block out framework components which may prevent removal of the framework from the cast. (C) The impression is poured using improved stone in the occlusal areas.

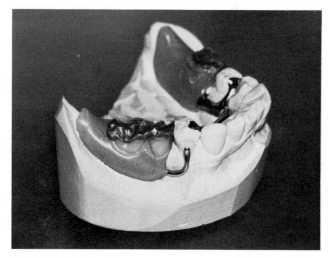

Fig. 21-4 The prosthesis is removed from the remount cast and a pressure-free centric record made. Softened wax is an acceptable recording material which permits repeated confirmation of the record during the procedure. The prosthesis is repositioned on the cast.

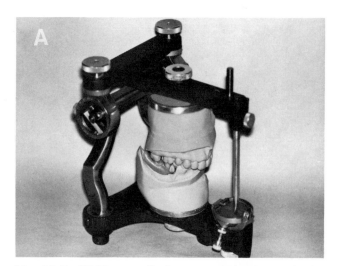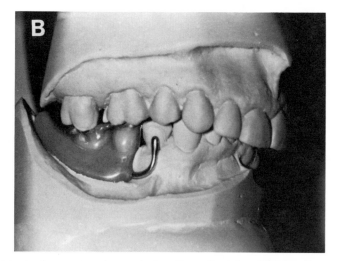

Fig. 21-5 (A) The mandibular remount cast is attached to the opposing cast and mounted on the articulator. (B) Note that the record is made at a vertical dimension slightly greater than the occlusal vertical dimension to eliminate rigid interferences in mandibular closure. The incisal pin is lengthened slightly to compensate for the increased vertical dimension of the record.

Chapter XXII

ATTACHMENTS

Attachments are indicated in esthetically demanding situations when conventional designs would not be satisfactory. Most tooth borne RPDs may be designed to satisfy esthetic requirements without attachments. Attachments usually require the placement of cast restorations on the abutment teeth which incorporate a part of the mechanism. A second portion of the mechanical element is incorporated in the adjacent denture base. An attachment serves as a substitute for a conventional clasp and must satisfy the basic requirements of clasp design. The primary advantage of an attachment is the elimination of visible clasp arms. This chapter does not provide technical information on the many attachment systems available today. The emphasis here is on those principles of design which contribute to a successful removable partial denture when attachments are utilized.

DEFINITION

An attachment is a mechanical device which contributes to the fixation, retention, stabilization, and support of a dental prosthesis.

TYPES OF ATTACHMENTS

A. PRECISION ATTACHMENT. A retainer used in fixed and removable prosthodontics consisting of a metal receptacle (matrix) and a close fitting part (patrix). The receptacle is usually contained within the normal or expanded contours of the crown of the abutment tooth and the close fitting part is attached to a pontic or the denture framework. (Fig. 22–1)

B. RIGID ATTACHMENT. An attachment which does not permit movement or flexion between the matrix and patrix. (Fig. 22–1)

C. NONRIGID ATTACHMENT. An attachment which permits movement between the matrix and patrix through the incorporation of a spring-loaded mechanism, hinge, ball and socket mechanism, or flexible elements. (Fig. 22–2)

D. INTRACORONAL ATTACHMENT. An attachment that is contained within the normal contours of the crown portion of a natural tooth. (Fig. 22–1)

E. EXTRACORONAL ATTACHMENT. An attachment that extends outside or external to the crown portion of a natural tooth. (Fig. 22–2)

ADVANTAGES OF ATTACHMENTS

Elimination of visible clasp arms.

DISADVANTAGES OF ATTACHMENTS

A. ADDITIONAL EXPENSE.

B. INCREASED FREQUENCY OF ADJUSTMENT AND FAILURE.

C. INCREASED TECHNICAL EXPERTISE REQUIRED.

D. UNPREDICTABLE OR UNFAVORABLE DISTRIBUTION OF FORCES.

1. Rigid attachments may direct excessive forces to the dento-alveolar segment, especially when used in tooth-mucosa borne RPDs. (Fig. 22–3)

2. Non-rigid attachments are often unpredictable, unfavorable or inequitable in terms of relative

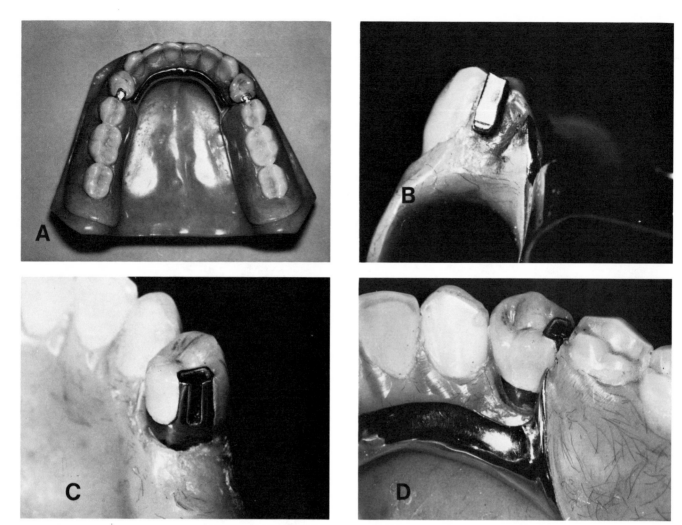

Fig. 22-1 (A) Intracoronal rigid precision attachments are incorporated in this prosthesis. One side is circular, the other rectangular in occlusal outline form. (B) The patrix is parallel sided and rectangular from the proximal view, incorporating an expandable gingival portion. (C) The matrix is contained within the normal contours of a cast restoration fabricated for the abutment tooth. (D) The patrix fits into the matrix intimately and satisfies the basic requirements of clasp design.

force distribution between the dento-alveolar and muco- osseous segments (Fig. 22–4).

3. Some non-rigid attachments direct excessive forces to the muco-osseous segment minimizing the forces directed to the dento-alveolar segment. (Fig. 22–5)

INDICATION FOR ATTACHMENTS.

When the esthetics demands of the patient cannot be satisfied with conventional partial dentures.

CONTRAINDICATIONS FOR ATTACHMENTS

A. When esthetic demands may be satisfied utilizing conventional clasp designs or the rotational path design. This applies to most tooth borne RPDs.

B. When control of the relative distribution of functional forces to the dento-alveolar and muco-osseous segments is critical to their preservation.

C. When financial constraints exist.

D. When professional recall and maintenance may be compromised. Patient follow-up is especially important when attachments are utilized.

RIGID ATTACHMENTS

A. ADVANTAGES.

1. Less susceptible to failure due to the absence of mobile elements.

2. Reduced bulk or thickness due to simplicity of design.

186

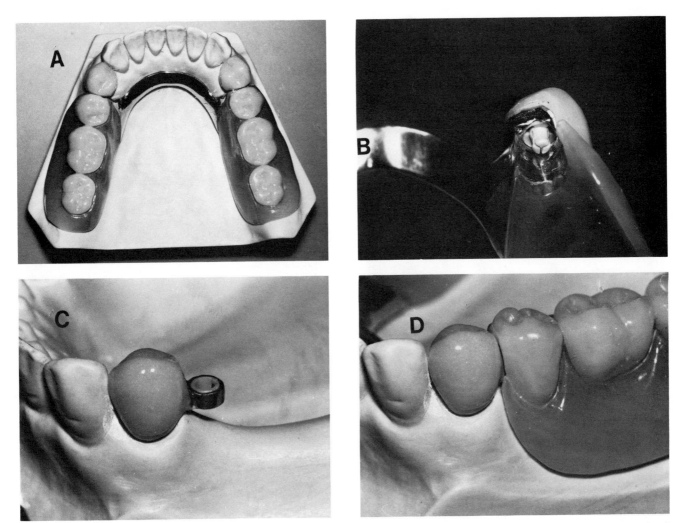

Fig. 22-2 (A) Extracoronal nonrigid precision attachments are incorporated in this prosthesis. (B) The patrix is comprised of a flexible extension which is designed to permit movement during function. (C) The matrix is attached to the cast restoration fabricated for the abutment tooth. It extends over the ridge area beyond the contours of the crown. (D) The patrix fits into the matrix intimately and satisfies the basic requirements of clasp design. (Models in Figs. 22-1 & 2 courtesy of Mr. Peter Staubli, C.D.T.)

3. Effective apically-directed load transfer to abutment teeth in tooth borne RPDs. (Fig. 22–6)

4. May be used to provide effective splinting and cross arch stabilization. (Fig. 22–6)

B. DISADVANTAGES.

1. Potential to torque abutment teeth in tooth-mucosa borne RPDs. (Fig. 22–3)

2. Usually requires placement of a cast restoration on the abutment tooth to accommodate the matrix.

3. Usually requires paralleling device to determine exact path of placement. (See technique for rigid intracoronal attachments)

C. INDICATIONS. High esthetic demands in the following situations.

1. Tooth borne RPDs when conventional designs are unacceptable.

2. Tooth-mucosa borne RPDs when favorable muco-osseous support is available (high ridge resistance).

3. Tooth-mucosa borne RPDs when abutment teeth demonstrate the potential to tolerate increased forces (high abutment resistance).

4. Tooth-mucosa borne RPDs when high ridge resistance and high abutment resistance exist.

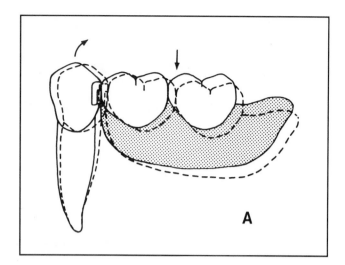

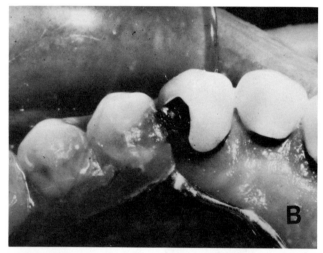

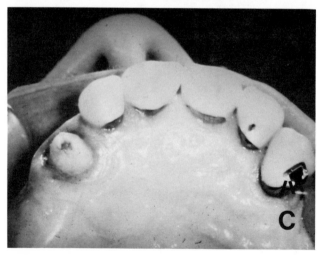

Fig. 22-3 (A) Demonstrates diagrammatically the potential torquing forces of a rigid attachment used in a tooth-mucosa borne RPD. (B) Excessive forces directed to the canine abutment from this distal extension RPD resulted in (C) fracture of the tooth.

NON RIGID ATTACHMENTS

A. ADVANTAGES.

1. May reduce forces directed to abutment teeth. (Fig. 22–5)

2. Usually does not require a paralleling device to determine exact path of placement.

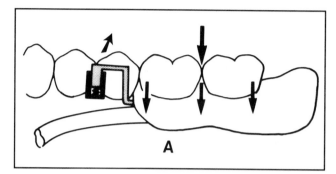

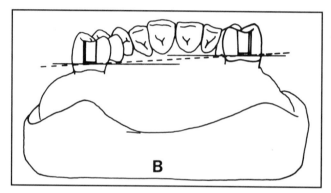

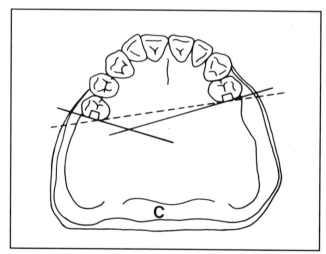

Fig. 22-4 (A) Some spring loaded varieties of stress director attachments may not move in function as they appear in a diagram if binding of the attachment apparatus occurs. This may lead to torquing of the abutment tooth as the curved arrow indicates. (B & C) Some types of attachments rely upon rotational or hinge type movement of the base area. If a common axis of rotation is not developed (dotted lines) the base areas may torque abutment teeth during function as the prosthesis cannot freely rotate around two separate axes simultaneously.

188

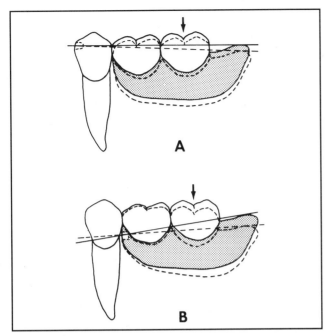

Fig. 22-5 Stress director attachments which permit freedom of movement of the base areas without binding may direct excessive forces to the muco-osseous supporting structures. Location of the rotational axis at the distogingival area of the abutment prevents a more even distribution of loading forces over the length of the ridge since movement of the base area is minimal adjacent to the attachment area. (A) Mesio-occlusal rotational center. (B) Distogingival rotational center.

3. May not require the placement of a cast restoration on the abutment teeth. (Fig. 22–7)

B. DISADVANTAGES.

   1. Increased rate of failure of the mobile or flexible elements.

   2. Usually increased expense.

   3. Usually increased bulk or thickness of the prosthesis to accommodate the components.

   4. Potential to increase forces directed to the muco-osseous segment. (Fig. 22–5)

C. INDICATIONS. High esthetic demands in the following situations.

   1. Tooth-mucosa borne RPDs. When reduced forces directed to the abutment teeth are required (low abutment resistance). Note, however, that in many situations nonrigid attachments are unpredictable in their functional force distribution. (Fig. 22–4)

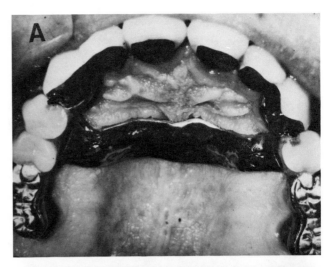

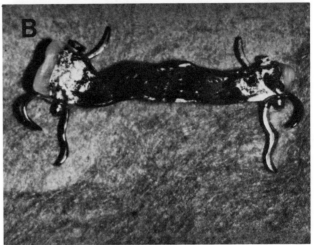

Fig. 22-6 (A & B) The placement of rests or rigid attachments providing dento-alveolar support adjacent to edentulous areas in tooth supported RPDs promotes apically directed force transmission during occlusal loading. The rigid intracoronal attachments may promote splinting and cross arch stabilization. Note the lingual cast bracing arms on the hemisected molars which rest on the ledged castings. Distobuccal roots of the molars were resected. Lateral incisors and canines are splinted bilaterally to reduce hypermobility and resist functional forces.

   2. Tooth-mucosa borne RPDs when favorable muco-osseous support is available (high ridge resistance).

   3. Tooth-mucosa borne RPDs when low abutment resistance and high ridge resistance exist.

INTRACORONAL ATTACHMENTS

A. ADVANTAGES.

   1. Usually permit abutment tooth and prosthesis contours conducive to periodontal health.

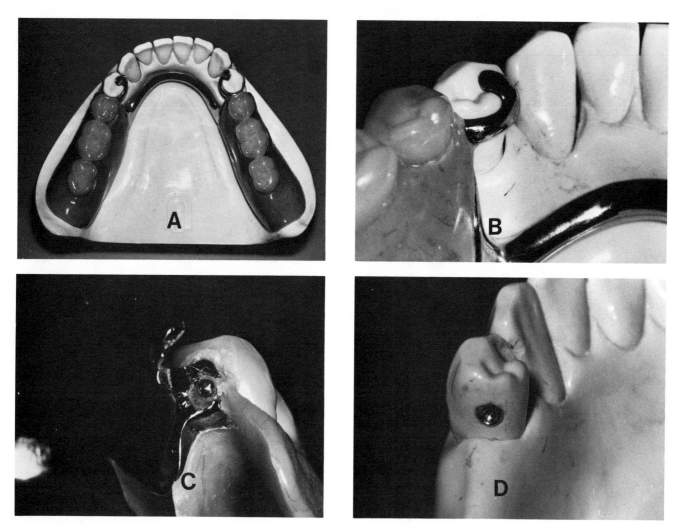

Fig. 22-7 (A) Several attachment systems do not require the placement of cast restorations on abutment teeth. (B) The mesial rest and lingual cast bracing arm provide bracing and support. (C) Retention is provided by a spring loaded flexible element which (D) engages a metal receptacle placed within the enamel of the abutment tooth. As with other attachment systems, unfavorable lateral forces may be developed if proper design is not provided.

2. May be used when less interarch distance is present to accommodate the attachment mechanism and position artificial teeth.

3. Usually promotes apically directed abutment tooth force transmission.

B. DISADVANTAGES.

1. May require increased tooth modification to incorporate attachment matrix. (Fig. 22–8)

2. Requires adequate occlusogingival dimensions of abutment tooth for effective fixation. Parallel sided intracoronal precision attachments usually require approximately 4 mm of occlusogingival dimension, necessitating a 7 mm crown height in order to provide adequate occlusal and gingival proximal embrasures. (Fig. 22–9)

EXTRACORONAL ATTACHMENTS

A. ADVANTAGES.

1. Usually requires less extensive tooth modification.

2. Reduced requirement of occlusogingival height of abutment tooth.

B. DISADVANTAGES.

1. Usually incorporates elements which result in contours of the abutment tooth or prosthesis which are not conducive to periodontal health.

2. Requires adequate interarch distance to accommodate the attachment mechanism and position artificial teeth.

3. Usually compromises the potential to direct forces along the long axis of the abutment

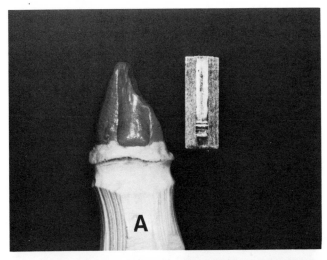

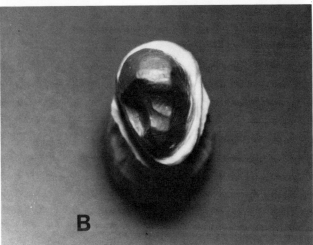

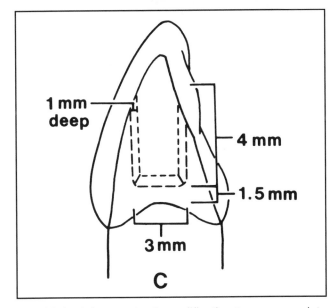

Fig. 22-8 Adequate tooth modification to accommodate the matrix of the attachment mechanism usually requires a proximal box preparation. (A & B) Dimensions of the proximal box are determined by the matrix. (C) The system presented requires a proximal box preparation with these approximate dimensions.

tooth. Vertical forces are directed external to the confines of the clinical crown of the abutment tooth.

TREATMENT PLANNING CONSIDERATIONS AND REQUIREMENTS

A. POTENTIAL FOR DENTO-ALVEOLAR SUPPORT. Adequate alveolar support is required since increased forces will usually be applied to abutment teeth.

1. Periodontal health and hygiene.
2. Alveolar bone index.
3. Root morphology.

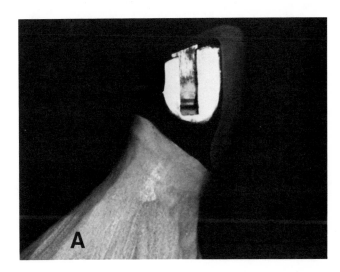

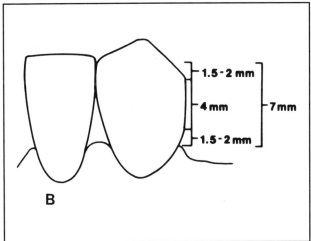

Fig. 22-9 (A) The completed crown demonstrates the incorporation of the matrix in addition to the preservation of occlusal and gingival embrasure space. (B) This diagram demonstrates the required seven millimeters or more occlusogingival crown length required to accommodate the matrix (4 mm minimum) and the occlusal and gingival embrasures.

4. Occlusogingival crown height.

5. Crown to root ratio.

6. Need for fixed splinting of abutment teeth.

B. POTENTIAL FOR MUCO-OSSEOUS SUPPORT. Adequate muco-osseous support is required to reduce the forces otherwise directed to the abutment teeth, especially in the tooth-mucosa borne RPD.

1. Basal and residual ridge bone index.

2. Mucosal health and hygiene.

3. Anatomic considerations. Attachments are generally most successful on the maxillary arch due to the support available with palatal coverage.

a. Palatal contours. A broad horizontal hard palate offers the most favorable support.

b. Residual ridge height and conformation.

C. POTENTIAL OF APPLIED FORCES. Excessive functional forces may increase the anticipated load on supporting tissues. (See Chapter III)

1. Opposing occlusion.

2. Muscular force potential.

3. Parafunctional habits.

4. Length of edentulous span.

5. History of prosthesis failure.

6. History of poor tissue tolerance.

D. TOOTH BORNE VERSUS TOOTH-MUCOSA BORNE. Unfavorable torquing forces are minimized in tooth borne attachment partial dentures.

DESIGN CONSIDERATIONS FOR THE TOOTH-MUCOSA BORNE RPD INCORPORATING A RIGID INTRACORONAL PRECISION ATTACHMENT

A. PREREQUISITES.

1. High esthetic demands.

2. Favorable dento-alveolar support (high abutment resistance).

3. Favorable muco-osseous support (high ridge resistance).

4. Normal potential of applied forces.

5. Potential for optimum post-insertion maintenance.

B. PROSTHESIS DESIGN AND TREATMENT PLANNING CONSIDERATIONS.

1. Optimum extension of denture bases to promote muco-osseous support for tooth-mucosa borne RPDs.

2. Utilization of selective pressure impression or reline procedures which maximize muco-osseous support for tooth-mucosa borne RPDs.

3. Major connector design. Maxillary major connector coverage of the horizontal hard palate to provide additional support for the tooth-mucosa borne RPD. (Fig. 22-12)

4. Splinting for force distribution. Abutment teeth usually are splinted to resist the increased functional forces. (Fig. 22-17)

5. Functional matrix-patrix relationship. This relationship is established while the framework is placed under a simulated functional loading to increase muco-osseous support and reduce tissueward movement of the denture base during function. (Fig. 22-17)

6. Clinical remount. The occlusion and articulation are adjusted utilizing a clinical remount procedure at delivery.

7. Reline procedures performed at recall, as indicated, in order to maintain muco-osseous support.

C. TECHNIQUE. Rigid intracoronal precision attachments. Note: The following procedure utilizing a Stern .070 GL is one example of the use of attachments in removable prosthodontics. Many other attachment systems are available and may be utilized.

1. Abutment teeth are prepared for crowns.

2. During preparation, sufficient reduction is completed to permit normal restoration contours in the area containing the matrix. (Fig. 22-8)

3. Complete arch impressions are made.

4. The crowns are waxed to normal anatomic contours. (Fig. 22-9)

5. A path of placement is determined, utilizing a surveyor. All involved abutment teeth are analyzed together incorporating all factors governing the determination of a path of placement. (Fig 22-10)

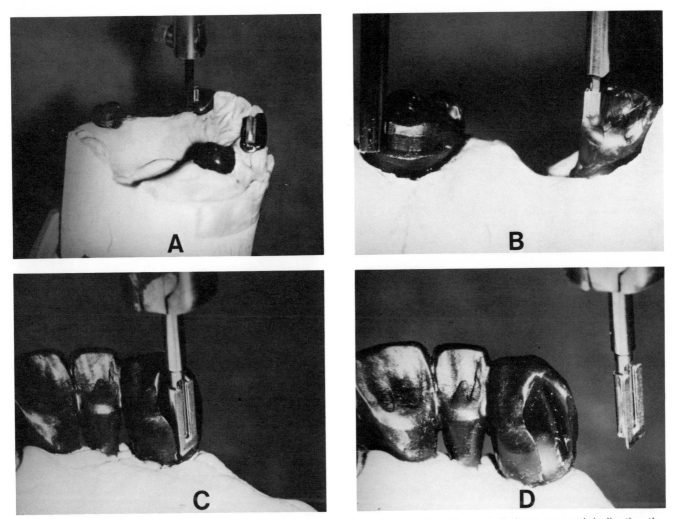

Fig. 22-10 (A) The surveyor aligns potential guiding planes of castings and matrices of all abutment teeth indicating the path of placement. (B) Features such as guiding planes and ledges are aligned in harmony with the matrices. (C & D) Adequate box form of the tooth preparation permits matrix placement at the required tilt. Note that an instrument usually available with rigid intracoronal attachment systems serves as a patrix analog which may be substituted for the surveyor analyzing rod to facilitate parallel alignment of the matrices with each other and with appropriate guiding planes.

6. The matrix is incorporated in the crown wax-ups, utilizing the surveyor to ensure alignment. (Fig. 22–10)

7. The lingual surfaces of crowns receiving attachment matrices are contoured to receive accessory cast circumferential retentive arms. The lingual ledge area opposing the terminal one third of the clasp arm is waxed parallel to the path of insertion. (Fig. 22–11)

8. The casting is made utilizing ceramometal.

9. A clinical metal try-in and a solder relation is usually necessary if abutments are to be splinted.

10. The porcelain is applied, contours are completed, and the crowns are polished. A final impression is completed with the crowns seated. The master cast is poured, and the framework is designed. (Fig. 22–12)

11. A lingual circumferential retentive arm and retentive mechanism are waxed to the patrix. The lingual accessory retentive arm is adapted to the previously contoured lingual ledge. The resin retentive mechanism extends over the ridge area to permit attachment to the base area of the framework. Relief of the tissue surface of the retentive mechanism is required to permit the metal band of the framework to be positioned. (Fig. 22–13)

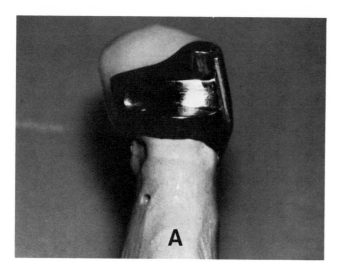

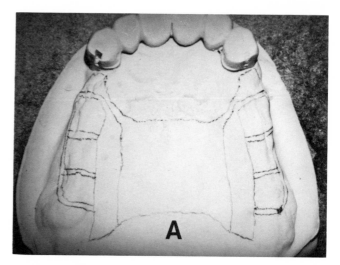

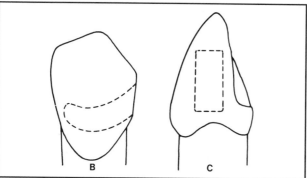

Fig. 22-11 (A) The completed crown demonstrates the contained proximal matrix and the lingual ledge. Diagrammatically the location of the lingual arm is demonstrated (B) from the lingual view and (C) from the proximal view. Note that the lingual surface of the crown is developed parallel to the facial and lingual walls of the matrix (dotted outline).

12. When interarch distance is limited, an additional transfer impression is necessary. The finished crowns and framework are seated in the mouth. A transfer impression is made, the castings are lubricated, resin dies are fabricated for the castings, and the cast is poured in stone. A more precise adaptation of the retentive mechanism to be attached to the patrix, and the metal band of the base area with its retentive mechanism, may be established to maximize the interarch distance available for artificial tooth placement. (Fig. 22–14)

13. The lingual retentive arm and retentive mechanism are cast to the patrix using ADA Class III or IV gold alloy. The patrix should be notched and roughened to enhance bonding of the cast alloy.

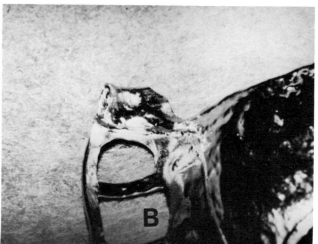

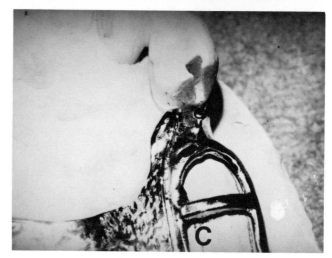

Fig. 22-12 For tooth-mucosa borne RPDs, maxillary major connectors should cover the horizontal hard palate to promote support. (A) Internal finish lines should be positioned to facilitate reline procedures. (B) Adjacent to abutment teeth the internal finish line should be located 5-7 mm from the gingival margin to increase the space available to develop the retentive mechanism (C) for the resin which attaches the patrix to the framework.

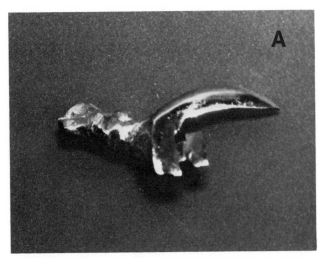
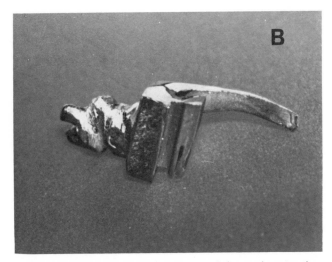

Fig. 22-13 (A) An occlusal view of the patrix with the attached lingual accessory retentive arm and the resin retentive network which permits attachment to the framework. (B) The lingual view demonstrates the expandable gingival lock.

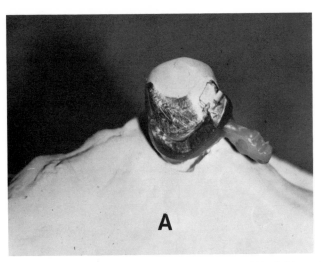
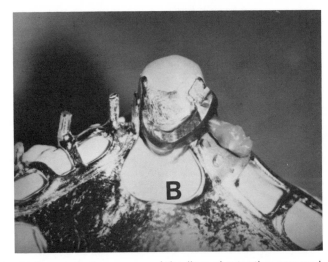

Fig. 22-14 The poured transfer impression (A) yields a cast which permits the wax-up of the lingual retentive arm and resin retentive mechanism to the patrix. (B) A close adaptation of the retentive mechanism to the framework is permitted through the use of this procedure. Without this additional cast the position of the retentive mechanism and the gingival relief must be determined arbitrarily.

14. The patrix is fitted to the matrix and adjusted, if necessary, to achieve the required degree of retention. A gingival lock, present in many systems, contributes to the adjustment of retention. (Fig. 22–15)

15. The crowns and framework are seated clinically. The presence of a space between the framework and the retentive mechanism of the patrix is confirmed. To establish optimum support, the framework is loaded to simulate functional forces by apically directing pressure on the major connector. The passive fitting of the patrix within the matrix (without binding) is again confirmed. (Fig. 22–16)

16. The retentive mechanism of the matrix is related to the base area of the framework during simulated occlusal loading utilizing a highly filled autopolymerizing polymethylmethacrylate acrylic resin. The resin is allowed to reach final polymerization. This resin may be trimmed to facilitate final wax up, but remains as a part of the final prosthesis. (Fig. 22–16)

17. Note that for bilateral extension base designs, an additional reference point may be required to assist in the accurate positioning of the framework during the luting of patrix to framework. (Fig. 22–17)

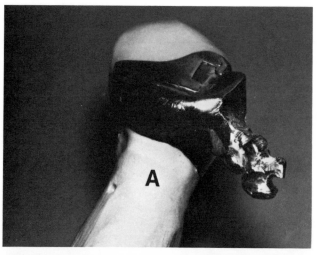

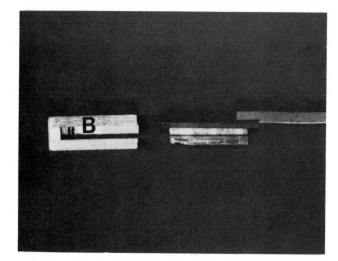

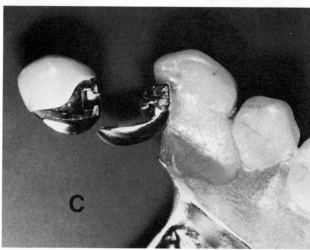

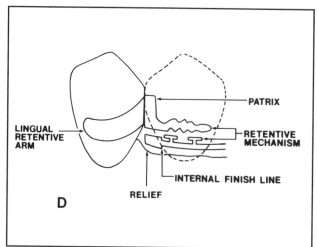

Fig. 22-15 (A) The lingual arm adapts to the lingual ledge of the casting. (B) The adjustable gingival lock located on the patrix may be expanded or compressed to increase or decrease mechanical retention. The expanded gingival portion of the patrix corresponds to a groove contained within the matrix. Following try-in of the framework and finished castings the patrix is inserted into the matrix and rigidly connected using autopolymerizing resin to the retentive elements of the frameworks in the mouth. (C) Acrylic resin bonds the retentive mechanisms of the patrix and the framework within the denture base. (D) Diagrammatically the artificial tooth (dotted outline) is positioned over the retentive mechanism which is connected to the patrix and attached with resin to the retentive mechanism of the framework.

18. The framework is repositioned on the master cast with space provided for the patrices to be seated without binding. The facio-proximal line angle of the abutment should be maintained to facilitate accurate artificial tooth placement. The resin should be adjusted to provide adequate space for tooth replacement. (Fig. 22–18)

19. Occlusion rims are fabricated. Horizontal and vertical maxillomandibular records are completed.

20. A set-up and wax try-in are completed.

21. The RPD is processed and finished. Care is taken not to process resin in or around the patrix. (Fig. 22–19)

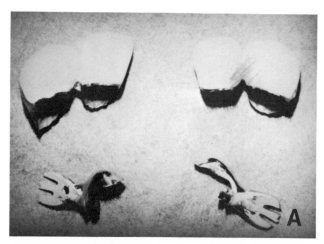

Fig. 22-16A Splinted castings and patrix complex completed.

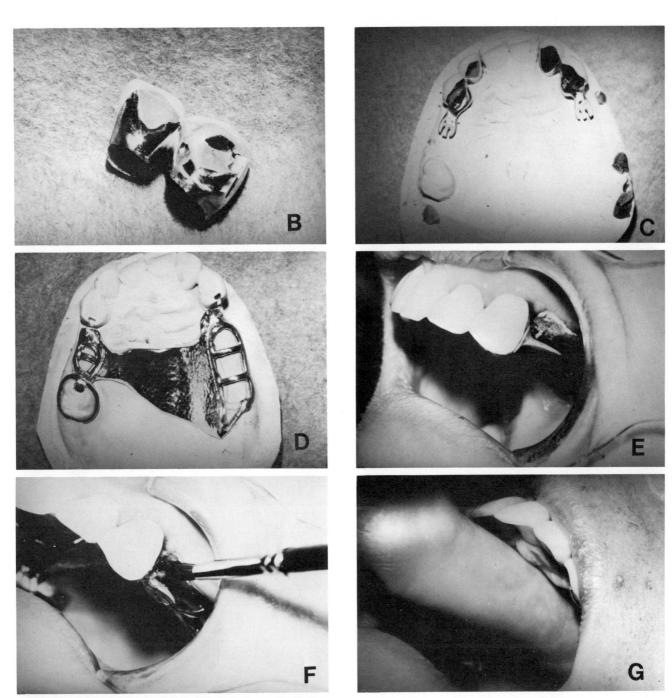

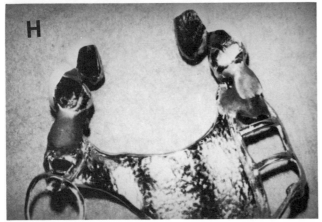

Fig. 22-16B - H (B) Lingual view of splinted castings containing matrix and lingual ledge. (C) Patrices positioned on working cast within matrices. (D) Framework positioned on appropriate master cast. (E) Crowns, framework, and patrix complex seated clinically confirming passive relationship. (F) Relating the patrix complex to the framework with autopolymerizing resin. (G) Simulated occlusal loading to be maintained during setting of the resin. (H) The framework and crowns related and removed from the mouth. A common path of withdrawal should be confirmed clinically at this time and at delivery prior to permanent crown cementation.

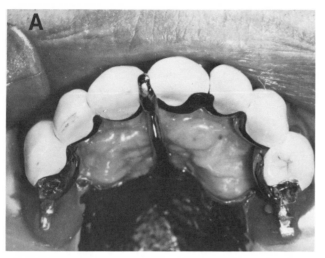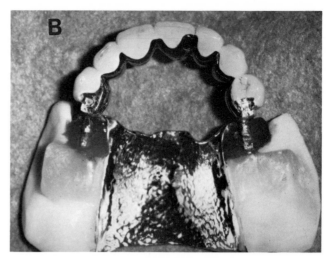

Fig. 22-17 (A) An incisal hook-type extension may facilitate the anteroposterior positioning of the framework during the relating of framework to patrix. (B) This extension is removed prior to the recording of maxillomandibular relations.

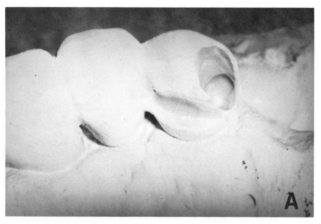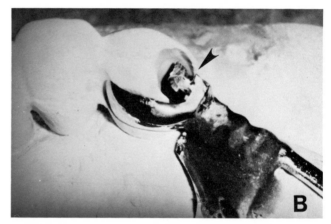

Fig. 22-18 (A) Complete seating of the framework with the attached patrix on the master cast requires meticulous relief of the matrix and lingual ledge areas of the abutment. (B) Maintenance of the distofacial line angle facilitates accurate artificial tooth placement.

22. A laboratory remount may be performed, accompanied by a procedure which preserves the facebow record.

23. A clinical remount is completed to finalize the occlusion and articulation. A transfer impression and maxillomandibular records are required to complete the clinical remount. (See Chapter XXI)

24. At delivery, the patient is taught to observe the precise path of placement and to seat the prosthesis with finger pressure (not biting pressure!)

25. Occasionally, it may be necessary to design slots or grooves in the base area to facilitate

removal of the prosthesis using a modified tooth brush handle or a dental instrument which is given to the patient. (Fig. 22–20)

26. Maintenance of an attachment prosthesis is very important

   i. Frequent periodontal recall.

   ii. Relining of the base areas as often as once a year is required to maintain optimum muco-osseous support. Frequency depends upon the rate of resorption.

   iii. Adjustment of retention by expanding the gingival lock and later by activating the frictional retention of the accessory lingual retentive arm. (Fig. 22–21)

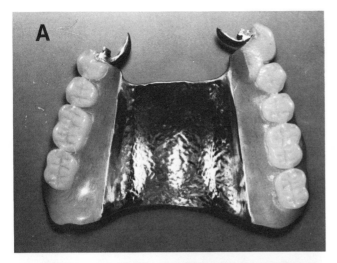

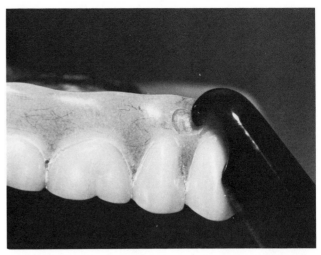

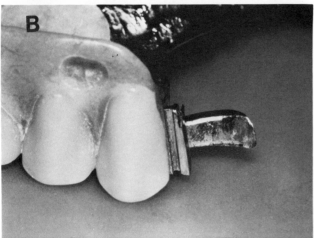

Fig. 22-20 A slot developed in the denture base may be engaged by a modified dental instrument or toothbrush handle to facilitate removal of the RPD by the patient.

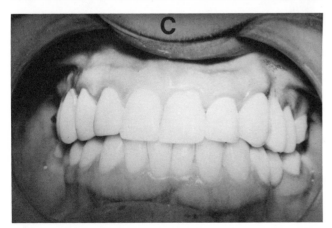

Fig. 22-19 The RPD is processed and polished. (A) The autopolymerized resin used to attach the matrix is maintained within the denture base. (B) Resin should not interfere with the patrix area. (C) Clinically seated.

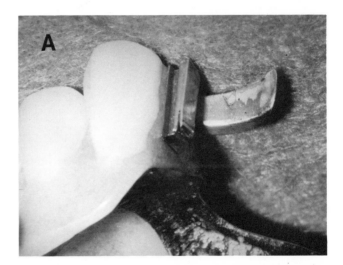

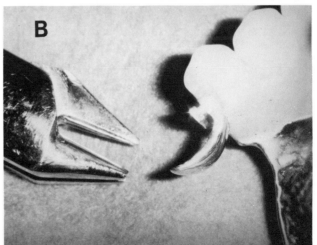

Fig. 22-21 (A) Retention may be increased by expanding the gingival lock or (B) by adjusting the lingual retentive arm.

27. Should the RPD require a remake, the patrix and its attached lingual retentive arm and resin retentive mechanism may be retrieved from the prosthesis and used in the new prothesis. This technique provides a patrix complex which demonstrates significant longevity due to the presence of both a gingival lock and an accessory lingual retentive arm which compensate for wear of the patrix following years of use. The use of acrylic resin as an attachment material facilitates retrieval of the complex, as required.

28. Should the acrylic resin bond fail between the patrix and the base area, it may be easily re-established during a clinical repair with acrylic resin. (Fig. 22–22)

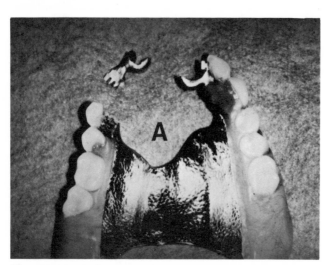 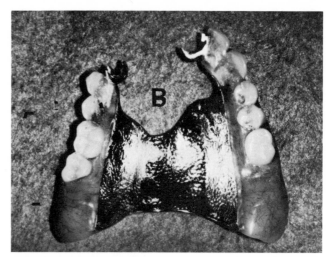

Fig. 22-22 (A) The patrix complex has fractured from the denture base. (B) The patrix may be luted again to the framework utilizing autopolymerizing acrylic resin.

Chapter XXIII

REMOVABLE PARTIAL OVERDENTURES

The roots of natural teeth may be retained to preserve alveolar bone. This may enhance the support, stability and retention for partial dentures. When a tooth cannot resist forces applied by clasps or rests, reducing its crown to root ratio for use as an overdenture abutment may be considered. The retained root should have a favorable periodontal prognosis. It will usually require endodontic therapy to permit the crown reduction. The patient should be instructed in appropriate oral hygiene procedures, including the daily use of fluoride on the overdenture abutment.

INDICATIONS

A. PRESERVING DENTO-ALVEOLAR SUPPORT.

   1. Support for tooth-mucosa borne partial dentures.

      a. Distal extension bases.
         (Figs. 23–1A, B, & C)

      b. Mesial extension bases (long-span anterior bases). (Figs. 23–2A & B)

   2. Support for long-span tooth borne partial dentures. (Fig. 23–3)

B. INADEQUATE PERIODONTAL SUPPORT. When the tooth cannot withstand the applied forces as a conventional abutment.

   1. Unfavorable crown to root ratio.

   2. Hypermobility.

C. INCREASING RETENTION OF THE PARTIAL DENTURE. The overdenture abutment tooth may be used with an attachment to augment retention. (Figs. 23-1B, 2B, & 3)

DESIGN CONSIDERATIONS

A. OVERDENTURE ABUTMENT.

   1. Contour.

      a. Tooth is reduced to a height of 1.5 to 3 mm above the free gingival margin.

      b. Contour should resemble adjacent residual ridge contour. It demonstrates a dome–shaped surface rounded mesiodistally and faciolingually.

      c. Prepared coronal surface should be smooth and highly polished.

   2. Endodontic treatment. Proper crown reduction usually requires endodontic therapy.

   3. Restorations.

      a. Amalgam. Amalgam is usually used to obturate the coronal portion of the canal. The presence of exposed dentin does not appear to increase the incidence of caries. (Fig. 23–4)

      b. Cast copings. Cast copings may be required to establish proper contour when excessive tooth structure is missing, or to retain an attachment component. Copings may introduce subgingival margins and inhibit caries detection. (Fig. 23–2A)

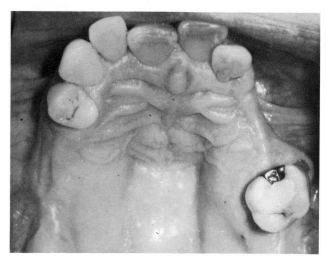

Fig. 23-1A Maxillary molar with severe periodontal disease involving both buccal roots.

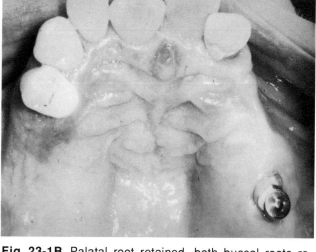

Fig. 23-1B Palatal root retained, both buccal roots resected. Metallic keeper for a magnet attachment in palatal root. Palatal root preserves dento-alveolar support and left side functions as a tooth borne base.

B. REMOVABLE PARTIAL DENTURE.

1. Contact of RPD with the overdenture abutment tooth.

   a. Resin. Easier to adjust or modify contact with tooth.

   b. Metal. More difficult to adjust or modify contact with tooth.

   c. Attachment. May be used to increase retention.

2. Artificial tooth placement. An overdenture abutment tooth usually requires extensive modification of the overlying artificial tooth for proper placement.

3. Framework design. The overdenture root preserves dento-alveolar support and may influence the fulcrum line axis in extension base partial dentures.

   a. Root located close to the abutment tooth. The root may act as a fulcrum point around which the denture base will tend to rotate. This rotation of the denture base will torque the abutment tooth regardless of the retainer used. (Fig. 23–5)

   b. Root located away from the abutment tooth. The root may support the extension base permitting it to function as a tooth borne base. A non-stress releasing clasp may be used on the abutment tooth. (Fig. 23–6)

4. Denture base. Grafted polymethylmethacrylate acrylic resins should be considered to increase strength. The base thickness is often compromised overlying the overdenture abutments.

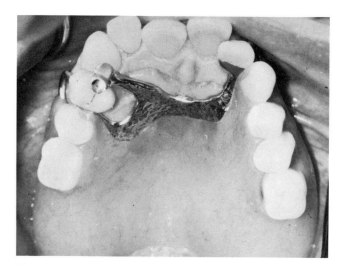

Fig. 23-1C Partial denture in place.

SELECTION CRITERIA FOR OVERDENTURE ABUTMENT TEETH

A. ENDODONTIC. Reduction to achieve proper contour usually necessitates endodontic therapy. Tooth should have a favorable endodontic prognosis.

B. PERIODONTAL. Tooth should have a favorable periodontal prognosis.

1. Alveolar bone support. Recontoured root should demonstrate adequate alveolar bone support, generally 5 mm or greater.

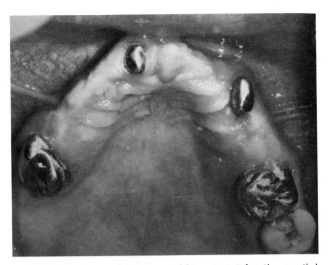

Fig. 23-2A Anterior roots provide support for the partial denture, and preserve alveolar bone. Roots are restored with cast copings.

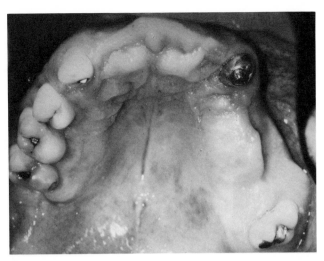

Fig. 23-2B Left maxillary canine is an overdenture abutment. Root is restored with a cast coping that retains an attachment component.

2. Mobility. Reduction of clinical crown height improves crown to root ratio and often reduces mobility.

3. Attached gingiva. Tooth should exhibit an adequate zone of attached gingiva.

C. RESTORATIVE. Tooth should be restorable to proper contour if caries or existing restorations are present.

D. POSITION. The position of the tooth and surrounding tissue should allow the required path of placement for the RPD. Retention of a root may result in an unfavorable tissue undercut in the denture base area.

E. PLAQUE CONTROL. The patient should demonstrate acceptable plaque control.

F. CARIES INDEX. The patient should demonstrate an acceptable caries index.

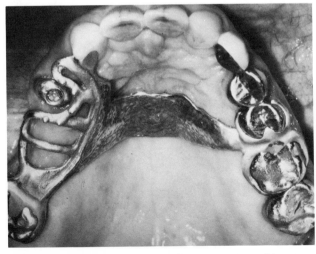

Fig. 23-3 Right premolar overdenture root provides support for the long-span base. An attachment will provide retention, eliminating the need for a clasp on the anterior abutment tooth.

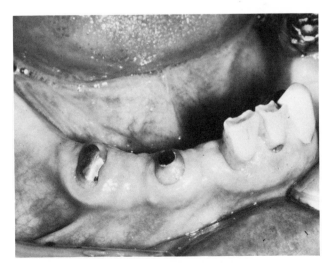

Fig. 23-4 Amalgam is used to obturate the coronal portion of the root canal.

MAINTENANCE

A. FLUORIDE TREATMENT

1. Daily. Apply stannous fluoride gel (0.4% SnF$_2$) to denture base adjacent to overdenture abutment and place RPD into mouth after tooth brushing. This procedure may be performed once or twice daily.

2. Periodontal recall appointments. Apply a fluoride compound to overdenture tooth after prophylaxis.

B. PERIODONTAL TREATMENT
   (See Chapter XIX)

C. RESTORATIVE TREATMENT
   (See Chapter XIX)

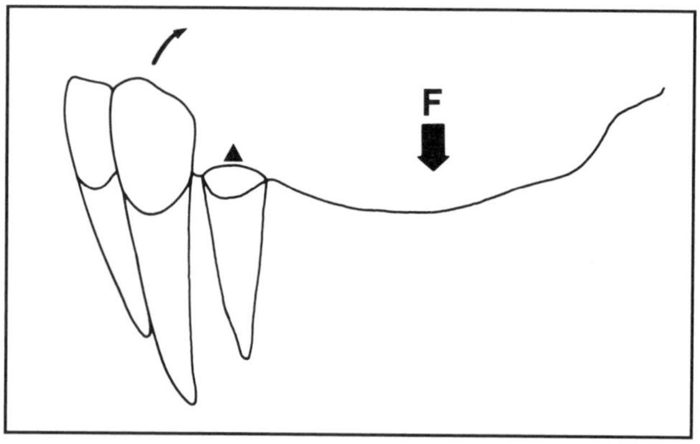

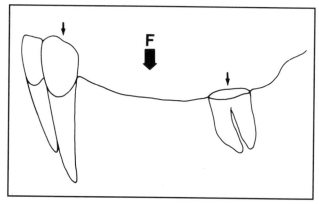

Fig. 23-5 Overdenture root located close to canine abutment tooth. When force (F) is applied to the base area, the root may act as a fulcrum point. A clasp on the canine will rotate occlusally, directing a torquing force to the tooth.

Fig. 23-6 Overdenture root located away from canine abutment tooth. When force (F) is applied to the base area, the root supports the base. Rotational movements are negligible. Clasp on canine does not torque tooth.

References

BIOMECHANICS

Atwood DA. Clinical Cephalometric and Densitometric Studies of Reduction of Residual Ridges. J Prosthet Dent 1971; 26:280.

Atwood DA. Some Clinical Factors Related to Rate of Resorption of Residual Ridges. J Prosthet Dent 1962; 12:441.

Barone JV. Physiologic Complete Denture Impressions. J Prosthet Dent 1963; 13:800.

Barrett, SF and Haines RW. Structure of the Mouth in the Mandibular Molar Region and Its Relation to the Denture. J Prosthet Dent 1962; 12:835.

Boucher CO. A Critical Analysis of Midcentury Impression Techniques for Full Dentures. J Prosthet Dent 1951; 1:472.

Boucher CO. Complete Denture Impressions Based Upon the Anatomy of the Mouth. J Am Dent Assoc 1944; 31:1174.

Carlsson GE and Perssin G. Morphologic Changes of the Mandible After Extraction and Wearing of Dentures. Odont Revy 1967; 18:27.

Cecconi BT. Effect of Rest Design on Transmission of Forces to Abutment Teeth. J Prosthet Dent 1974; 32:141-151.

Craddock FW. Prosthetic Dentistry, ed 2. St. Louis, 1951, The CV Mosby Co., pp 212-213.

Craddock FW. Retromolar Region of the Mandible. J Am Dent Assoc 1953; l47:453.

Craig RG and Farah JW. Stresses From Loading Distal-Extension Removable Partial Dentures. J Prosthet Dent 1978; 39:274-277.

DeVan MM. The Nature of the Partial Denture Foundation: Suggestions for its Preservation. J Prosthet Dent 1952; 2:2:210.

DeVan MM. An Analysis of Stress Concentration on the Part of Alveolar Bone with A View to Its Preservation. D Cosmos 1935; 77:109.

DiPietro GJ and Moergeli JR. Significance of the Frankfort-Mandibular Plane Angle to Prosthodontics. J Prosthet Dent 1976; 36:6:624.

Edwards LF and Boucher CO. Anatomy of the Mouth in Relation to Complete Dentures. J Am Dent Assoc 1942; 29:331.

Fleisch L. The Effect of Mechanical Loading on the Clear Cells of the Oral Epithelium. J Dent Res 1979; 58:1810.

Fleisch L and Austen JC. A Histologic Study of the Response of Masticatory and Lining Mucosa to Mechanical Loading in the Vervet Monkey. J Prosthet Dent 1978; 39:211-216.

Frechette AR. The Influence of Partial Denture Design on Distribution of Force to Abutment Teeth. J Prosthet Dent 1956; 6:195.

Frechette AR. Partial denture planning with Special Reference to Stress Distribution. J Prosthet Dent 1951; 1:710-724.

Friedman S. Edentulous Impression Procedures for Maximum Retention and Stability. J Prosthet 1957; 7:14.

Frost HM. Bone Remodelling Dynamics, Springfield, IL, CC Thomas, 1963.

Gibbs CH et al. Limits of Human Bite Strength. J Prosthet Dent 1986; 56:2:226.

Glickman I. Clinical Periodontology, ed 4, Philadelphia 1972, W.B. Saunders Co., pp 432-439.

Goodkind RJ. The Effects of Removable Partial Dentures on Abutment Tooth Mobility: A Clinical Study. J Prosthet Dent 1973; 30:139-146.

Jacobson TE and Krol AJ. A Contemporary Review of the Factors Involved in Complete Denture Retention, Stability and Support. Part I: Retention. J Prosthet Dent 1983; 49:1:5.

Jacobson TE and Krol AJ. A Contemporary Review of the Factors Involved in Complete Denture Retention, Stability and Support. Part II: Stability. J Prosthet Dent 1983; 49:2:165.

Jacobson TE and Krol AJ. A Contemporary Review of the Factors Involved in Complete Denture Retention, Stability and Support. Part III: Support. J Prosthet Dent 1983; 49:3:306.

Kaires AK. Effect of Partial Denture Design on Bilateral Force Distribution. J Prosthet Dent 1956a; 6:373-385.

Kaires AK. Effect of Partial Denture Design on Unilateral Force Distribution. J Prosthet Dent 1956b; 6:526-533.

Kaires AK. Partial Denture Design and its Relation to Force Distribution and Masticatory Performance. J Prosthet Dent 1956c; 6:672-683.

Kelly E. Changes Caused by a Mandibular Removable Partial Denture Opposing a Maxillary Complete Denture. J Prosthet Dent 1972; 27:2:140.

Kydd WL, Dutton DA, and Smith DW. Lateral Forces Exerted on Abutment Teeth by Partial Dentures. J Am Dent Assoc 1964; 68:859-863.

Kydd WL, Daly CH, and Nansen D. Variation in the Response to Mechanical Stress of Human Soft Tissues as Related to Age. J Prosthet Dent 1974; 32:493-500.

Kydd WL and Daly CH. The Biologic and Mechanical Effects of Stress on Oral Mucosa. J Prosthet Dent 1982; 47:317-329.

Ledley RS. Theoretical Analysis of Displacement and Force Distribution for the Tissue Bearing Surfaces of Dentures. J Dent Res 1968; 47:318-322.

MacGregor AR, Miller TG, and Farah JW. Stress Analysis of Partial Dentures. J Dent 1978; 6:125-132.

MacGregor AR, Miller TP, and Farah JW. Stress Analysis of Partial Dentures with Bounded and Free-End Saddles. J Dent 1980; 8:27-34.

Manderson RD, Wills DJ, Picton DCA. Biomechanics of Denture-Supporting Tissues. In: Lefkowitz W., ed. Proceedings of the Second International Prosthodontic Congress, St. Louis: The CV Mosby Co, 1979;99.

Maxfield JB, Nicholls JI, Smith DE. The Measurement of Forces Transmitted to Abutment Teeth of Removable Partial Dentures. J Prosthet Dent 1979; 41:134.

Melnick M. Prognostic Elements of the "Bone Factor" Analysis. J Periodontol, 1974; 48:815.

McCracken WL. A Comparison of Tooth-Borne and Tooth-Tissue-Borne Removable Partial Dentures. J Prosthet Dent 1953; 3:375-381.

Monteith BD. Management of Loading Forces on Mandibular Distal-Extension Prostheses. Part II: Classification for Matching Modalities to Clinical Situations. J Prosthet Dent 1984; 52:6:832.

Nishimura I, Flynn E, and Atwood DA. A Local Pathophysiologic Mechanism of the Resorption of Residual Ridges: Protaglandin. J Prosthet Dent 1988; 60:3:381.

Orban B. Oral Histology and Embryology, ed 3, St. Louis, 1953, The CV Mosby Co.

Picton DCA and Wills DJ. Viscoelastic Properties of the Periodontal Ligament and Mucous Membrane. J Prosthet Dent 1978; 40:263-272.

Preiskel HW. The Posterior Lingual Extension of Complete Lower Dentures. J Prosthet Dent 1968; 19:452.

Swoope CC and Frank RP. Stress Control and Design, *Clinical Dentistry*, Chapter II, Vol 5, pp1-12.

Tallgren A. The Continuing Reduction of the Residual Alveolar Ridges in Complete Denture Wearers: A Mixed-Longitudinal Study Covering 25 Years. J Prosthet Dent 1972; 27:120.

Warren AB and Caputo AA. Load Transfer to Alveolar Bone as Influenced by Abutment Designs for Tooth Supported Dentures. J Prosthet Dent 1975; 33:137-148.

Thompson WD, Kratochvil FJ, and Caputo AA. Evaluation of Photoelastic Stress Patterns Produced by Various Designs of Bilateral Distal Extension Removable Partial Dentures. J Prosthet Dent 1977; 38:261-273.

Van Scotter DE and Boucher LJ. The Nature of Supporting Tissues for Complete Dentures. J Prosthet Dent 1965; 15:285.

Watt DM and Likeman PR. Morphological Changes in the Denture Bearing Area Following the Extraction of the Maxillary Teeth. Br Dent J 1974; 136:225.

Wills DJ and Manderson RD. Biomechanical Sspects of the Support of Partial Dentures. J Dent 1977; 5:310-318.

Wirthlin MR. Review of Bone Biology in Periodontal Disease. J West Soc Perio, 1986; 34:4:125.

Wood WW. A Review of Masticatory Muscle Function. J Prosthet Dent 1987; 57:2:222.

Wright WH. The Importance of Tissue Changes Under Artificial Dentures. J Am Dent Assoc 1929; 16:1027.

CLASPS AND INDIRECT RETAINERS

Bates JF. Retention of Partial Dentures. Brit Dent J 1980; 149:171-174.

Browning JP et al. Effect of Positional Loading of Three Removable Partial Denture Clasp Assemblies on Movement of Abutment Teeth. J Prosthet Dent 1986; 55:3:347.

Browning JD, Meadors LW, Eick JD. Movement of Three Removable Partial Denture Clasp Assemblies Under Occlusal Loading. J Prosthet Dent 1986; 55:69-74.

Brudvik JS and Morris HF. Stress-Relaxation Testing. Part III Influence of Wire Alloys, Gauges and Lengths on Clasp Behavior. J Prosthet Dent 1981; 46:4:374.

Brudvik JS and Wormley JH. Construction Techniques for Wrought Wire Retentive Clasp Arms as Related to Clasp Flexibility. J Prosthet Dent 1973; 30:769.

Cecconi B, Asgar K, and Dootz E. The effect of Partial Denture Clasp Design on Abutment Tooth Movement. J Prosthet Dent 1971; 25:44-56.

Cecconi B, Asgar K, and Dootz E. Clasp Assembly Modifications and Their Effect on Abutment Tooth Movement. J Prosthet Dent 1972; 27:160-167.

Cecconi BT, Asgar K, Dootz E. The Effect of Partial Denture Clasp Design on Abutment Tooth Movement. J Prosthet Dent 1971; 25:44-56.

Christidou L, Osborne J, and Chamberlain JB. The Effect of Partial Denture design on the Mobility of Abutment Teeth. J Prosthet Dent 1972; 27:160-167.

Clayton JA, Jaslow C. A Measurement of Clasp Forces on Teeth. J Prosthet Dent 1971; 25:21-43.

Crispin BJ and Watson JF. Margin Placement of Esthetic Veneer Crowns. Part I: Anterior Tooth Visibility. J Prosthet Dent 1981; 45:3:278.

DeBoer J. The Effects on Function of Distal Extension Removable Partial Dentures as Determined by Occlusal Rest Position. J Prosthet Dent 1988; 60:6:693.

Demer WJ. An Analysis of Mesial Rest-I-Bar Clasp Designs. J Prosthet Dent 1976; 36:243-253.

DeVan MM. Preserving Natural Teeth Through the Use of Clasps. J Prosthet Dent 1955; 6:208-214.

Firtell DN, Grisius RJ, and Muncheryan AM. Reaction of the Anterior Abutment of a Kennedy Class II Removable Partial Denture to Various Clasp Arm Designs: An In Vitro Study. J Prosthet Dent 1985; 1:77.

Eliason CM. RPA Clasp Design for Distal-Extension Removable Partial Dentures. J Prosthet Dent 1983; 49:25.

Firtell DN. Effect of Clasp Design Upon Retention of Removable Partial Dentures. J Prosthet Dent 1968; 20:43-52.

Frank RP, Brudvik JS and Nicholls JI. A Comparison of the Flexibility of Wrought Wire and Cast Circumferential Clasps. J Prosthet Dent 1983; 48-471.

Frank RP and Nicholls JI. A Study of the Flexibility of Wrought Wire Clasps. J Prosthet Dent 1981; 45:259.

Frank RP, Nicholls JI. An Investigation of the Effectiveness of Indirect Retainers. J Prosthet Dent 1977; 38:494-506.

Frank RP. Direct Retainers for Distal-Extension Partial Dentures. J Prosthet Dent 1986; 56:5:562.

Goodkind RJ. The Effects of Removable Partial Dentures on Abutment Tooth Mobility: A Clinical Study. J Prosthet Dent 1973; 30:139-146.

Ko SH, McDowell GC, Kotowicz WE. Photoelastic Stress Analysis of Mandibular Removable Partial Dentures with Mesial and Distal Occlusal Rests. J Prosthet Dent 1986; 56:454-60.

Kotowicz WE, Fisher RL, Reed RA, Jaslow C. The Combination Clasp and the Distal Extension Removable Partial Denture. Dent Clin No Am 1973; 17:651-660.

Kratochvil FJ and Caputo AA. Photoelastic Analysis of Pressure on Teeth and Bone Supporting Removable Partial Dentures. J Prosthet Dent 1972; 32:52.

Kratochvil FJ. Influence of Occlusal Rest Position and Clasp Design on Movement of Abutment teeth. J Prosthet Dent 1963; 13:114.

Kratochvil FJ, Davidson PN, Guijt J. Five Year Survey of Treatment with Removable Partial Dentures, Part I. J Prosthet Dent 1982; 48:237-244.

Krol AJ. Clasp Design for Extension Base Removable Partial Dentures. J Prosthet Dent 1973; 29:408-415.

Krol AJ. RPI Clasp Retainer and its Modifications. Dent Clin No Am 17:631, 1973.

LaVere AM. Analysis of Facial Surface Undercuts to Determine Use of RPI or RPA Clasps. J Prosthet Dent 1986; 56:6:741.

Matheson GR, Brudvik JS and Nicholls JI. Behavior of Wrought Wire Clasps After Repeated Permanent Deformation. J Prosthet Dent 1986;, 55:2:226.

McDowell GC. Force Transmission by Indirect Retainers During Unilateral Loading., J Prosthet Dent 1978;, 39:616-21.

McDowell GC. Force Transmission by Indirect Retainers When a Unilateral Dislodging Force is Applied. J Prosthet Dent 1982;, 47:360-5.

Nelson DR, VonGonten AS, and Kelly TW. The Cast Round RPA Clasp. J Prosthet Dent 1985;, 54:2:307.

Pezzoli M, Rossetto M, and Calderal PM. Evaluation of Load Transmission by Distal-Extension Removable Partial Dentures by Using Reflection Photoelasticity. J Prosthet Dent 1986;, 56:3:329.

Robinson C. Clasp Design and Rest Placement for the Distal Extension Removable Partial Denture. Dent Clin No. Am 1970; 14:583 (July).

Schneider R. Significance of Abutment Tooth Angle of Gingival Convergence on Removable Partial Denture Retention. J Prosthet Dent 1987;, 58:2:194.

Shohet H. Relative Magnitudes of Stress on Abutment Teeth with Different Retainers. J Prosthet Dent 1969; 21:267-282.

Stade EH, Stewart GP, Morris HF and Pesavento JR. Influence of Fabrication Technique on Wrought Wire Clasp Flexibility. J Prosthet Dent 1985; 54:4:532.

Stone E. Tripping Action of Bar Clasps. J Am Dent Assn 1936;, 23:596.

Tebrock OC, Rohen RM, Fenster RK, Pelleu GB. The Effect of Various Clasping Systems on the Mobility of Abutment Teeth for Distal-Extension Removable Partial Dentures. J Prosthet Dent 1979; 41:511-516.

Thompson WD, Kratochvil FJ, and Caputo AA. Evaluation of Photoelastic Stress Patterns Produced by Various Designs of Bilateral Distal-Extension Removable Partial Dentures. J Prosthet Dent 1977; 38:261.

Zach GA. Advantages of Mesial Rests for Removable Partial Dentures. J Prosthet Dent 1975; 33:32-35.

IMPRESSION PROCEDURES

Applegate OC. Essentials of Removable Partial Denture Prosthesis. 3rd ed. Philadelphia: WB Saunders Co., 1966; 253-89.

Applegate OC. An Evaluation of the Support for the Removable Partial Denture. J Prosthet Dent 1960; 10:112-123.

Applegate OC. The Partial Denture Base. J Prosthet Dent 1955; 5:636-648.19.McLean, DW. The Partial Denture as a Vehicle for Function. J Am Dent Assoc 1936; 23:171-178.

Calverley, MJ and Moergeli JR. Effect on the Fit of Removable Partial Denture Frameworks When Master Casts are Treated with Cyanoacrylate Resin. J Prosthet Dent 1987; 58:3:327.

Carlyle LW. Compatibility of Irreversible Hydrocolloid Impression Materials with Dental Stone. J Prosthet Dent 1983; 49:3:434.

Cummer WE. Impression in Partial Denture Service. D Cosmos 1928; 70:278-292.

El-Khudary NM, Shaaban NA and Abdel-Hakim AM. Effect of Complete Denture Impression Technique on the Oral Mucosa. 1985; 53:4:543.

Fehling AW, Hesby RA and Pelleu GB. Dimensional Stability of Autopolymerizing Acrylic Resin Impression Trays. J Prosthet Dent 1986; 55:5:592.

Frank RP. Analysis of Pressure Produced During Maxillary Edentulous Impression Procedures. J Prosthet Dent 1969; 22:400.

Holmes JB. The Altered Cast Impression Procedure for the Distal Extension Removable Partial Denture. Dent Clin No Am 1970; 14:569.

Holmes JB. Influence of Impression Procedure and Occlusal Loading on Partial Denture Movement. J Prosthet Dent 1965; 15:474-481.

Jasim FA, Brudvik JS and Nicholls, JI. Impression Distortion from Abutment Tooth Inclination in Removable Partial Dentures. J Prosthet Dent 1985; 54:4:532.

Kaiser DA. A Study of Distortion and Surface Hardness of Improved Artificial Stone Casts. J Prosthet Dent 1976; 36:373.

Kramer HM. Impression Techniques for Removable Partial Dentures. J Prosthet Dent 1961; 11:84-92.

Leupold RJ, Kratochvil FJ. An Altered Cast Procedure to Improve Tissue Support for Removable Partial Dentures. J Prosthet Dent 1965; 15:672-678.

Leupold RJ. A Comparative Study of Impression Procedures for Distal Extension Removable Partial Dentures. J Prosthet Dent 1966; 16:708-720.

Lytle RB. Soft Tissue Displacement Beneath Removable Partial and Complete Dentures. J Prosthet Dent 1962; 12:34.

Lytle RB. Complete Denture Construction Based on a Study of the Deformation of the Underlying Soft Tissues. J Prosthet Dent 1959; 9:539.

Maxfield JB, Nicholls JI, and Smith DE. The Measurements of Forces Transmitted to Abutment Teeth of Removable Partial Dentures. J Prosthet Dent 1979; 40:134.

Metley AC. Obtaining Efficient Soft Tissue Support for the Partial Denture Base. J A D A 1958; 56:679-688.

Morrow RM and Brown CE. Compatibility of Alginate Impression Material and Dental Stone. J Prosthet Dent 1971; 25:556.

Mundez AJ. The Influence of Impression Trays on the Accuracy of Stone Casts Poured from Irreversible Hydrocolloid Impressions. J Prosthet Dent 1985; 54:3:383.

Schneider RL and Taylor TD. Compressive Stregnth and Surface Hardness of Tyep IV Die Stone When Mixed with Water Substitutes. J Prosthet Dent 1984; 52:4:510.

Stuart LM and Elliott RW. A Comparative Study of the Tissue Surface Contours on Casts Fabricated by Using Two Impression Techniques for Mandibular Distal Extension Removable Partial Dentures. Newsletter of American College of Prosthodontists 1983; p 16-18.

Vahidi F. Vertical Displacement of Distal-Extension Ridges by Different Impression Techniques. J Prosthet Dent 1978; 40:374.

MAJOR CONNECTORS

Addy M, and Bates JF. Plaque Accumulation Following the Wearing of Different Types of Removable Partial Dentures. J Oral Rehabil 1979; 6:111-117.

Bergman B. Periodontal Reactions in Connection with Removable Partial Dentures. In: Proceedings of European Prosthodontic Association. Fourth Meeting, Warsaw, Poland, 1980.

Bergman B, Hughson A, Olson CO. Caries, Periodontal and Prosthetic Findings in Patients with Removable Partial Dentures. A Ten Year Longitudinal Study. J Prosthet Dent 1982; 48:506-514.

Bergman B, Hughson A, Olsson CO. Periodontal and Prosthetic Conditions in Patients Treated with Removable Partial Dentures and Artificial Crowns. A Longitudinal Two-Year Study. Acta Odontol Scand 1971; 29:621-638.

Bergman B, Hughson A, Olsson CO. Caries and Periodontal Status in Patients Fitted with Removable Partial Dentures. J Clin Periodontol 1977; 4:134-146.

Campbell LD. Subjective Reactions to Major Connector Designs for Removable Partial Dentures. J Prosthet Dent 1977; 37:507.

Carlsson GE, Bergman B, Hedegard B. Changes in Contour of the Maxillary Alveolar Process Under Immediate Dentures. Acta Odontol Scand 1967; 25:45-47.

Carlsson GE, Hedegard B, and Koivumaa KK. Studies in Partial Denture prosthesis. II. An Investigation of Manidublar Partial Dentures with Double Extension Saddles. Acta Odontol Scand 1961; 19:215-237.

Carlsson GE, Hedegard B, and Koivumaa KK. Studies in Partial Denture prosthesis. III. An Investigation of Manidublar Partial Dentures with Double Extension Saddles. Acta Odontol Scand 1962; 19:95-119.

Carlsson GE, Hedegard B, Koivumaa KK. Studies in Partial Dental Prosthesis. IV. Final Results of a 4 Year Longitudinal Investigation of Dentogingivally Supported Partial Dentures. Acta Odontol Scand 1965; 23:443-472.

Derry A and Bertram U. A Clinical Survey of Removable Partial Dentures After 2 Years Usage. Acta Odontol Scand 1970; 28:581-598.

Koivumaa KK. Changes in Periodontal Tissues and Supporting Structures Connected with Partial Dentures. Suom Hammaslaak Toim 1956; 52(Suppl 1): 1-188.

Lavere AM and Krol AJ. Selection of a Major Connector for the Distal Extension-Base Removable Partial Denture. J Prosthet Dent 1973; 30:102.

Meyer JR and Krol AJ. Selection and Design of Major Connectors for Removable Partial Dentures. Gen Dent 1985; 33:508-512.

Schwalm CA, Smith DE, Erickson JD. A Clinical Study of Patients 1 to 2 Years After Placement of Removable Partial Dentures. J Prosthet Dent 1977; 38:380-319.

Tomlin HR and Osborne J. Cobalt-chromium Partial Dentures. A Clinical Survey. Br Dent J 1961; 110:307-310.

Tryde G and Bratenberg F. The Sublingual Bar. Tandlaegebladet 1965; 69:873-885.

Wagner AG and Traweek FC. Compairson of Major Connectors for Removable Partial Dentures. J Prosthet Dent 1982; 47:242.

MOUTH PREPARATION

Axinn S. Preparation of retentive areas for clasps in enamel. J Prosthet Dent 1975, 34:405-407.

Cecconi BT. Effect of Rest Design on Transmission of Forces to Abutment Teeth. J Prosthet Dent 1974; 32:141.

Chandler HT, Brudvik JS, Fisher WT. Surveyed crowns. J Prosthet Dent 1973, 30:775-780.

Gaston GW. Rest area preparations for removable partial dentures. J Prosthet Dent 1960, 10:124-134.

Glann GW, Appleby RC. Mouth preparation for removable partial dentures. J Prosthet Dent 1960, 10:698-706.

Holmes JB. Preparation of abutment teeth for removable partial dentures. J Prosthet Dent 1968, 20:396-406.

Holt JE. Guiding Planes: When and Where. J Prosthet Dent 1981; 46:4-6.

Janus CE et al. The Use of Custom Cast-Metal Resin-Bonded Cingulum Rest Seats Under Removable Dentures. Comp Cont Ed 1985, 6:5:364.

Jenkins CBG, Berry DC. Modification of tooth contour by acid-etch retained resins for prosthetic purposes. Brit Dent J 1976, 141:89-90.

Jochen DG. Achieving planned parallel guiding planes for removable partial dentures. J Prosthet Dent 1972, 27:654-661.

Krikos AA. Artificial undercuts for teeth which have unfavourable shapes for clasping. J Prosthet Dent 1969, 22:301-306.

Krikos AA. Preparing guide planes for removable partial dentures. J Prosthet Dent 1975, 34:152-155.

Leopold RJ and Faraone KL. Etched Castings as an Adjunct to Mouth Preparation for Removable Partial Dentures. J Prosthet Dent 1985, 53:5:655.

Lyon HE. Resin-Bonded Etched-Metal Rest Seats. J Prosthet Dent 1985; 53:336.

McCracken WL. Mouth preparation for partial dentures. J Prosthet Dent 1956, 6:39-52.

Meyers RE, Pfeifer DL, Mitchell DL, and Pelleu GB. A Photoelastic Study of Rests of Solitary Abutments for Distal-Extension Removable Partial Dentures. J Prosthet Dent 1986, 56:6:702.

Mills ML. Mouth preparation for the removable partial denture. J Am Dent Assoc 1960, 60:154-159.

Sansom BP et al. Rest Seat Designs for Inclined Posterior Abutments. A Photoelastic Comparison. J Prosthet Dent 1987, 58:1:57.

Schorr L, Clayman LH. Reshaping abutment teeth for reception of partial denture clasps. J Prosthet Dent 1954, 4:625-633.

Seely PW, Windeler SE, and Norling BK. An Investigation of Shear Bond Strengths of Various Resin-Bonded Inner Surface Rest Seat Designs for Removable Partial Dentures. J Prosthet Dent 1987, 58:2:186.

Seiden A. Occlusal rests and rest seats. J Prosthet Dent 1958, 8:431-440.

Seto BG and Caputo AA. Photoelastic Analysis of Stresses in Resin-Bonded Cingulum Rest Seats. J Prosthet Dent 1986, 56:4:460.

Stern WJ. Guiding planes in clasp reciprocation and retention. J Prosthet Dent 1975, 34:408-414.

Stern MA, Brudvik JS, and Frank RP. Clinical Evaluation of Removable Partial Denture Rest Seat Adaptation. J Prosthet Dent 1985, 53:5:658.

Toth RW et al. Load Cycling of Lingual Rest Sets Prepared in Bonded Composite. J Prosthet Dent 1986, 56:2:239.

Toth RW, Fiebiger GE, Mackert JR, and Goldman BM. Shear Strength of Lingual Rest Seats Prepared in Bonded Composite. J Prosthet Dent 1986. 56:1:99.

Wong R, Nicholls JI, Smith DE. Evaluation of Prefabricated Lingual Rest Seats for Removable Partial Dentures. J Prosthet Dent 1982, 48:521

PERIODONTAL CONSIDERATIONS

Addy M and Bates JF. Plaque Accumulation Following the Wearing of Different Types of Removable Partial Dentures. J Oral Rehab 1979; 7:2:147.

Anderson JN and Lammie GA. A Clinical Survey of Partial Dentures. Brit Dent J 1952; 92:59-67.

Basker RM and Tryde G. Connectors for Mandibular Partial Dentures: Use of the Sublingual Bar. J of Oral Rehab 1977; 4:389.

Bates JF and Addy M. Partial Dentures and Plaque Accumulation. J Dent 1978; 6:285-293.

Bergman BO, et al. Caries, Periodontal and Prosthetic FIndings in Patients with Removable Partial Dentures: A Ten-Year Longitudinal Study. J Prosthet Dent 1982; 48:506.

Bergman, BO. Periodontal Reactions to Removable Partial Dentures: A Literature Review. J Prosthet Dent 1987; 58:4:454.

Bergman BO and Ericson G. Cross Sectional Study of the Periodontal Status of Removable Partial Denture Patients. J Prosthet Dent 1989; 61:2:208.

Bergman B, Hugoson A, and Olsson CO. Periodontal and Prosthetic Conditions in Patient Treated with Removable Partial Dentures and Artificial Crowns. Acta Odont Scand 1971; 29B:621-638.

Bergman B, Hugoson A, and Olsson CO. Caries and Periodontal Status in Patients Fitted with Removable Partial Dentures. J Clin Periodontol 1977; 4:134-146.

Bergman B. Periodontal Reactions in Connection with Removable Partial Dentures. In Proceedings of European Prosthodontic Assoc, Fourth Meeting. Warsaw, Poland. 1980.

Bissada NF, Ibramham ST, and Barsoun WM. Gingival Response to Various Types of Removable Partial Dentures. J Periodontol 1974; 45:651-659.

Bollman F and Hlavacek J. Position of the Sublingual Arch Bar. Quintess of Dent Tech 1978; 2:21.

Bollman FL and Hlavacek J. Die Lage Des Unterzunger Bugels, Dtsch, Zahnarztl 1975; 30:726.

Brill N et al. Ecologic Changes in the Oral Cavity Caused by Removable Partial Dentures. J Prosthet Dent 1977; 38:2:138.

Campbell LD. Subjective Reactions to Major Connector Designs for Removable Partial Dentures. J Prosthet Dent 1977; 32:5:507.

Carlsson GE, Hedegard B, and Koivumaa KK. Studies in Partial Denture Prosthesis. IV Final Results of a 4-year Longitudinal Investigation of Dentogingivally supported Partial Dentures. Acta Odont Scand 1965; 23:443-472.

Casey DM and Lauciello FR. A Method for Working the Functional Depth of the Floor of the Mouth. J Prosthet Dent 1980; 43:1:108.

Chandler JA and Brudvik JA. Clinical Evaluation of Patients 8 to 9 Years After Placement of Removable Partial Dentures. J Prosthet Dent 1984; 51:6:736.

Derry A and Bertram UA. Clinical Survey of Removable Partial Dentures After Two Years Usage. Acta Odontol Scand 1970; 28:581.

El-Ghamrawy E. Quantative Changes in Dental Plaque Formation Related to Removable Partial Dentures. J Oral Rehabil 1976; 3:115-120.

El-Ghamrawy E. Qualitative Changes in Dental Plaque Formation Related to Removable Partial Dentures. J Oral Rehabil 1979a; 6:183-188.

El-Ghamrawy E. A Tooth-Brush Designed for Proximal Surfaces Adjacent to Toothless Spaces in the Partially Edentulous Patient. J Oral Rehabil 1979b; 6:323-325.

El-Ghamrawy E. Quantitative Changes in Dental Plaque Formation Related to Removable Partial Dentures. J Oral Rehab 1979; 3:183.

El-Ghamrawy E. Plaque Recordings as a Guide to the Prognosis for Partial Denture Treatment. J Oral Rehab 1980; 7:117.

El-Ghamrawy E. Plaque Recordings as a Guide to the Prognosis for Partial Denture Treatment. J Oral Rehabil 1980; 7:117-121.

El-Ghamrawy E. Plaque Formation: Crevicular Temperature Related to Minor Connector Position. IADR 1982, Ab. 387. J Dent Res 1982; 61:221.

El-Ghamrawy E and Runov J. Offsetting the Increased Plaque Formation in Partial Denture Wearers by Toothbrushing. J Oral Rehabil 1979; 6:399-403.

El-Ghamrawy E and Runov J. Proximal Plaque Accumulation with Two Minor Connectors. J Oral Rehabil 1980; 7:27-30.

Farrel J. Partial Denture Tolerance. Dent Pract 1969; 19:5:162.

Gattozzi, et al. Evaluating the Floor of the Mouth for Lingual Bar Major Connector Positioning of a Removable Partial Denture. J Ky Dent Assoc 1979; 5:33.

Glantz PO and Stafford GD. The Effect of Some Components on the Rigidity of Mandibular Bilateral Free End Saddle Dentures. J Oral Rehab 1980; 7:6.

Hansen CA and Campbell DJ. Clinical Comparison of Two Mandibular Major Connector Designs. J Prosthet Dent 1985; 54:6:805.

Hobkirk JA and Strahan JD. The Influence on the Gingival Tissues of Prostheses Incorporating Gingival Relief. J Dent 1979; 7:15-21.

Jacobson T. Educating Denture Patients. J Cal Dent Assoc, Apr 1982, p 81.

Jacobson TE. Periodontal Considerations in Removable Partial Denture Design. Comp of Cont Ed 1987; 8:7:530.

Kerschbaum T, et al. The Dimensions of Cast Bar Dentures. Dtsch. Zahnarztl 1979; 34:8:635.

Koivumaa KK. Changes in Periodontal Tissues and Supporting Structures Connected With Partial Dentures. Proc Finn Dent Soc 1956; 52:Sp.I.

Kratochvil FJ. 5 year Survey of Treatment with Removable Partial Dentures, Part I. J Prosthet Dent 1982; 48:237.

Lechner SK. Partial Dentures and Gingival Health. Aust Dent J 1965; 10:223-226.

Lindhe J and Nyman S. The Effect of Plaque Control and Surgical Pocket Elimination on the Establishment and Maintenance of Periodontal Health. A Longitudinal Study of Periodontal Therapy in Cases of Advanced disease. J Clin Periodontol 1975; 2:67.

Lindhe J and Nyman S. The Role of Occlusion in Periodontal Disease and the Biological Rationale for Splinting in Treatment of Periodontitis. Oral Science Rev 1977; 10:11.

Maeda T, El-Ghamrawy E, Kroone HB, Runov J, Stoltze K, and Brill N. Crevicular Temperature Rise Stimulated by Plaque Formation. J Oral Rehabil 1979; 6:229-234.

Mkil E, Koivumaa KK, and Jansson H. Clinical Investigations of Skeletal partial Dentures with Lingual Splints. 1. Periodontal and Dental Changes. Proc Finn Dent Soc 1971; 67:312-324.

Marinello CP. The Sublingual Bar: Planning and Realization. Comp of Cont Ed 1985; 6:8:559.

Merijohn GK. Perio Access. Perio Access Publishing, San Francisco, 1988.

Nakazawa I. A Clinical Survey of Removable Partial Dentures - A Follow Up Examination Over a 16 Year Period. Bull Tokyo Med Dent Univ 1977; 24:125-137.

Nyman S and Lindhe J. A Longitudinal Study of Combined Periodontal and Prosthetic Treatment of Patients with Advanced Periodontal Disease. J Periodontal 1979; 50:4:163.

Nyman S and Lindhe, J. Persistent Tooth Hypermobility Following Completion of Periodontal Treatment. J of Clin Perio 1976; 3:81.

Nyman S et al. The Role of Occlusion for the Stability of Fixed Bridges in Patients with Reduced Periodontal Tissue Support. J of Clin Perio 1975; 2:53-66.

Perlitsh MJ. A Systematic Approach to the Interpretation of Tooth Mobility and its's Clinical Implications. Symposium in Perio Rest Inter-relationships. Dent Clin No Amer 1980; 24:2:177.

Pietrokovski J and Chapman RJ. The Form of the Mandibular Anterior Lingual Alveolar Process in Partially Edentulous Patients. J Prosthet Dent 1981; 45:4:371.

Rantanen T, Siirila HS, and Lehvila P. Effect of Instruction and Motivation on Dental Knowledge and Behaviour Among Wearers of Partial Dentures. Acta Odontol Scand 1979; 38:9-15.

Ramfjord SP and Ash, Jr. MM. Significance of Occlusion in the Etiology and Treatment of Early, Moderate, and Advanced Periodontitis. J Periodontol 1981; 52:511.

Rissin L, et al. Six Year Report of the Periodontal Health of Fixed and Removable Partial Denture Abutment Teeth. J Prosthet Dent 54:4:461, 1985.

Rissin L et al. Effect of Age and Removable Partial Dentures on Gingivitis and Periodontal Disease. J Prosthet Dent 1979; 42:2:217.

Runov J et al. Host Response to Two Different Designs of Minor Connectors. J Oral Rehab 1980; 20:7.

Schwalm CA, Smith DE and Erickson JD. A Clinical Study of Patients 1 to 2 Years After Placement of Removable Partial Dentures. J Prosthet Dent 1977; 38:380.

Seemann SK. A Study of the Relationship Between Periodontal Disease and the Wearing of Partial Dentures. Aust Dent J 1963; 8:206-208.

Sekine H et al. Studies on Physical Factors of Major Connectors in Partial Dentures: The Rigidity of the Lingual Bar for Buccal-Lingual Rotating Forces of the Saddle. Shikwa Gakoo 1979; 79:9:1881.

Stipho H et al. The Effect of Oral Prostheses on Plaque Accumulation. Br Dent J 1978; 145:47.

Thayer HH and Kratochvil FJ. Periodontal Considerations with Removable Partial Dentures. Dent Clin N Amer 1980; 24:357-368.

Tryde, G and Bratenberg F. The Sublingual Bar. Tandlaegebladet 1965; 69:11:873.

Vafa M and Kotowicz WE. Plaque Retention with Lingual Bar and Lingual Plate Major Connectors. IADR, Ab. 609. J Dent Res 1980; 59:(Sp.Iss.A.)

Waerhaug J. Justification for Splinting in Periodontal Therapy. J Prosthet Dent 1969; 22:2:201.

ROTATIONAL PATH DESIGN

Bauman R. Rotational Path Partial Dentures: Problems and Potential. Compendium Cont Ed 1986, 7:356-362.

Brien N, Lamarche C, Tache R: Les plans d'insertion multidirectionnels: leur application aux ponts papillon. J Dent Que' 1985; 22:69-76.

Brien N, Champagne P, Cote S. Comparison Entre Deux Types de Crochets Utilises sur les Prostheses Partielles Amovibles a Plan d'insertion Multidirectionnel. J Dent Que 1985; 22:495-501.

Firtell DN, Jacobson TE. Removable partial dentures with rotational paths of insertion: problem analysis. J Prosthet Dent 1983; 50:8-15.

Garver DG. A new clasping system for unilateral distal extension removable partial dentures. J Prosthet Dent 1978; 39:268-273.

Jacobson TE. Satisfying Esthetic Demands with Rotational Path Partial Dentures. J Am Dent Assoc 1982; 104:460-465.

Jacobson TE and Krol AJ. Rotational Path Removable Partial Denture Design. J Prosthet Dent 1982; 48:370-376.

King GE. Dual Path Design for Removable Partial Dentures. J Prosthet Dent 1978; 39:392-395.

King GE, Barco MT, Olson RJ. Inconspicuous Retention for Removable Partial Dentures. J Prosthet Dent 1978; 39:505-507.

Krol AJ and Finzen FC. Rotational Path Removable Partial Dentures: Part I. Replacement of Posterior Teeth. Int J Prosthodont 1988; 1:17-27.

Krol AJ and Finzen FC. Rotational Path Removable Partial Dentures: Part II. Replacement of Posterior Teeth. Int J Prosthodont 1988; 1:135-142.

Krol AJ. Partial Denture Design, An Outline Syllabus, ed 2. University of the Pacific School of Dentistry, San Francisco, 1976, p 22.

Sanson BP, Flinton RJ, Parks VJ, Pelleu GB, Kingman A. Rest seat designs for inclined posterior abutments: A photoelastic comparison. J Prosthet Dent 1987; 50:8.

Schwartz RS, Murchison DG. Design Variations of the Rotational Path Partial Denture. J Prosthet Dent 1987; 58:336-338.

ADDITIONAL REFERENCES

Brown DR, Desjardins RP and Chao YS. Fatigue Failure in Acrylic Resin Retaining Minor Connectors. J Prosthet Dent 1987, 58:3:329.

Dunny JA, and King GE. Minor Connector Designs for Anterior Acrylic Resin Bases: A Preliminary Study. J Prosthet Dent 1975; 34:496.

Elarbi EA et al. Radiographic Detection of Porosities in Removable Partial Denture Castings. J Prosthet Dent 1985, 54:5:674.

Fisher RL. Factors that Influence the Base Stability of Mandibular Distal-Extension Removable Partial Dentures: A Longitudinal Study. J Prosthet Dent 1983; 50:167-71.

Frechette AR. The Influence of Partial Denture Design on Distribution of Force to Abutment Teeth. J Prosthet Dent 1956; 6:195-212.

Jacobson TE, Chang JC, Kerig PP and Watanabe LG. Bond Strength of 4-META Acrylic Resin Denture Base to Cobalt Chromium Alloy. J Prosthet Dent 1988; 60:5:570.

Jacobson TE, Chang JC, Kerij PP, and Watanabe LG. Bond Strength of 4-META Acrylic Resin Denture Base to Cobalt Chromium Alloy. J Prosthet Dent 1988, 60:5:570.

Kaplan P. Metal Cingulum and Loop Technique for Retaining Resin Base Material and Mandibular Incisors. J Prosthet Dent 1988; 59:1:111.

LaVere AM, Freda A. A simplified procedure for survey and design of diagnostic casts. J Prosthet Dent 1977; 37:680-683.

Lewis AJ. Radiographic Evaluation of Porosities in Removable Partial Denture Castings. J Prosthet Dent 1978; 39:278.

Pascoe DR, Wimmer J. A Radiographic Technique for Detection of Internal Defects in Dental Castings. J Prosthet Dent 1978; 39:150.

Wictorin L, Julin P, Mollersten L. Roentgenological Detection of Casting Defects in Cobalt-Chromium Frameworks. J Oral Rehabil 1979; 6:137.

Wise HB, Kaiser DA. A Radiographic Technique for Examination of Internal Defects in Metal Frameworks. J Prosthet Dent 1979; 42:594.

Zurasky JE and Duke ES. Improved Adhesion of Denture Acrylic Resins to Base Metal Alloys. J Prosthet Dent 1987; 57:4:520.

Glossary

A

ABUTMENT. A tooth, a portion of a tooth or that portion of an implant that serves to support, stabilize or retain a prosthesis.

ACTION DISTANCE. The distance through which the retentive clasp arm travels from its initial contact with the tooth to its final position.

ACRYLIC RESIN. Any of a group of thermoplastic resins made by polymerizing esters of acrylic or methacrylic acids.

AKERS CLASP. obj. See " CIRCLET CLASP ".

ALGINATE, IRREVERSIBLE HYDROCOLLOID. An hydrocolloid consisting of salts of alginic acid. Used as an impression material.

ALLOY. A metal that is composed of elements that are mutually soluble in the liquid state.

ALTERED CAST, MODIFIED CAST. A master cast that is altered before processing a denture base.

ALTERED CAST IMPRESSION. A negative likeness of a portion or portions of the edentulous area(s) made independently of and following the initial impression of the teeth.

ALVEOLAR BONE. The bone of the maxillae or mandible that surrounds and supports the teeth.

ALVEOLAR RIDGE. The bony ridge (alveolar process) of the maxillae or mandible which contains the alveoli (sockets of the teeth).

ANATOMIC CROWN. The portion of a natural tooth which extends from its dentoenamel junction to the occlusal surface or incisal edge.

ANATOMIC IMPRESSION. An impression which records the tissues at rest.

ANATOMIC TEETH. 1. Artificial teeth which duplicate the anatomic forms of natural or artificial teeth. 2. Teeth that have prominent cusps on the masticating surfaces and are designed to articulate with the teeth of the opposing natural or artificial dentition.

ANTERIOR PALATAL STRAP. A palatal strap that covers a portion of the anterior hard palate.

ANTEROPOSTERIOR PALATAL STRAP. A major connector that consists of an anterior and posterior palatal strap.

APPROACH ARM. That portion of an infrabulge clasp arm that arises from the denture base area and extends to the retentive portion of the clasp arm.

ARCH FORM. The geometric shape of the dental arch.

ARTIFICIAL CROWN. A metal, plastic or ceramic restoration that covers three or more axial surfaces and the occlusal surface of a tooth.

ARTICULATION. The contact relationships of maxillary and mandibular teeth as they move against each other.

ATROPHY. A diminution in size of a cell, tissue, organ or part.

ATTACHMENT. A mechanical device for the support, retention and stabilization of a dental prosthesis.

AUTOPOLYMERIZING RESIN, ACTIVATED R, SELF CURE R, COLD CURE R. A resin which can be polymerized by an activator and a catalyst without use of external heat.

AXIS. A straight line around which a body may rotate.

B

BACKING. A metal support that attaches a facing to a prosthesis.

BACK ACTION CLASP. A clasp consisting of a remote rest and a circumferential retentive clasp arm encircling the tooth.

BALANCED ARTICULATION. The bilateral, simultaneous, anterior and posterior occlusal contact of teeth in centric and eccentric positions.

BALL REST. A rigid extension of a partial denture that contacts the lingual surface of an anterior tooth in a prepared ball shaped rest seat.

BAR CLASP, INFRABULGE CLASP. The retentive clasp arm originates from the major connector or from within the denture base and approaches the area of contact on the tooth from a gingival direction.

BAR CLASP ARM. A clasp arm which has its origin in the denture base or major connector. It consists of the arm which traverses the gingival structures and a terminal end which appoaches the tooth in a gingivo-occlusal direction.

BAR CONNECTOR. A metal component of greater length than width that serves to connect the parts of a removable partial denture.

BASAL BONE. The osseous tissue of the mandible and maxillae exclusive of the alveolar processes.

BASAL SEAT. That surface of the oral mucosa covered by the denture base.

BASE METAL ALLOY. An alloy composed of metals that are not precious.

BIOMECHANICS, BIOPHYSICS. 1. The study of biology from the functional point of view. 2. An application of the principles of engineering design as implemented in living organisms.

BONE ATROPHY. Bone resorption both internally in density and externally in form.

BONE INDEX, BONE FACTOR. Assesment of the relative response of bone to stmulation or irritation. The ratio of osteogenesis to osteolysis.

BRACING, STABILITY. The resistance to horizontal components of force.

BRACING COMPONENT. Any component of a removable partial denture that offers resistance to horizontal forces.

BUCCAL SHELF. A primary force bearing anatomic area which is comprised of cortical bone and extends from the base of the residual ridge in the posterior part of the mandible to the external oblique ridge.

C

CANCELLOUS BONE. Refers to the spongy tissue located in the medulla of bone. This bone is composed of a variable trabecular network containing interstitial tissue which may be hematopoietic.

CAST. A positive likeness of some desired form.

CAST CLASP ARM. A clasp arm that consists of cast metal.

CINGULUM REST. A rigid extension of a partial denture which contacts the lingual surface of an anterior tooth in a prepared inverted "V" or "U" shaped rest seat.

CIRCLET CLASP. A clasp which consists of a rest, a cicumferential retentive clasp arm and a circumferential bracing clasp arm, both originating from the minor connector in the area of the rest. Previously known as an "Akers" clasp.

CIRCUMFERENTIAL CLASP, SUPRABULGE CLASP. 1. A clasp that encircles a tooth by more than 180 degrees, including opposite angles and which generally contacts the tooth throughout the extent of the clasp, with at least one terminal located in an undercut area. 2. A clasp whose retentive clasp arm originates from a minor connector or proximal plate usually near the occlusal surface and approaches the undercut from an occlusal direction.

CIRCUMFERENTIAL CLASP ARM. A clasp arm which has its origin in a minor connector or proximal plate and which follows the contour of the tooth in a plane approximately perpendicular to the path of placement of the partial denture.

CIRCUMFERENTIAL "C" CLASP. A clasp which consists of a rest, a circumferential "C" retentive clasp arm, and a circumferential bracing clasp arm, both originating from a minor connector in the area of the rest.

CLASP. An extracoronal direct retainer that engages an abutment tooth for retention, stability and support of a partial denture.

CLINICAL CROWN. The portion of the tooth which extends occlusally or incisally from the junction of the tooth and the alveolar bone.

COMBINATION CLASP. A clasp that incorporates two different types of clasp arms.

COMPLETE PALATAL PLATE. A palatal plate which covers the entire hard palate.

CONNECTOR. That part of a partial denture which unites its components.

CONTINUOUS BAR CONNECTOR, KENNEDY BAR CONNECTOR. A metal bar usually resting on the lingual surfaces of mandibular anterior teeth which may aid in their stabilization and may act as an indirect retainer in distal extension removable partial dentures.

CORTICAL BONE. A peripheral layer of compact osseous tissue.

CUSTOM TRAY. An individualized impression tray made from a cast recovered from a preliminary impression. It is used in making a final impression.

CROWN. See Anatomic c., Artificial c., Clinical c.

D

DEFINITIVE PROSTHESIS. A prosthesis to be used over an extended period of time.

DENTAL CAST. A positive likeness of a part or parts of the oral cavity.

DENTAL IMPLANT. A material or device placed in or on oral tissues to support an oral prosthesis.

DENTITION, NATURAL DENTITION. The natural teeth as considered collectively in the dental arch.

DENTO-ALVEOLAR SEGMENT. That portion of the maxillary or mandibular arch which contains the abutment tooth and its investing structures.

DENTULOUS. A condition in which natural teeth are present in the mouth.

DENTURE. An artificial substitute for missing natural teeth and adjacent tissues.

DENTURE BASE. That component of a partial denture which contacts the oral mucosa and to which artificial teeth are attached.

DENTURE FOUNDATION AREA. The surfaces of the oral structures available to support a denture.

DENTURE BASAL SURFACE, IMPRESSION S. INTAGLIO S. The portion of the denture surface that has its contour determined by the impression of the underlying soft tissue.

DENTURE OCCLUSAL SURFACE. The portion of the surface of a denture that makes contact or near contact with its antagonist.

DENTURE POLISHED SURFACE, CAMEO S. The portion of the surface of a denture that extends in an occlusal direction from the border of denture and includes the facial, lingual and palatal surfaces. It is the part of the denture base that is usually polished, and includes the buccal and lingual surfaces of the teeth.

DIAGNOSIS. The determination of the nature of a disease.

DIAGNOSTIC CAST. A likeness of a part or parts of the oral cavity or facial structures for the purpose of study and treatment planning.

DIRECT RETAINER. A clasp or attachment applied to an abutment tooth for the purpose of retaining a removable partial denture.

DISPLACEABILITY OF TISSUE. The quality of oral tissues that permits them to be placed in other than a relaxed position.

DISTAL EXTENSION PARTIAL DENTURE. A removable partial denture that is retained by natural teeth at the anterior ends of the denture base segments and in which a portion of the functional load is carried by the muco-osseous segment(s).

DUAL PATH OF PLACEMENT. A path of placement whereby the segment with the rigid retainers is seated first along a straight path to gain access to the rotational centers, then the prosthesis is rotated into place.

E

ELONGATION. The ratio of increase in length after the fracture of a material to its original length.

EMBRASURE CLASP. Two circlet clasps originating from a common minor connector.

ENDOSTEAL IMPLANT. An implant which is placed into the bone to provide an abutment for a fixed or removable denture.

EXTENDED OCCLUSAL REST. A rigid extention of a partial denture that contacts the occlusal surface of a posterior tooth in a prepared rest seat which extends more than one half the mesiodistal width of the tooth.

EXTENSION BASE PARTIAL DENTURE. A removable partial denture that is supported and retained by natural teeth only at one end of the denture base segments and in which a portion of the functional load is carried by the muco-osseous segment.

EXTERNAL FINISH LINE. The line of demarcation between the metal and resin which exists on the polished surface of a removable partial denture.

EXTRACORONAL ATTACHMENT. An attachment which is outside or external to the crown portion of a natural tooth.

EXTRUSION. The movement of teeth beyond the natural occlusal plane which may be accompanied by similar movement of their supporting tissues.

F

FABRICATION. The building, making or constructing of a restoration.

FACING. A veneer of restorative material used on a prosthesis or as a restoration to simulate a natural tooth.

FINISH LINE. 1. The peripheral extension of tooth preparation. 2. The planned junction of different materials.

FIXED PARTIAL DENTURE. A partial denture that is cemented to natural teeth or roots or affixed to dental implants that furnish the primary support for the prosthesis.

FLANGE. The part of the denture base that extends from the cervical ends of the teeth to the border of the denture.

FORCE. An influence that, when exerted upon a body, tends to set the body into motion or to alter its present state of motion. Force applied to any material causes deformation of that material.

FRAMEWORK. The skeletal portion of a prosthesis (usually metal) around which and to which are attached the remaining portions of the prosthesis to produce the finished restoration.

FREE GINGIVAL MARGIN. The edge or summit of the free type gingival tissue.

FULCRUM LINE AXIS. An imaginary line passing through or near the primary rests of an extension base partial denture around which the removable partial denture tends to rotate during function.

FUNCTIONAL FORCE. The force applied by the muscles during function (e.g. mastication, speech).

FUNCTIONAL RANGE OF MOVEMENT. The distance through which the mandible moves during normal speech, swallowing, mastication, yawning and other associated movements.

FUSION TEMPERATURE. The temperature at which the alloy fractures under stress.

G

GUIDING PLANES, GUIDING SURFACES. Vertical parallel surfaces of abutment teeth oriented so as to contribute to the direction of the path of placement and dislodgment of removable partial dentures.

H

HAMULAR NOTCH. See "PTERYGOMAXILLARY NOTCH."

HARDNESS. The resistance to indentation.

HARD PALATE. The bony portion of the roof of the mouth.

HEIGHT OF CONTOUR, SURVEY LINE. A line encircling a tooth designating its greatest circumferance at a selected position as determined by a dental surveyor.

HORIZONTAL HARD PALATE. A primary force bearing anatomic area comprised of cortical bone of the palatine bones and maxillae and extends between the vertical inclines of the maxillary posterior ridges.

HYDROCOLLOID. The materials described as colloid sols with water that are used in dentistry as elastic impression materials. Hydrocolloid can be reversible or irreversible.

I

IATROGENIC. Resulting from the activity of the clinician; applied to disorders in the patient induced by the clinician.

IMMEDIATE DENTURE. A complete or removable partial denture fabricated for placement immediately after the removal of natural teeth.

IMPLANT DENTURE. A denture that receives its stability, support and retention from a substructure that is partially or wholly implanted under the soft tissues of the denture basal seat.

IMPRESSION, DENTAL. An imprint or negative likeness of the teeth, edentulous areas and adjacent tissues.

INCISAL REST. A rigid extension a partial denture which contacts the incisal surface of an anterior tooth.

INCISIVE PAPILLA. The elevation of soft tissue covering the incisive or nasopalatine canal.

INDIRECT RETAINER. A component of a tooth-mucosa borne removable partial denture that contacts an abutment tooth on the opposite side of the fulcrum line assisting the direct retainers in preventing displacement of an extension base through mechanical leverage.

INFRABULGE. That portion of the crown of a tooth apical to the survey line.

INFRABULGE CLASP. See "BAR CLASP".

INFRAERUPTION. Failure of eruption of a tooth to the occlusal plane.

INTERARCH DISTANCE, INTERRIDGE DISTANCE. The vertical distance between the maxillary and mandibular dentate or edentate arches under conditions that must be specified.

INTERDENTAL PAPILLA. A projection of the gingiva filling the space between the proximal surfaces of two adjacent teeth.

INTERIM PROSTHESIS. A fixed or removable device designed to serve for a short period of time, after which it is to be replaced by a more definitive restoration.

INTERNAL FINISH LINE. The line of demarcation between metal and resin which exists on the tissue surface of a removable partial denture.

INTRACORONAL ATTACHMENT. An attachment which is within the normal contours of the crown portion of the natural tooth.

INTRUSION. Movement of a tooth in an apical direction.

IRREVERSIBLE HYDROCOLLOID, ALGINATE. A hydrocolloid consisting of sols of alginic acid having a physical state which is changed by an irreversible chemical reaction forming an insoluble calcium alginate.

INVESTMENT CAST, REFRACTORY CAST. A cast made of a material that will withstand high temperature wihout disintegrating.

L

LABIAL BAR. A major connector located labial to the dental arch joining two or more bilateral parts of a mandibular removable partial denture.

LINGUAL BAR. A major connector located lingual to the dental arch joining two or more bilateral parts of a removable partial denture.

LINGUAL PLATE. A major connector located lingual to the dental arch which covers the gingival tissue and contacts the lingual surfaces of the teeth joining two or more parts of a removable partial denture.

LINGUAL REST. A rigid extension of a partial denture which contacts the lingual surface of an anterior tooth in a rest seat preparation.

LONGITUDINAL AXIS. An imaginary line extending anteroposteriorly along the crest of the posterior ridge around which the partial denture tends to rotate in function when chewing unilaterally.

M

MAJOR CONNECTOR. A plate, strap or bar that connects the components on one side of the arch to those on the opposite side.

MASTER CAST. A replica of the tooth surfaces, residual ridge areas and other parts of the dental arch and facial structures used to fabricate a dental restoration or prosthesis.

MASTICATORY FORCE. The force applied by the muscles of mastication during function.

MATRIX. 1. A mold or impression in which something is formed. 2. The portion of an attachment system that receives the patrix.

METAL STOP. A small projection of metal at the distal end of an extension base frame that contacts the cast and prevents downward movement of the plastic retention area during packing with resin.

METHYL METHACRYLATE RESIN. A transparent thermoplastic acrylic resin that is used in dentistry by mixing the liquid methyl methacrylate monomer with the polymer powder.

MIDPALATAL STRAP, POSTERIOR PALATAL STRAP. A palatal strap that covers a portion of the posterior hard palate. The mid-palatal strap is generally used as a single palatal major connector. The posterior palatal strap is generally used together with an anterior palatal strap and is located more posteriorly.

MINOR CONNECTOR. A rigid component which links the major connector or base and other components of the partial denture such as rests, indirect retainers and clasps.

MODULOUS OF ELASTICITY. The ratio between stress and strain within the elastic range of a material.

MODIFIED PALATAL PLATE. A palatal plate that covers a portion of the hard palate. It is wider than a palatal strap, but covers less tissue than a complete palatal plate.

MODIOLUS. The structure near the corner of the mouth, where eight muscles converge, that functionally separates the labial vestibule from the buccal vestibule.

MONOMER. Any molecule that can be bound to a similar molecule to form a polymer.

MUCO-OSSEOUS SEGMENT. The portion of the residual ridge, basal bone and their soft tissue covering.

MUCOSA. A mucous membrane comprised of epithelium, basement membrane and lamina propria.

MUCOSITIS. Inflammation of the mucous membrane.

MYLOHYOID RIDGE. An oblique ridge on the lingual surface of the mandible which extends from the level of roots of the last molar teeth posteriorly to the symphysis anteriorly and which serves as a bony attachment for the mylohyoid muscles forming the floor of the mouth.

N

NECROSIS. Tissue death.

NONANATOMIC TEETH. Artificial teeth with occlusal surfaces lacking anatomic form.

NONRIGID ATTACHMENT. An attachment which permits movement between the matrix and the patrix through the incorporation of a spring loaded mechanism, hinge, ball and socket mechanism or flexible elements.

O

OCCLUSAL BALANCE. A condition in which there are simultaneous contacts of opposing teeth or tooth analogues (e.g. occlusion rims) on both sides of the opposing dental arches during eccentric movements within the functional range.

OCCLUSAL FORCE. The result of muscular activity applied on opposing teeth.

OCCLUSAL PREMATURITY. Any contact of opposing teeth that occurs before the planned intercuspation.

OCCLUSAL REST. A rigid extension of a partial denture which contacts the occlusal surface of a posterior tooth in a prepared rest seat.

OCCLUSAL VERTICAL DIMENSION. The distance between two selected points, one on the fixed and one on the movable member (maxillae and mandible) when the occluding members are in contact.

OCCLUSION. The static relationship between the incising or masticating surfaces of the maxillary or mandibular teeth or tooth analogues.

OSSEOINTEGRATION. An apparent direct connection of an implant surface and host bone without intervening connective tissue.

OVERDENTURE, OVERLAY PARTIAL DENTURE. A removable partial denture that covers and rests on one or more remaining natural teeth, roots or dental implants.

OVERLAY REST. A rigid extension of a patial denture that contacts the majority of the occlusal surface of a posterior tooth.

P

PALATAL PLATE. A major connector that covers a portion of the palatal surface and whose anteroposterior width exceeds 12 mm.

PALATAL STRAP. A major connector that covers a portion of the palatal surface and whose width is within the 8-12 mm range.

PAPILLA. Any small, nipple shaped elevation.

PARAFUNCTIONAL FORCE. The force applied by the muscles during parafunction (e.g. bruxism, clenching).

PARTIAL DENTURE. A dental prosthesis that restores one or more but not all of the natural teeth and associated parts and is supported by the teeth and/or mucosa; it may be removable or fixed.

PARTIAL DENTURE IMPRESSION. A negative likeness of a part or all of a partially edentulous arch.

PASSIVITY. The quality or condition of inactivity or rest assumed by the teeth, tissues and denture when a removable partial denture is in place but not under masticatory force.

PATRIX. The extension of an attachment system that fits into the matrix.

PATH OF DISLODGEMENT. The specific direction in which a partial denture may be dislodged.

PATH OF PLACEMENT, PATH OF INSERTION. The specific direction in which a prosthesis is placed upon abutment teeth.

PEAR-SHAPED PAD. The most distal extension of attached keratinized mucosa overlying the mandibular ridge crest formed by the scarring pattern following extraction of the most posterior molar. It should be differentiated from the retromolar pad.

PERIDENTAL. The structures surrounding the teeth, including the gingiva, periodontal ligament and alveolar bone.

POLYMER. A chemical compound consisting of a large organic molecule built by repetition of smaller monomeric units.

POLYMERIZATION. The forming of a compound by the joining together of molecules of small molecular weights into a compound of large molecular weights.

PONTIC. An artificial tooth on a partial denture that replaces a missing natural tooth, restores its function and usually fills the space previously filled by the natural crown.

POSTERIOR PALATAL STRAP, MIDPALATAL STRAP. A palatal major connector that covers a portion of the posterior hard palate and whose width (anteroposterior) dimension is 12 mm or less. The strap is located either in the middle of the hard palate or further posteriorly.

PRECIOUS ALLOY. An alloy predominantly composed of elements considered precious, that is, gold, the six metals of the platinum group (platinum, osmium, iridium, palladium, ruthenium and rhodium), and silver.

PRECISION ATTACHMENT, FRICTIONAL ATTACHMENT. A retainer used in fixed or removable prosthodontics consisting of a metal receptacle (matrix) and a closely fitting part (patrix); the receptacle is usually contained within the normal or expanded contours of the crown of the abutment tooth and the closely fitting part is attached to a pontic or to the denture framework.

PRELIMINARY IMPRESSION, PRIMARY IMPRESSION. An impression made for the purpose of diagnosis, treatment planning or for the fabrication of an impression tray.

PRIMARY OCCLUSAL TRAUMATISM. Pathologic periodontal tissue changes induced by occlusal forces not produced by normal masticatory function.

PROGNOSIS. A forecast as to the probable result of a disease or a course of therapy.

PROPORTIONAL LIMIT. The unit of stress beyond which deformations are no longer proportional to applied loads.

PROSTHESIS. 1. An artificial replacement of an absent part of the human body. 2. A therapeutic device to improve or alter function.

PROSTHODONTICS. The branch of dentistry pertaining to the restoration and maintenance of oral function, comfort, appearance and health of the patient by the restoration of natural teeth or the replacement of missing teeth and contiguous oral and maxillofacial tissues with artificial substitutes.

PROVISIONAL PROSTHESIS. An interim prosthesis designed to be used for varying periods of time.

PROXIMAL PLATE. A plate of metal in contact with the proximal surface of an abutment tooth.

PROXIMATE REST, ADJACENT REST. A rest on a removable partial denture abutment tooth which is located adjacent to the edentulous span.

PTERYGOMAXILLARY NOTCH, HAMULAR NOTCH. The palpable notch formed by the junction of the maxilla and the pterygoid hamulus of the sphenoid bone.

R

REBASE. The laboratory process of replacing the entire denture base material on an existing prosthesis.

RECIPROCAL COMPONENT. A rigid component which contacts the abutment tooth and counteracts the force exerted by a flexible retentive component.

RECIPROCATION. The resistance to horizontal components of force directed toward an abutment tooth by an active retentive element.

RECORD BASE, TRIAL BASE. A material or device representing the base of a denture. It is used for making maxillomandibular relation records and for the arrangement of teeth.

RELIEF. 1. The reduction or elimination of undesirable pressure or force from a specific area under a denture base. 2. The space that exists between the tissue surface of the prosthesis and the adjacent or underlying tissue. 3. The space in an impression tray for impression material.

RELIEF AREA. That portion of the denture or custom impression tray which is reduced to eliminate excessive pressure or contact.

RELINE. The procedures used to resurface the tissue side of a denture with new base material to produce an accurate adaptation to the denture foundation area.

REMODELING. The morphologic change in bone as an adaptive response to altered environmental demands. Progressive remodeling occurs where there is a proliferation of tissue and regressive remodeling occurs when osteoclastic resorption is evident.

REMOTE REST. A rest on a removable partial denture that is located in a prepared rest seat on the occlusal or incisal surface opposite the edentulous span.

REMOUNT CAST. A cast formed in a prosthesis for the purpose of mounting the prosthesis on an articulator.

REMOUNT PROCEDURE. A method used to relate restorations to an articulator for refinement of the occlusion.

REMOVABLE PARTIAL DENTURE. A partial denture that can be removed at will; often referred to as an RPD.

RESIDUAL RIDGE. The portion of the alveolar ridge and its soft tissue covering which remains following the removal of teeth.

RESIDUAL RIDGE CREST. The highest continuous surface of the residual ridge comprised of cancellous bone not necessarily coincident with the center of the of the ridge.

RESIN. A broad term used to describe natural or synthetic substances that form plastic materials after polymerization. They are named according to their chemical composition, physical sructure and means for activation of polymerization.

RESORPTION. Loss of tissue substance by physiologic or pathologic processes.

REST. A rigid extension of a partial denture which contacts a remaining tooth in a prepared rest seat to transmit vertical and horizontal forces.

REST SEAT. That portion of a natural tooth or a cast restoration prepared to receive a rest.

RETAINER. Any type of device used for the fixation or retention of a prosthesis.

RETENTION. Resistance to vertical dislodging forces.

RETENTIVE CLASP ARM. A clasp arm whose terminal portion engages an undercut area of an abutment tooth.

RETENTIVE FULCRUM LINE. An imaginary line connecting the retentive points of clasp arms of an extension base partial denture around which the denture tends to rotate when subjected to vertical dislodging forces.

RETROMOLAR PAD. A mass of tissue consisting of non-keratinized mucosa located posterior to the retromolar papilla and overlying loose glandular connective tissue. This freely movable area should be differentiated from the pear-shaped pad.

RETROMOLAR PAPILLA. The gingival papilla located distal to and in contact with the distal surface of the third molar or second molar if the third molar is congenitally missing.

REVERSIBLE HYDROCOLOID. Colloidal gel that is gelled by cooling and returned to the sol condition by sufficiently increasing the temperature.

RIDGE. A long narrow, raised portion or crest.

RIGID ATTACHMENT. An attachment which does not permit movement or flexion between the matrix and the patrix.

RING CLASP. A clasp consisting of a rest(s), a long circumferential clasp arm encircling the tooth and an optional reinforcing element.

ROTATIONAL PATH OF PLACEMENT. A path of placement of a removable partial denture that incorporates a curved or dual path allowing one or more of the rigid components of the framework to gain access to and engage undercut areas.

ROTATIONAL PATH REMOVABLE PARTIAL DENTURE. A removable partial denture that incorporates a rotational path of placement.

RII CLASP. A clasp consisting of a rest, an " I " bar retentive clasp arm and an " I " bar bracing clasp arm.

RPA CLASP. A clasp consisting of a rest, promimal plate and an Akers clasp arm. See " RPC " clasp. In this syllabus the term " Akers " has been replaced by the term " circlet ".

RPC CLASP. A clasp consisting of a rest, proximal plate and a circumferential retentive clasp arm. Same clasp as "RPA."

RPI CLASP. A clasp consisting of a rest, proximal plate and an " I " bar retentive clasp arm.

S

SECONDARY OCCLUSAL TRAUMATISM. Pathologic periodontal tissue changes induced by occlusal forces produced by normal masticatory function on teeth with decreased attachment apparatus.

SELECTIVE PRESSURE IMPRESSION. An impression which incorporates varying degrees of pressure on the denture bearing areas.

SEMIPRECIOUS ALLOY. An alloy composed of precious and base metals.

SHOULDER. The rigid portion of a circumferential clasp arm.

SOFT PALATE. The moving part of the palatal structure posterior to the hard palate.

STABILITY, BRACING. The resistance to horizontal components of force.

STABILIZED RECORD BASE. A record base lined with a material to improve its fit and adaptation to the underlying supporting tissues.

STRESS BREAKER. Objectionable. See "STRESS DIRECTOR."

STRESS DIRECTOR. A device or system that relieves specific dental structures of part or all of the occlusal forces and redirects those forces to other bearing structures or areas.

STUDY CAST. Objectionable. See " DIAGNOSTIC CAST."

SUBLINGUAL BAR. A mandibular major connector located lingual to the dental arch whose horizontal dimension exceeds its vertical dimension. It is essentially a lingual bar turned on its side.

SUBPERIOSTEAL IMPLANT. A device that is placed under the periosteum and overlying the cortex.

SUPPORT. Resistance to vertical seating forces.

SUPPORTIVE FULCRUM LINE. An imaginary line that passes through or near the primary rests of an extension base partial denture around which the denture tends to rotate when subjected to vertical seating forces.

SUPRABULGE. The portion of a tooth crown that converges toward the occlusal surface, i.e., above the height of contour.

SUPRAERUPTION. Movement of teeth beyond the normal occlusal plane.

SURVEYING. An analysis and comparison of the prominence of intraoral contours associated with the fabrication of a prosthesis.

SURVEY LINE. A line produced on a cast by a surveyor or scriber marking the greatest prominence of contour in relation to the planned path of placement of a partial denture.

SURVEYOR, DENTAL SURVEYOR. A paralleling instrument used in the fabrication of a removable partial denture. It is used to locate and delineate the contours and relative positions of abutment teeth and associated structures.

T

TENSILE STRESS. The internal induced force that resists the elongation of a material in a direction parallel to the direction of the stresses.

TENSILE STRENGTH. The maximal tensile stress a material can withstand before rupture.

TISSUE. 1. The various cellular combinations that make up the body. 2. An aggregation of similarly specialized cells united in the performance of a particular function.

TISSUE DISPLACEABILITY. 1. The quality of oral tissues which permits them to be placed in other than a relaxed position. 2. The degree to which tissues permit displacement.

TISSUE DISPLACEMENT. The change in the form or position of tissues as the result of pressure.

TOOTH BORNE, DENTO-ALVEOLAR SUPPORTED. A term used to describe a prosthesis which depends entirely upon the abutment teeth for support.

TOOTH BORNE BASE. The denture base restoring an edentulous region which has abutment teeth at each end for support. The mucosal tissue which it covers is not ordinarily used for support.

TOOTH-MUCOSA BORNE, DENTO-ALVEOLAR AND MUCO-OSSEOUS SUPPORTED. A term used to describe a prosthesis or part of a prosthesis which depends upon abutment teeth and mucosa of the residual ridge and basal bone areas for support.

TORQUE. A twisting or rotary force.

TOUGHNESS. The ability of a material to withstand stresses and strain without breaking.

TRANSITIONAL DENTURE. A removable partial denture serving as a temporary prosthesis to which artificial teeth will be added as natural teeth are lost and which will be replaced after post extraction tissue changes have occured.

TREATMENT PLAN. The sequence of procedures planned for the treatment of a patient following diagnosis.

TRIPOD MARKINGS. Marks or lines drawn on a cast to assist with repositioning the cast on a dental surveyor in a previously defined orientation.

TRIPODIZING. The procedure of placing the tripod markings.

TRIPPING ACTION. The action attributed to an infrabulge clasp arm that engages the undercut directly from a gingival direction. Such a clasp arm has a "push" type effect along the tooth surface when the partial denture is being removed or dislodged. It is contrasted with other types of infrabulge and suprabulge clasp arms that engage the undercut from an occlusal direction and have a "pull" type effect. An "I" bar infrabulge clasp arm is an example of a "push" type clasp arm with tripping action.

U

UNDERCUT. 1. That portion of the surface of an object which is beyond the height of contour in relation to the path of placement. 2. To create areas that provide mechanical retention for materials.

UNILATERAL REMOVABLE PARTIAL DENTURE. A dental prosthesis restoring missing teeth on one side only.

V

VERTICAL AXIS. An imaginary vertical line around which the partial denture tends to rotate on a horizontal plane in function.

VESTIBULE. The portion of the oral cavity bounded on one side by the teeth, gingivae and alveolar ridge (in the edentulous mouth, the residual ridge) and on the opposite side by the lips, cheeks or tongue.

VERTICAL DIMENSION. The distance between two selected points, one on the fixed and one on the movable member (maxilllae and mandible).

W

WROUGHT WIRE CLASP ARM. A clasp arm which consists of wrought metal.

Y

YIELD STRENGTH. The stress at which a material exhibits a deviation from the proportionality of stress to strain. The onset of plastic strain.

Z

ZERO DEGREE TEETH. Posterior denture teeth having no cusp angles in relation to the horizontal occlusal surface.